Keto Diet Cookbook:

The Complete guide 2021 for beginners 1000 easy recipes to Lose Weight, Boost Your Metabolism and Stay Healthy Lifestyle to Burn Fat Quickly

Gary Volgel

Table of Contents

Introduction

Under the ketogenic diet, the body is pushed to the state of ketosis wherein it uses up fat bodies called ketones as its main source of energy instead of glucose. Unlike other short-lived fad diets, the ketogenic diet has been around for more than ninety years as it was first used to treat patients who suffered from epilepsy. Today, it is still used to minimize the effects of epileptic seizures, but it is also used for weight loss. People who follow the ketogenic diet limit the intake of carbohydrates to around 20 to 30 net grams daily or 5% of the daily diet. Net grams refer to the number of carbohydrates that remain after subtracting the grams of dietary fiber. Since the carbohydrate intake is limited, dieters are encouraged to consume more fat and protein in amounts of 80% and 20%; respectively. The ketogenic diet is often referred to as a low-carb diet, but it is important to take note that it [ketogenic diet] is entirely different from the other low-carb diets that encourage protein loading. Protein is not as important as fat is in the ketogenic diet. The reason is that the presence of a higher amount of protein pushes the body to the process called gluconeogenesis wherein protein is converted into glucose. If this happens, the body is not pushed to a state of ketosis. This is the reason why it is so crucial to consume more fat under the ketogenic diet than protein. When we eat, the carbohydrates found in the food that we consume is converted into a simple sugar called glucose. Alongside converting carbs to glucose, the pancreas also manufactures insulin, which is a hormone responsible for pushing glucose into the cells to be used up as energy. Keto Diet Cookbook As glucose is used up as the main source of energy, the fats that you also consume from food is not utilized thus they are immediately stored in the liver and adipocytes (specialized fat cells). Moreover, if you consume too many carbohydrates, the glucose that is not used up is converted into glycogen and is stored in the liver and muscles as standby energy source. If not used up, it is processed and converted to fat and stored all over the body, thus you gain weight. However, the body is working in a brilliant system that allows us to use up and burn off fats from our body. The ability of the body to produce ketones is part of the millions of years of the human evolution. It protected our ancestors during times of starvation in the past. During periods of famines in the past wherein the body cannot consume carbohydrates over long periods of time, the body uses up fats as a source of energy, as it does in ketosis. This process has helped our ancestors survived for millions of years. Amazing, right? So, when does ketosis happen? People usually enter the state of ketosis after 3 to 4 days consuming little amounts of carbohydrates. But to undergo the state of ketosis, some people think that you must stop eating altogether—but not with the ketogenic diet. The ketogenic diet bypasses starvation by encouraging you to eat more fats and adequate amounts of protein so that you don't have to undergo starvation. So, what food should you eat? This diet regimen encourages people to consume more fats sourced from healthy and whole food ingredients. That way, the body is pushed to a pure state of ketosis without ever feeling hungry.

Pork, Beef & Lamb Recipes

1. Mom's Meatballs in Creamy Sauce

(Ready in about 30 minutes | Servings 6) Per serving: 378 Calories; 29.9g Fat; 2.9g Carbs; 23.4g Protein; 0.3g

Ingredients

For the Meatballs: 2 eggs 1 tablespoon steak seasoning 1 tablespoon green garlic, minced 1 tablespoon scallions, minced 1 pound ground pork 1/2 pound ground turkey For the Sauce: 3 teaspoons ghee 1 cup double cream 1 cup cream of onion soup Salt and pepper, to your liking 1/2 teaspoon dried rosemary

Directions

Preheat your oven to 365 degrees F. In a mixing bowl, combine all ingredients for the meatballs. Roll the mixture into 20 to 24 balls and place them on a parchment-lined baking sheet. Roast for about 25 minutes or until your meatballs are golden-brown on the top. While your meatballs are roasting, melt the ghee in a preheated sauté pan over a moderate flame. Gradually add in the remaining ingredients, whisking constantly, until the sauce has reduced slightly. Bon appétit!

2. Easy Pork Tenderloin Gumbo

(Ready in about 35 minutes | Servings 6) Per serving: 427 Calories; 16.2g Fat; 3.6g Carbs; 33.2g Protein; 4.4g

Ingredients

1 pound pork tenderloin, cubed 8 ounces New Orleans spicy sausage, sliced 1 tablespoon Cajun spice mix 1 medium-sized leek, chopped 2 tablespoons olive oil 5 cups bone broth 1/2 cup celery, chopped 1 teaspoon gumbo file 1/4 cup flaxseed meal 3/4 pound okra 2 bell peppers, deveined and thinly sliced

Directions

In a heavy-bottomed pot, heat the oil until sizzling. Sear the pork tenderloin and New Orleans sausage for about 8 minutes or until browned on all sides; set aside. In the same pot, cook the leek and peppers until they softened. Add in the gumbo file, Cajun spice and broth. Bring it to a rolling boil. Turn the heat to medium-low and add in celery. Let it simmer for 18 to 20 minutes longer. Stir in the flax seed meal and okra along with the reserved meat. Then, continue to simmer for 5 to 6 minutes or until heated through. Enjoy!

3. Bacon Blue Cheese Fat Bombs

(Ready in about 5 minutes | Servings 4) Per serving: 232 Calories; 17.6g Fat; 2.9g Carbs; 14.2g Protein; 0.6g

Ingredients

1 ½ tablespoons mayonnaise 1/2 cup bacon, chopped 3 ounces blue cheese, crumbled 3 ounces cream cheese 2 tablespoons chives, chopped 2 teaspoons tomato puree

Directions

Mix all ingredients until everything is well combined. Shape the mixture into 8 equal fat bombs. Serve well chilled!

4. German Pork Rouladen

(Ready in about 1 hour + marinating time | Servings 6) Per serving: 220 Calories; 6g Fat; 2.8g Carbs; 33.3g Protein; 0.4g

Ingredients

1 ½ pounds boneless pork loin, butterflied 2 garlic cloves, pressed 1 tablespoon ghee, room temperature 1 tablespoon Mediterranean herb mix 1 teaspoon mustard seeds 1/2 teaspoon cumin seeds 1 cup roasted vegetable broth 1 large-sized onion, thinly sliced Salt and black peppercorns, to taste 1/2 cup Burgundy wine

Directions

Boil the pork loin for about 5 minutes; pat it dry. Now, combine the Mediterranean herb mix, mustard seeds, cumin seeds, garlic and ghee. Unfold the pork loin and spread the rub all over the cut side. Roll the pork and secure with kitchen string. Allow it to sit at least 2 hours in your refrigerator. Place the pork loin in a lightly greased baking pan. Add on wine, broth, onion, salt, and black peppercorns. Roast in the preheated oven at 390 degrees F approximately 1 hour. Bon appétit!

5. Pork and Vegetable Souvlaki

(Ready in about 20 minutes + marinating time | Servings 6) Per serving: 267 Calories; 10.6g Fat; 5.3g Carbs; 34.9g Protein; 1.3g

Ingredients

1 tablespoon Greek spice mix 2 cloves garlic, crushed 3 tablespoons coconut aminos 3 tablespoons olive oil 1 tablespoon stone-ground mustard 2 tablespoons fresh lemon juice 1 pound brown mushrooms 2 bell peppers, cut into thick slices 1 red bell pepper, cut into thick slices 1 zucchini, cubed 1 shallot, cut into wedges 2 pounds pork butt, cubed Bamboo skewers, soaked in cold water for 30 minutes

Directions

Mix the Greek spice mix, garlic, coconut aminos, olive oil, mustard, and lemon juice in a ceramic dish; add in pork cubes and let it marinate for 2 hours. Thread the pork cubes and vegetables onto the soaked skewers. Salt to taste. Grill for about 15 minutes, basting with the reserved marinade. Bon appétit!

6. Pork and Broccoli Stew

(Ready in about 2 hours | Servings 6) Per serving: 326 Calories; 13.9g Fat; 6g Carbs; 23.5g Protein; 1.2g

Ingredients

2 tablespoons lard, at room temperature 1 ½ pounds pork shoulder, cubed 1 teaspoon smoked paprika Sea salt and ground black pepper to taste 1 brown onion, chopped 1 stalk celery, chopped 1 teaspoon garlic, finely minced 1/4 cup dry red wine 3 cups water 2 bay leaves 1/2 teaspoon celery seeds 2 bell peppers, chopped 1 chili pepper, chopped 1 cup broccoli, broken into florets 1 tablespoon beef bouillon granules 1 tablespoon flax seed meal

Directions

Melt the lard in a heavy-bottomed pot over a moderate flame. Now, cook the pork for 5 to 6 minutes or until browned on all sides. Season with paprika, salt, and black pepper; reserve. In the same pot, sauté the onion, celery and garlic until they've softened. Add a splash of dry red wine to scrape up any browned bits from the bottom of your pot. Add in the water, bay leaves, celery seeds, bell peppers, and chili pepper. Reduce the temperature to simmer and add in the reserved pork. Continue to simmer for 1 hour 20 minutes. Add in the broccoli and beef bouillon granules and cook an additional 15 minutes. Add in the flax seed meal to thicken the cooking liquid. Taste and adjust the seasonings. Bon appétit!

7. Italian Pork Soup

(Ready in about 1 hour | Servings 4) Per serving: 331 Calories; 17.6g Fat; 4.4g Carbs; 37.4g Protein; 0.9g

Ingredients

1 shallot, chopped 4 cups beef bone broth 1 tomato, crushed 1 Pepperoncini, seeded and cut into very thin strips with scissors 1 tablespoon Italian herb mix 1 teaspoon green garlic, minced 1/2 cup Marsala wine 1 carrot, thinly sliced 2 tablespoons olive oil 1 ½ pounds pork stew meat, cubed 1 Italian pepper, thinly sliced Salt and black pepper, to taste

Directions

In a soup pot, heat the oil over a moderately high flame. Brown the pork for about 6 minutes until no longer pink; set aside. In the same pot, cook the shallot until tender and fragrant. Stir in the garlic and continue to sauté for 30 seconds more or until aromatic. Add in wine to deglaze the bottom of the soup pot. Add in the remaining ingredients along with the reserved pork; bring to a rapid boil. Reduce the heat to medium-low; continue to simmer, partially covered, for about 45 minutes. Bon appétit!

8. Barbecue Saucy Pork

(Ready in about 2 hours | Servings 8) Per serving: 561 Calories; 34g Fat; 1.7g Carbs; 52.7g Protein; 0.4g

Ingredients

2 tablespoons olive oil 1 teaspoon fresh garlic, halved 2 pounds pork butt Sea salt and freshly ground black pepper, to taste 1/3 teaspoon hot paprika A few drops of liquid smoke 1/3 teaspoon ground cumin 1/2 cup marinara sauce 1 teaspoon hot sauce 1 teaspoon stone-ground mustard

Directions

Rub the pork with the olive oil and garlic. Sprinkle with salt, pepper, and hot paprika. Roast the pork at 410 degrees F for 20 minutes. Turn the heat to 340 degrees F and roast for about 1 hour. In a mixing bowl, whisk the remaining ingredients. Spoon the sauce over the pork and continue to roast an additional 20 minutes. Enjoy!

9. Polish Sausage and Sauerkraut

(Ready in about 35 minutes | Servings 6) Per serving: 309 Calories; 20.6g Fat; 4.2g Carbs; 19.3g Protein; 3.8g

Ingredients

4 slices Polish bacon, chopped 2 pork sausages, sliced 1 onion, chopped 1/3 cup dry white wine 1 Serano pepper, finely minced 1 teaspoon garlic, finely minced 1/2 teaspoon fennel seeds, ground 1/2 teaspoon mustard seeds 1 cup vegetable broth 1 ½ pounds prepared sauerkraut, drained

Directions In a saucepan, fry the bacon over medium-high heat for 7 to 8 minutes; reserve. In the same pan, cook the sausage until no longer pink for 4 to 5 minutes; reserve. Then, cook the onions until tender and translucent for 5 to 6 minutes. Add a splash of wine to deglaze the pan. Add in the remaining ingredients and bring to a boil; turn the heat to simmer and continue to cook for 15 to 18 minutes or until everything is cooked through.Bon appétit!

10. Breakfast Mug Muffin

(Ready in about 10 minutes | Servings 2) Per serving: 327 Calories; 16.6g Fat; 5.8g Carbs; 40g Protein; 1.2g

Ingredients

1/2 cup marinara sauce 1/2 cup cheddar cheese, shredded 1/2 pound ground pork 1 teaspoon garlic paste 1/2 teaspoon shallot powder Salt and ground black pepper, to taste 1/2 teaspoon paprika

Directions

In a mixing bowl, combine all ingredients until everything is well incorporated. Spoon the mixture into two microwave-safe mugs. Microwave for 5 minutes until set but still moist.Bon appétit!

11. Baked Pork Meatballs in Pasta Sauce

Ready in about: 45 minutes | Serves: 6 Per serving: Kcal 590, Fat 46.8g, Net Carbs 4.1g, Protein 46.2g

Ingredients

2 lb ground pork 1 tbsp olive oil 1 cup pork rinds, crushed 2 cloves garlic, minced ½ cup coconut milk 2 eggs, beaten ½ cup Parmesan cheese, grated ½ cup asiago cheese, grated Salt and black pepper to taste 2 jars sugar-free marinara sauce 1 cup Italian blend kinds of cheeses 3 tbsp fresh basil, chopped Preheat oven to 400°F.

Directions

Combine the coconut milk and pork rinds in a bowl. Mix in the ground pork, garlic, asiago cheese, Parmesan cheese, eggs, salt, and pepper and stir. Form balls of the mixture and place them in a greased baking pan. Bake in the oven for 20 minutes. Transfer the meatballs to a plate. Pour half of the marinara sauce into the baking pan. Place the meatballs back in the pan and pour in the remaining marinara sauce. Sprinkle with the Italian blend cheeses and drizzle with the olive oil. Cover the pan with foil and put it back in the oven. Bake for 10 minutes. After, remove the foil, and cook for 5 minutes. Once ready, take out the pan and garnish with basil. Serve on a bed of squash spaghetti.

12. Charred Tenderloin with Lemon Chimichurri

Ready in about: 64 minutes | Serves: 4 Per serving: Kcal 388, Fat 18g, Net Carbs 2.1g, Protein 28g

Ingredients

13. Lemon Chimichurri

1 lemon, juiced ¼ cup mint leaves, chopped ¼ cup fresh oregano, chopped 2 cloves garlic, minced ¼ cup olive oil Salt to taste

Pork

1 (4 lb) pork tenderloin Salt and black pepper to taste 1 tbsp olive oil Make the lemon chimichurri to have the flavors incorporate while the pork cooks.

Directions

In a bowl, mix the mint, oregano, and garlic. Then, add the lemon juice, olive oil, and salt, and combine well. Set aside. Preheat the charcoal grill to 450°F, creating a direct heat area and indirect heat area. Rub the pork with olive oil and season with salt and pepper. Place the meat over direct heat and sear for 3 minutes on each side, moving to the indirect heat area. Close the lid and cook for 25 minutes on one side Next, open, turn the meat, and grill for 20 minutes on the other side. Remove the pork from the grill and let it sit for 5 minutes before slicing. Spoon lemon chimichurri over the pork and serve with fresh salad.

14. Pork Goulash with Cauliflower

Ready in about: 15 minutes | Serves: 4 Per serving: Kcal 475, Fat 37g, Net Carbs 4.5g, Protein 44g

Ingredients

1 red bell pepper, chopped 2 tbsp olive oil 1 ½ lb ground pork Salt and black pepper to taste 2 cups cauliflower florets 1 onion, chopped 14 oz canned diced tomatoes ¼ tsp garlic powder 1 tbsp tomato puree

Directions

Heat olive oil in a pan over medium heat. Add in the pork and brown for 5 minutes. Mix in the bell pepper and onion and cook for 4 minutes. Stir in 1 cup water, tomatoes, and cauliflower. Bring to a simmer and cook for 5 minutes. Pour in tomato paste, salt, pepper, and garlic powder and stir for 5 minutes. Serve.

15. Pork Wraps

Ready in about: 40 minutes | Serves: 6 Per serving: Kcal 435, Fat 37g, Net Carbs 2g, Protein 34g

Ingredients

6 bacon slices 2 tbsp fresh parsley, chopped 1 lb pork tenderloin, sliced ⅓ cup ricotta cheese 3 tbsp coconut oil ¼ cup onions, chopped 3 garlic cloves, minced 2 tbsp Parmesan cheese, grated 15 oz canned diced tomatoes ⅓ cup vegetable stock Salt and black pepper to taste ½ tsp Italian seasoning

Directions

Use a meat pounder to flatten the pork pieces. Set the bacon slices on top of each piece and divide the parsley, ricotta cheese, and Parmesan cheese between them. Roll each pork piece and secure it with a toothpick. Set a pan over medium heat and warm oil. Cook the pork rolls until browned. Remove. Add onions and garlic in the pan and cook for 5 minutes. Place in the stock and cook for 3 minutes. Get rid of the toothpicks from the rolls and return to the pan. Stir in pepper, salt, tomatoes, and Italian seasoning. Bring to a boil, reduce the heat, and cook for 20 minutes covered. Split among bowls to serve.

16. Pulled Pork with Avocado

Ready in about: 2 hours 55 minutes | Serves: 6 Per serving: Kcal 567, Fat 42.6g, Net Carbs 4.1g, Protein 42g

Ingredients

2 lb pork shoulder 1 tbsp avocado oil ½ cup vegetable stock 1 tsp taco seasoning 1 avocado, sliced Preheat oven to 350°F.

Directions

Rub the pork with taco seasoning and set in a greased baking dish. Pour in the vegetable stock. Place in the oven, cover with aluminium foil, and cook for 1 hour 45 minutes. Discard the foil and cook for another 10-15 minutes until brown on top. Leave to rest for 15-20 minutes. Shred it with 2 forks. Serve topped with avocado slices.

17. BBQ Pork Pizza with Goat Cheese

Ready in about: 30 minutes | Serves: 4 Per serving: Kcal 344, Fat 24g, Net Carbs 6,5g, Protein 18g

Ingredients

1 low carb pizza bread 1 tbsp olive oil 1 cup Manchego cheese, grated 2 cups leftover pulled pork ½ cup sugar-free BBQ sauce 1 cup goat cheese, crumbled Preheat oven to 400°F.

Directions

Put the pizza bread on a pizza pan. Brush with olive oil and sprinkle the Manchego cheese all over. Mix the pork with BBQ sauce and spread over the cheese. Drop goat cheese on top and bake for 25 minutes until the cheese has melted. Slice the pizza with a cutter and serve.

18. Easy Pork Bistek

(Ready in about 30 minutes | Servings 4) Per serving: 305 Calories; 20.6g Fat; 3.7g Carbs; 22.5g Protein; 0.6g

Ingredients

1 red onion, peeled and chopped 1 garlic clove, minced 2 tablespoons olive oil 1 ½ pounds pork blade steak 1/4 cup dry red wine 1/2 teaspoon salt 1/2 teaspoon freshly ground black pepper 1/2 teaspoon cayenne pepper 1 teaspoon mustard seeds

Directions

In a frying pan, heat 1 tablespoon of the olive oil over a moderate heat. Now, sear the pork steaks for 8 to 9 minutes per side. Pour in a splash of wine to deglaze the pot. Sprinkle with spices and continue to cook for 10 minutes more, adding additional water if necessary; reserve. In the same frying pan, heat the remaining tablespoon of olive oil and cook the onions and garlic until they have softened. Bon appétit!

19. Italian-Style Pork Casserole

(Ready in about 50 minutes | Servings 6) Per serving: 478 Calories; 36g Fat; 4.9g Carbs; 33.5g Protein; 0.3g

Ingredients

1 ¼ pounds ground pork 6 eggs, lightly beaten 2 tablespoons fresh Italian parsley 2 ½ cups almond meal 1 Italian peppers, thinly sliced 1 cup double cream 1/2 teaspoon celery seeds 1 stick butter, melted Salt and pepper, to the taste

Directions

Start by preheating your oven to 350 degrees F Thoroughly combine the eggs, almond meal, and melted until well combined. Press the mixture into a lightly oiled baking dish. In a nonstick skillet, cook the ground pork for about 4 minutes, breaking apart with a wide spatula; season with salt and pepper to taste. Add in the remaining ingredients and stir to combine well. Spread this mixture over the crust, using a wide spatula. Bake in the preheated oven at 350 degrees F for about 40 minutes. Let it stand for 10 minutes before slicing. Bon appétit!

20. Roasted Pork Rib Chops

(Ready in about 30 minutes + marinating time | Servings 4) Per serving: 452 Calories; 34.8g Fat; 4.7g Carbs; 26.3g

Ingredients

4 (2- 1 1/2"-thick) pork bone-in pork rib chops 1 teaspoon mustard seeds 2 tablespoons fresh lime juice 1/2 teaspoon celery salt 1/2 teaspoon freshly ground black pepper 1 garlic clove 2 tablespoons butter, room temperature 1 cup leeks, sliced 2 carrots, sliced 1 celery stalk, diced

Directions

Place the pork, mustard seeds, fresh lime juice, celery salt, salt, pepper, and garlic in a ceramic dish. Cover and let them marinate in your refrigerator for about 3 hours. In an oven-safe skillet, melt the butter over medium-high heat. Sear the pork cutlets until bottom side is golden brown, about 2 minutes. Flip them over and cook on other side about 2 minutes. Repeat the process, turning about every 1 to 2 minutes, until an instant-read thermometer inserted into the thickest part registers 150 degrees F. Add in the leeks, carrots, and celery and continue to cook, partially covered, for 5 minutes more. Transfer the skillet to the oven and roast the pork with the vegetables for about 10 minutes. Bon appétit!

21. Mom's Signature Pork Meatloaf

(Ready in about 45 minutes | Servings 6) Per serving: 251 Calories; 7.9g Fat; 4.5g Carbs; 34.6g Protein; 1.4g

Ingredients

1 cup tomato puree, no sugar added 1 ½ tablespoons Swerve 1 tablespoon champagne vinegar 1/2 teaspoon dried rosemary 1 teaspoon fresh coriander 1/3 cup almond meal 1 large egg Sea salt and ground black pepper 1 teaspoon celery seeds 1 ½ pounds ground pork 1/4 cup pork rinds, crushed 1 large onion, chopped 2 cloves garlic, finely minced

Directions

In a mixing dish, thoroughly combine the almond meal, egg, salt, black pepper, celery seeds, ground pork, pork rinds, onion, and garlic. Press the meatloaf mixture into a lightly greased loaf pan. In a saucepan, cook the remaining ingredients until the sauce has thickened and reduced slightly. Spread the sauce evenly over the top of your meatloaf. Roast in the preheated oven at 365 degrees F for 35 minutes. Place under the preheated broiler for 5 to 6 minutes. Bon appétit!

22. Pork Rib Soup with Avocado

(Ready in about 20 minutes | Servings 6) Per serving: 423 Calories; 31.8g Fat; 6g Carbs; 25.9g Protein; 3.2g

Ingredients

1 ¼ pounds pork spare ribs, boneless and cut into chunks 2 tablespoons butter, room temperature Sea salt and ground black pepper, to taste A pinch of dried Mexican oregano 2 vine-ripened tomatoes, undrained 1 celery, chopped 1 onion, peeled and chopped 1 teaspoon garlic, crushed 1 teaspoon habanero pepper, seeded and minced 3 cups beef broth, less-sodium 1/4 cup fresh coriander, roughly chopped 1 medium-sized avocado, pitted and sliced

Directions

Melt the butter in a heavy-bottomed pot over a moderate heat. Sauté the onion, garlic, pepper and celery approximately 3 minutes. Then, sear the pork for 4 to 5 minutes, stirring continuously to ensure even cooking. Add in the broth, salt, black pepper, oregano, tomatoes, and coriander. Continue to simmer, partially covered, for about 12 minutes. Bon appétit!

23. Creamed Pork Soup

(Ready in about 25 minutes | Servings 4) Per serving: 490 Calories; 44g Fat; 6.1g Carbs; 24.3g Protein; 2.2g Fiber

Ingredients

3/4 pound pork chops, cubed 2 tomatoes, pureed 1 cup double cream 1/2 teaspoon Tabasco sauce 1 tablespoon chicken bouillon granules 4 cups water 2 tablespoons butter, melted 1 white onion, chopped 1 celery stalk, chopped 1 carrot, chopped Seasoned salt and freshly cracked black pepper, to taste 1/2 teaspoon red pepper flakes 1/2 cup avocado, pitted, peeled and diced

Directions

In a soup pot, melt the butter over medium-high heat. Cook the onion, celery, and carrot until tender and fragrant or about 6 minutes. Heat the remaining tablespoon of butter and sear the pork for 4 to 5 minutes, stirring periodically to ensure even cooking. Add in the water, pureed tomatoes, chicken bouillon granules, salt, black pepper, and red paper flakes, salt, and pepper. Partially cover and continue to simmer for 10 to 12 minutes. Fold in the double cream and Tabasco sauce. Let it simmer for 5 minutes until cooked through .Bon appétit!

24. Saucy Boston Butt

(Ready in about 1 hour 20 minutes | Servings 8) Per serving: 369 Calories; 20.2g Fat; 2.9g Carbs; 41.3g Protein; 0.7g Fiber

Ingredients

1 tablespoon lard, room temperature 2 pounds Boston butt, cubed Salt and freshly ground pepper 1/2 teaspoon mustard powder A bunch of spring onions, chopped 2 garlic cloves, minced 1/2 tablespoon ground cardamom 2 tomatoes, pureed 1 bell pepper, deveined and chopped 1 jalapeno pepper, deveined and finely chopped 1/2 cup unsweetened coconut milk 2 cups chicken bone broth

Directions

In a wok, melt the lard over moderate heat. Season the pork belly with salt, pepper and mustard powder. Sear the pork for 8 to 10 minutes, stirring periodically to ensure even cooking; set aside, keeping it warm. In the same wok, sauté the spring onions, garlic, and cardamom. Spoon the sautéed vegetables along with the reserved pork into the slow cooker. Add in the remaining ingredients, cover with the lid and cook for 1 hour 10 minutes over low heat. Bon appétit!

25. Pork in Blue Cheese Sauce

(Ready in about 30 minutes | Servings 6) Per serving: 348 Calories; 18.9g Fat; 1.9g Carbs; 40.3g Protein; 0.3g Fiber

Ingredients

2 pounds pork center cut loin roast, boneless and cut into 6 pieces 1 tablespoon coconut aminos 6 ounces blue cheese 1/3 cup heavy cream 1/3 cup port wine 1/3 cup roasted vegetable broth, preferably homemade 1 teaspoon dried hot chile flakes 1 teaspoon dried rosemary 1 tablespoon lard 1 shallot, chopped 2 garlic cloves, chopped Salt and freshly cracked black peppercorns, to taste

Directions

Rub each piece of the pork with salt, black peppercorns, and rosemary. Melt the lard in a saucepan over a moderately high flame. Sear the pork on all sides about 15 minutes; set aside. Cook the shallot and garlic until they've softened. Add in port wine to scrape up any brown bits from the bottom. Reduce the heat to medium-low and add in the remaining ingredients; continue to simmer until the sauce has thickened and reduced. Bon appétit!

26. Mediterranean-Style Cheesy Pork Loin

(Ready in about 25 minutes | Servings 4) Per serving: 476 Calories; 35.3g Fat; 6.2g Carbs; 31.1g Protein; 1.4g Fiber

Ingredients

1 pound pork loin, cut into 1-inch-thick pieces 1 teaspoon Mediterranean seasoning mix Salt and pepper, to taste 1 onion, sliced 1 teaspoon fresh garlic, smashed 2 tablespoons black olives, pitted and sliced 2 tablespoons balsamic vinegar 1/2 cup Romano cheese, grated 2 tablespoons butter, room temperature 1 tablespoon curry paste 1 cup roasted vegetable broth 1 tablespoon oyster sauce

Directions

In a frying pan, melt the butter over a moderately high heat. Once hot, cook the pork until browned on all sides; season with salt and black pepper and set aside. In the pan drippings, cook the onion and garlic for 4 to 5 minutes or until they've softened. Add in the Mediterranean seasoning mix, curry paste, and vegetable broth. Continue to cook until the sauce has thickened and reduced slightly or about 10 minutes. Add in the remaining ingredients along with the reserved pork. Top with cheese and cook for 10 minutes longer or until cooked through.Enjoy!

27. Oven-Roasted Spare Ribs

(Ready in about 3 hour 40 minutes + marinating time | Servings 6) Per serving: 385 Calories; 29g Fat; 1.8g Carbs; 28.3g Protein; 0.1g Fiber

Ingredients

2 pounds spare ribs 1 garlic clove, minced 1 teaspoon dried marjoram 1 lime, halved Salt and ground black pepper, to taste

Directions

Toss all ingredients in a ceramic dish. Cover and let it refrigerate for 5 to 6 hours. Roast the foil-wrapped ribs in the preheated oven at 275 degrees F degrees for about 3 hours 30 minutes. Bon appétit!

28. Peanut Butter Pork Stir-Fry

Ready in about: 23 minutes | Serves: 4 Per serving: Kcal 571, Fat 49g, Net Carbs 1g, Protein 22.5g

Ingredients

2 tbsp ghee 2 lb pork loin, cut into strips Pink salt to taste 2 tsp ginger-garlic paste ¼ cup chicken broth 5 tbsp peanut butter, softened 2 cups mixed stir-fry vegetables ½ tsp chili pepper

Directions

Melt the ghee in a wok over high heat. Rub the pork with salt, chili pepper, and ginger-garlic paste. Place it into the wok and cook for 6 minutes until no longer pink. Mix peanut butter and broth until smooth. Pour in the wok and stir for 6 minutes. Add in the mixed veggies and simmer for 5 minutes. Adjust the taste with salt and black pepper and spoon the stir-fry to a side of cilantro cauli rice.

29. Pork Lettuce Cups

Ready in about: 20 minutes | Serves: 6 Per serving: Kcal 311, Fat 24.3g, Net Carbs 1g, Protein 19g

Ingredients

2 lb ground pork 1 tbsp ginger-garlic paste Pink salt and black pepper to taste 3 tbsp butter Leaves from 1 head Iceberg lettuce 2 green onions, chopped 1 red bell pepper, chopped ½ cucumber, finely chopped ½ tsp cayenne pepper

Directions

Melt the butter in a pan over medium heat. Rub the pork with ginger-garlic paste, salt, pepper, and cayenne pepper and add it to the pan. Cook for 10 minutes until the pork is no longer pink. Remove and let it cool. Pat the lettuce leaves dry with paper towels. Spoon two to three tablespoons of the pork mixture in each leaf. Top with green onions, bell pepper, and cucumber. Serve with soy drizzling sauce.

30. Pork & Mushroom Bake

Ready in about: 1 hour 15 minutes | Serves: 6 Per serving: Kcal 403, Fat: 32.6g, Net Carbs: 8g, Protein: 19.4g

Ingredients

1 onion, chopped 2 (10.5-oz) cans mushroom soup 6 pork chops ½ cup sliced mushrooms Salt and black pepper to taste Preheat oven to 370°F.

Directions

Season the pork with salt and pepper. Place on a baking dish. Combine the mushroom soup, mushrooms, and onion in a bowl and stir. Pour it over the pork. Bake for 45 minutes.

31. Pork Chops with Mint & Parsley Pesto

Ready in about: 3 hours 10 minutes | Serves: 4 Per serving: Kcal 567, Fat 40g, Net Carbs 5.5g, Protein 37g

Ingredients

1 cup parsley 1 cup mint 1 ½ onions, chopped ⅓ cup pistachios, chopped 3 tbsp avocado oil Salt to taste 4 pork chops 2 garlic cloves, minced 1 lemon, juiced and zested

DirectionsIn a food processor, combine the parsley with avocado oil, mint, pistachios, salt, lemon zest, and half of the onions. Rub the pork with this mixture, place In a bowl, and refrigerate for 1 hour while covered. Remove the chops and set them to a baking dish. Top with the remaining onions and garlic. Sprinkle with lemon juice. Pour in 1 cup of water. Bake for 2 hours in the oven at 250°F. Serve warm.

32. Bacon Smothered Pork Chops

Ready in about: 25 minutes | Serves: 6 Per serving: Kcal 435, Fat 37g, Net Carbs 3g, Protein 22g

Ingredients

6 strips bacon, chopped 6 pork chops Pink salt and black pepper to taste 2 sprigs fresh thyme ¼ cup chicken broth ½ cup heavy cream

Directions

Cook bacon in a large skillet on medium heat for 5 minutes. Remove with a slotted spoon onto a paper towel-lined plate to soak up excess fat. Season the pork chops with salt and black pepper and brown in the bacon fat for 4 minutes on each side. Remove to the bacon plate. Stir the thyme, chicken broth, and heavy cream in the skillet and simmer for 5 minutes. Return the chops and bacon and cook further for another 2 minutes. Serve chops with a generous ladle of sauce.

33. Pancetta & Kale Pork Sausages

Ready in about: 30 minutes | Serves: 4 Per serving: Kcal 386, Fat 29g, Net Carbs 5.4g, Protein2 1g

Ingredients

2 cups kale 4 cups chicken broth 2 tbsp olive oil 1 cup heavy cream 3 pancetta slices, chopped ½ lb radishes, chopped 2 garlic cloves, minced Salt and black pepper to taste ½ tsp red pepper flakes 1 onion, chopped 1 ½ lb hot pork sausage, chopped

Directions

Warm the olive oil in a pot over medium heat. Stir in garlic, onion, pancetta, and sausage and cook for 5 minutes. Pour in the broth, radishes, and kale and simmer for 10 minutes. Sprinkle with salt, red pepper flakes, and black pepper. Add in the heavy cream, stir, and cook for about 5 minutes. Serve.

34. Juicy Pork Medallions

Ready in about: 30 minutes | Serves: 4 Per serving: Kcal 325, Fat 18g, Net Carbs 6g, Protein 36g

Ingredients

1 lb pork tenderloin, cut into medallions 2 onions, chopped 6 bacon slices, chopped ½ cup vegetable stock

Directions

Set a pan over medium heat. Add in the bacon and cook until crispy, about 5 minutes; remove to a plate. Add onions to the pan and cook for 3 minutes; set aside. Add the pork medallions to the pan Brown for 3 minutes on each side, turn, and reduce the heat. Add in the vegetable stock and cook for 10 minutes. Return the bacon and onions to the pan and cook for 1 minute. Serve warm.

35. Lemon Pork Chops with Buttered Brussels Sprouts

Ready in about: 35 minutes | Serves: 6 Per serving: Kcal 549, Fat 48g, Net Carbs 2g, Protein 26g

Ingredients

3 tbsp lemon juice 3 cloves garlic, pureed 2 tbsp olive oil 6 pork loin chops 1 tbsp butter 1 lb Brussels sprouts, trimmed, halved 2 tbsp white wine Salt and black pepper to taste Preheat oven to 400°F.

Directions

Mix the lemon juice, garlic, salt, black pepper, and oil in a bowl. Brush the pork with the mixture. Place in a baking sheet and brown in the oven for 15 minutes, turning once. Remove. Melt butter in a small wok and cook the Brussels sprouts for 5 minutes until tender. Drizzle with white wine, sprinkle with salt and black pepper, and cook for another 5 minutes. Serve them with the chops.

36. Greek Pork with Olives

Ready in about: 35 minutes | Serves: 4 Per serving: Kcal 415, Fat 25.2g, Net Carbs 2.2g, Protein 36g

Ingredients

4 pork chops, bone-in Salt and black pepper to taste 2 garlic cloves, minced ½ cup Kalamata olives, pitted, sliced 2 tbsp olive oil 1 cup vegetable broth Season pork chops with black pepper and salt.

Directions

Add them to a roasting pan. Add in garlic, olives, olive oil, and vegetable broth. Roast in the oven for 10 minutes at 425°F. Serve warm.

37. Pork Nachos

Ready in about: 15 minutes | Serves: 4 Per serving: Kcal 452, Fat 25g, Net Carbs 9.3g, Protein 22g

Ingredients

1 bag low carb tortilla chips 2 cups leftover pulled pork 1 red bell pepper, chopped 1 red onion, diced 2 cups Monterey Jack cheese, grated Preheat oven to 350°F.

Directions

Arrange the chips on a baking pan, scatter pork over, followed by red bell pepper and onion, and sprinkle with the cheese. Place the pan in the oven and cook for 10 minutes until the cheese has melted. Allow cooling for 3 minutes and serve.

38. Balsamic Grilled Pork Chops

Ready in about: 20 minutes + marinating time | Serves: 6 Per serving: Kcal 418, Fat 26.8g, Net Carbs 1.5g, Protein 38g

Ingredients

6 pork loin chops, boneless 1 tbsp erythritol ¼ cup balsamic vinegar 3 cloves garlic, minced ¼ cup olive oil Salt and black pepper to taste Put the pork in a plastic bag.

Directions

In a bowl, mix the erythritol, balsamic vinegar, garlic, olive oil, salt, pepper, and pour the mixture over the pork. Seal the bag, shake it, and place it in the refrigerator for 2 hours. Preheat the grill to medium heat, remove the pork when ready, and grill covered for 10 minutes on each side. Remove and let sit for 4 minutes. Serve with sautéed parsnips.

39. Pork Stew with Bacon & Cauliflower

Ready in about: 40 minutes | Serves: 6 Per serving: Kcal 331, Fat 14.2g, Net Carbs 2.9g, Protein 43.8g

Ingredients

2 lb pork tenderloin, cubed 2 cups chicken broth 3 tbsp olive oil 1 onion, chopped Salt and black pepper to taste 2 garlic cloves, minced 1 cup canned diced tomatoes 1 cup bacon, chopped 1 head cauliflower, cut into florets

Directions

Warm the olive oil in a saucepan over medium heat. Add in the bacon, pork, onion, and garlic and sauté for 3-4 minutes until the onion is tender. Pour in the chicken stock and tomatoes and simmer for 20-25 minutes. Add in the cauliflower and cook for 10 more minutes. Season with salt and pepper. Serve warm.

40. Beef Mushroom Meatloaf

Ready in about: 1 hour and 15 minutes | Serves: 12 Per serving: Kcal 294, Fat: 19g, Net Carbs: 6g, Protein: 23g

Ingredients 3 pounds ground beef ½ cup chopped onions ½ cup almond flour 2 garlic cloves, minced 1 cup sliced mushrooms 3 eggs ¼ tsp pepper 2 tbsp chopped parsley ¼ cup chopped bell peppers ⅓ cup grated Parmesan cheese 1 tsp balsamic vinegar 1 tsp salt Glaze 2 cups balsamic vinegar 1 tbsp sweetener 2 tbsp sugar-free ketchup

DirectionsCombine all meatloaf ingredients in a large bowl. Press this mixture into a greased loaf pans. Bake in the oven for 30 minutes at 370ºF. Combine all the glaze ingredients in a saucepan over medium heat. Simmer for 20 minutes until the glaze is thickened. Pour ¼ cup of the glaze over the meatloaf. Save the extra for future use. Put the meatloaf back in the oven and cook for 20 more minutes.

41. Beef & Cheddar Stuffed Eggplants

Ready in about: 30 minutes | Serves: 4 Per serving: Kcal 574, Fat 27.5g, Net Carbs 9.8g, Protein 61,8g

Ingredients

2 eggplants 2 tbsp olive oil 1 ½ lb ground beef 1 medium red onion, chopped 1 roasted red pepper, chopped Pink salt and black pepper to taste 1 cup yellow cheddar cheese, grated 2 tbsp dill, chopped Preheat oven to 350ºF.

DirectionsLay the eggplants on a flat surface, trim off the ends, and cut in half lengthwise. Scoop out the pulp from each half to make shells. Chop the pulp. Heat oil in a skillet over medium heat. Add the ground beef, red onion, pimiento, and eggplant pulp and season with salt and pepper. Cook for 6 minutes while stirring to break up lumps until beef is no longer pink. Spoon the beef into the eggplant shells and sprinkle with cheddar cheese. Place on a greased baking sheet and cook to Melt the cheese for 15 minutes until eggplant is tender. Serve warm topped with dill.

42. Melt-in-Your-Mouth Ribs

(Ready in about 4 hours 30 minutes | Servings 4) Per serving: 412 Calories; 14g Fat; 4.3g Carbs; 43.3g Protein; 0.7g

Ingredients

1 ½ pounds spare ribs 1 tablespoon olive oil, at room temperature 2 cloves garlic, chopped 1 Italian pepper, chopped Salt and black peppercorns, to taste 1/2 teaspoon ground cumin 2 bay leaves A bunch of green onions, chopped 3/4 cup beef bone broth, preferably homemade 2 teaspoons erythritol

Directions Heat the olive oil in a saucepan over medium-high heat. Sear the ribs for 6 to 7 minutes on each side. Whisk the broth, erythritol, garlic, Italian pepper, green onions, salt, pepper, and cumin until well combined. Place the spare ribs in your crock pot; pour in the pepper/broth mixture. Add in the bay leaves. Cook for about 4 hours on Low setting.

43. Old-Fashioned Stew with Pork Butt

Butt (Ready in about 25 minutes | Servings 4) Per serving: 295 Calories; 15.6g Fat; 6.3g Carbs; 17.3g Protein; 1.1g

Ingredients

3/4 pound boneless pork butt, cubed 1 ½ cups vegetable stock 1 tablespoon lard, room temperature 1 teaspoon Serrano pepper, deveined and minced 2 garlic cloves, minced 1/2 teaspoon ground cloves 1 yellow onion, chopped 1 carrot, chopped 1 tablespoon fresh coriander, chopped 2 ounces cream cheese, full-fat Himalayan salt and ground black pepper, to taste

Directions

Melt the lard in a soup pot over medium-high heat. Now, sauté the onion, carrot, and Serrano pepper for about 4 minutes or until tender and fragrant. Add in the boneless pork butt and cook for a father 5 to 6 minutes, stirring continuously to ensure even cooking. Add in the garlic, vegetable stock, ground cloves, salt, black pepper, and coriander; bring to a rapid boil. Now, reduce the temperature to medium-low. Cook for 15 to 20 minutes or until everything is thoroughly cooked. Bon appétit!

44. Pork and Carrot Mini Muffins

(Ready in about 35 minutes | Servings 6) Per serving: 303 Calories; 17g Fat; 6.2g Carbs; 29.6g Protein; 1.7g

Ingredients

1 egg, whisked 1 ounce envelope onion soup mix Kosher salt and ground black pepper, to taste 2 cloves of garlic, minced 1 cup carrots, shredded 1 cup tomato puree 1 tablespoon coconut aminos 1 tablespoon stone-ground mustard 1 ½ teaspoons dry basil 1 cup Romano cheese, grated 1 pound pork, ground 1/2 pound turkey, ground

Directions In a mixing bowl, combine all ingredients until everything is well incorporated. Press the mixture into a lightly-oiled muffin tin. Bake in the preheated oven at 355 degrees F for 30 to 33 minutes; let it cool slightly before unmolding and serving. Bon appétit!

45. Creole-Style Pork Shank

(Ready in about 30 minutes + marinating time | Servings 6) Per serving: 335 Calories; 24.3g Fat; 0.8g Carbs; 26.4g Protein; 0.4g

Ingredients

1 ½ pounds pork shank, cut into 6 serving portions 1 tablespoon Creole seasoning A few drops of liquid smoke Salt and cayenne pepper, to taste 3 teaspoons vegetable oil 2 clove garlic, minced 1 ½ tablespoons coconut aminos

Directions Blend the salt, cayenne pepper, vegetable oil, garlic, liquid smoke, Creole seasoning, and coconut aminos until you get a uniform and creamy mixture. Massage the pork shanks on all sides with the prepared rub mixture. Let it marinate for about 2 hours in your refrigerator. Grill for about 20 minutes until cooked through. Enjoy!

46. Rich Pork and Bacon Meatloaf

(Ready in about 1 hour 10 minutes | Servings 6) Per serving: 396 Calories; 24.1g Fat; 5.1g Carbs; 38.1g Protein; 0.5g

Ingredients

1 ¼ pounds ground pork 1/2 pound pork sausage, broken up 6 strips bacon 2 garlic cloves, finely minced 1 teaspoon celery seeds Salt and cayenne pepper, to taste 1 bunch coriander, roughly chopped 1 egg, beaten 2 ounces half-and-half 1 teaspoon lard 1 medium-sized leek, chopped

Directions Melt the lard in a frying pan over medium-high heat. Cook the leek and garlic until they have softened or about 3 minutes. Add in the ground pork and sausage; cook until it is no longer pink, about 3 minutes. Add in the half-and-half, celery seeds, salt, cayenne pepper, coriander, and egg. Press the mixture into a loaf pan. Place the bacon strips on top of your meatloaf and bake at 390 degrees F about 55 minutes. Bon appétit!

47. Pork Cutlets with Kale

(Ready in about 25 minutes + marinating time | Servings 6) Per serving: 234 Calories; 11g Fat; 2g Carbs; 29.8g Protein; 0.9g

Ingredients

Sea salt and ground black pepper, to taste 2 teaspoons olive oil 1/4 cup port wine 2 garlic cloves, smashed 2 tablespoons oyster sauce 2 tablespoons fresh lime juice 1 medium leek, sliced 2 bell peppers, chopped 2 cups kale 1 ½ pounds pork cutlets

Directions

Sprinkle the pork with salt and black pepper. Then, make the marinade by whisking 1 teaspoon of olive oil, wine, garlic, oyster sauce, and lime juice. Let the pork marinate for about 2 hours in your refrigerator Heat the remaining teaspoon of olive oil in a frying pan. Fry the leek and bell peppers for 4 to 5 minutes, stirring continuously, until they have softened slightly; set aside. In the same pan, sear the pork along with the marinade until browned on all sides. Stir the reserved vegetables into the frying pan along with the kale. Continue to cook for 5 to 6 minutes more. Bon appétit!

48. Cheesy Chinese-Style Pork

(Ready in about 20 minutes | Servings 6) Per serving: 424 Calories; 29.4g Fat; 3.8g Carbs; 34.2g Protein; 0.6g Fiber

Ingredients

1 tablespoon sesame oil 1 ½ pounds pork shoulder, cut into strips Himalayan salt and freshly ground black pepper, to taste 1/2 teaspoon cayenne pepper 1/2 cup shallots, roughly chopped 2 bell peppers, sliced 1/4 cup cream of onion soup 1/2 teaspoon Sriracha sauce 1 tablespoon tahini (sesame butter) 1 tablespoon soy sauce 4 ounces gouda cheese, cut into small pieces

Directions

Heat he sesame oil in a wok over a moderately high flame. Stir-fry the pork strips for 3 to 4 minutes or until just browned on all sides. Add in the spices, shallots and bell peppers and continue to cook for a further 4 minutes. Stir in the cream of onion soup, Sriracha, sesame butter, and soy sauce; continue to cook for 3 to 4 minutes more. Top with the cheese and continue to cook until the cheese has melted.

49. Breakfast Muffins with Ground Pork

(Ready in about 25 minutes | Servings 6) Per serving: 330 Calories; 30.3g Fat; 2.3g Carbs; 19g Protein; 1.2g Fiber

Ingredients

1 stick butter 3 large eggs, lightly beaten 2 tablespoons full-fat milk 1/2 teaspoon ground cardamom 3 ½ cups almond flour 2 tablespoons flaxseed meal 1 teaspoon baking powder 2 cups ground pork Salt and pepper, to your liking 1/2 teaspoon dried basil

Directions

In the preheated frying pan, cook the ground pork until the juices run clear, approximately 5 minutes. Add in the remaining ingredients and stir until well combined. Spoon the mixture into lightly greased muffin cups. Bake in the preheated oven at 365 degrees F for about 17 minutes. Allow your muffins to cool down before unmolding and storing. Bon appétit!

50. Brie-Stuffed Meatballs

(Ready in about 25 minutes | Servings 5) Per serving: 302 Calories; 17.3g Fat; 1.9g Carbs; 33.4g Protein; 0.3g Fiber

Ingredients

2 eggs, beaten 1 pound ground pork 1/3 cup double cream 1 tablespoon fresh parsley Kosher salt and ground black pepper 1 teaspoon dried rosemary 10 (1-inch) cubes of brie cheese 2 tablespoons scallions, minced 2 cloves garlic, minced

Directions

Mix all ingredients, except for the brie cheese, until everything is well incorporated. Roll the mixture into 10 patties; place a piece of cheese in the center of each patty and roll into a ball. Roast in the preheated oven at 380 degrees F for about 20 minutes. Bon appétit!

51. Ground Pork Stuffed Peppers

(Ready in about 40 minutes | Servings 4) Per serving: 290 Calories; 20.5g Fat; 8.2g Carbs; 18.2g Protein; 1.5g Fiber

Ingredients

6 bell peppers, deveined 1 tablespoon vegetable oil 1 shallot, chopped 1 garlic clove, minced 1/2 pound ground pork 1/3 pound ground veal 1 ripe tomato, chopped 1/2 teaspoon mustard seeds Sea salt and ground black pepper, to taste

Directions

Parboil the peppers for 5 minutes. Heat the vegetable oil in a frying pan that is preheated over a moderate heat. Cook the shallot and garlic for 3 to 4 minutes until they've softened. Stir in the ground meat and cook, breaking apart with a fork, for about 6 minutes. Add the chopped tomatoes, mustard seeds, salt, and pepper. Continue to cook for 5 minutes or until heated through. Divide the filling between the peppers and transfer them to a baking pan. Bake in the preheated oven at 365 degrees F approximately 25 minutes.Bon appétit!

52. Pork Pie with Cauliflower

Ready in about: 1 hour and 30 minutes | Serves: 6 Per serving: Kcal 485, Fat: 41g, Net Carbs: 4g, Protein: 29g

Ingredients

Crust 1 egg ¼ cup butter 2 cups almond flour ¼ tsp xanthan gum ¼ cup shredded mozzarella A pinch of salt Filling 2 lb ground pork ⅓ cup pureed onion ¾ tsp allspice 1 cup mashed cauliflower 1 tbsp ground sage 2 tbsp butter Preheat oven to 350°F.

Directions

Whisk together all the crust ingredients in a bowl. Make two balls out of the mixture and refrigerate for 10 minutes. Combine ½ cup water, meat, and salt, in a pot over medium heat. Cook for about 15 minutes. Place the meat along with the other ingredients in a bowl. Mix with your hands to combine. Roll out the pie crusts and place one at the bottom of a greased pie pan. Spread the filling over the crust. Top with the other coat. Bake in the oven for 50 minutes. Serve.

53. Grilled Pork Loin Chops with Barbecue Sauce

Ready in about: 15 minutes + marinating time | Serves: 4 Per serving: Kcal 363, Fat 26.6g, Net Carbs 0g, Protein 34.1g

Ingredients

4 thick-cut pork loin chops, boneless ½ cup sugar-free BBQ sauce 1 tsp black pepper 1 tbsp erythritol ½ tsp ginger powder 2 tsp sweet paprika

Directions

In a bowl, mix pepper, erythritol, ginger powder, and sweet paprika, and rub the pork on all sides with the mixture. Cover the pork chops with plastic wrap and place them in the fridge to marinate for 2 hours. Preheat the grill to 450°F. Unwrap the meat, place on the grill grate, and cook for 2 minutes per side. Reduce the heat and brush the BBQ sauce on the meat, cover, and grill for 5 minutes. Open the lid, turn the meat, and brush again with barbecue sauce. Continue cooking covered for 5 minutes. Serve.

54. Pork Osso Bucco

Ready in about: 1 hour 55 minutes | Serves: 6 Per serving: Kcal 590, Fat 40g, Net Carbs 6.1g, Protein 34g

Ingredients

3 tbsp butter, softened 6 (16 oz) pork shanks 2 tbsp olive oil 2 cloves garlic, minced 1 cup diced tomatoes Salt and black pepper to taste 1 onion, chopped ½ celery stalk, chopped ½ cup chopped carrots 1 cups Cabernet Sauvignon wine 3 cups vegetable broth 2 tsp lemon zest

Directions

Melt the butter in a large saucepan over medium heat. Season the pork with salt and black pepper and brown it for 12 minutes; remove to a plate. In the same pan, sauté the onion for 3 minutes. Return the pork shanks. Stir in the wine, carrots, celery, tomatoes, broth, salt, and pepper and cover the pan. Let simmer on low heat for 1 ½ hours, basting the pork every 15 minutes with the sauce. In a bowl, mix the garlic, parsley, and lemon zest to make a gremolata, and stir the mixture into the sauce when it is ready. Turn the heat off and dish the Osso Bucco. Serve with creamy turnip mash.

55. Spicy Pork Ribs

Ready in about: 8 hours 45 minutes | Serves: 6 Per serving: Kcal 580, Fat 36.6g, Net Carbs 0g, Protein 44.5g

Ingredients

3 racks pork ribs, silver lining removed 2 cups sugar-free BBQ sauce 2 tbsp erythritol 2 tsp chili powder 2 tsp cumin powder 2 tsp smoked paprika 2 tsp garlic powder Salt and black pepper to taste 1 tsp mustard powder

DirectionsPreheat a smoker to 400°F, using mesquite wood to create flavor in the smoker. In a bowl, mix the erythritol, chili powder, cumin powder, black pepper, smoked paprika, garlic powder, salt, and mustard powder. Rub the ribs and let marinate for 30 minutes. Place on the grill grate and cook at reduced heat of 225°F for 4 hours. Flip the ribs after and continue cooking for 4 hours. Brush the ribs with bbq sauce on both sides and sear them in increased heat for 3 minutes per side. Remove and let sit for 4 minutes before slicing. Serve with red cabbage coleslaw.

56. Oregano Pork Chops with Spicy Tomato Sauce

Ready in about: 50 minutes | Serves: 4 Per serving: Kcal 410, Fat 21g, Net Carbs 3.6g, Protein 39g

Ingredients

4 pork chops 1 tbsp fresh oregano, chopped 2 garlic cloves, minced 2 tbsp canola oil 15 oz canned diced tomatoes 1 tbsp tomato paste Salt and black pepper to taste ¼ cup tomato juice 1 red chili, finely chopped

DirectionsWarm the olive oil a pan over medium heat. Season the pork with salt and pepper. Add it to the pan and cook for 6 minutes on both sides; remove to a bowl. Sauté the garlic in the same fat for 30 seconds. Stir in tomato paste, tomatoes, tomato juice, and chili. Bring to a boil and reduce the heat. Place in the pork chops and simmer everything for 30 minutes. Sprinkle with fresh oregano and serve.

57. Jamaican Pork Oven

Roast Ready in about: 4 hours and 20 minutes | Serves: 4 Per serving: Kcal 282, Fat: 24g, Net Carbs: 0g, Protein: 23g

Ingredients

2 lb pork roast 1 tbsp olive oil 1 tsp jerk spice blend 2 cups chicken stock Salt and black pepper to taste Rub the pork with olive oil, spice blend, salt, and pepper.

Directions

Heat a dutch oven over medium heat and sear the meat well on all sides. Add in the chicken stock. Cover the pot and cook for 4 hours on low heat. Shred the pork with 2 forks and serve with green salad.

58. Swiss-Style Italian Sausage

Ready in about: 25 minutes | Serves: 6 Per serving: Kcal 567, Fat 45g, Net Carbs 7.6g, Protein 34g

Ingredients

¼ cup olive oil 2 lb Italian pork sausage, chopped 1 onion, sliced 4 sun-dried tomatoes, sliced thin Salt and black pepper to taste ½ lb Gruyere cheese, grated 3 yellow bell peppers, chopped 3 orange bell peppers, chopped 1 tsp red pepper flakes

Directions

Set a pan over medium heat and warm oil. Place in the sausage slices and cook each side for 3 minutes. Remove to a bowl and set aside. Stir tomatoes, bell peppers, and onion in the pan and cook for 5 minutes. Season with black pepper, pepper flakes, and salt and mix well. Cook for 1 minute and remove from heat. Lay sausage slices onto a baking dish, place the bell pepper mixture on top and scatter with the Gruyere cheese. Place in the preheated to 340°F oven. Bake for 10 minutes until the cheese melts. Serve warm.

59. Smoked Pork Sausages with Mushrooms

Ready in about: 1 hour 10 minutes | Serves: 6 Per serving: Kcal 525, Fat 32g, Net Carbs 7.3g, Protein 29g

Ingredients

3 yellow bell peppers, chopped 2 lb smoked sausage, sliced Salt and black pepper to taste 2 lb portobello mushrooms, sliced 2 sweet onions, chopped 1 tbsp swerve sugar 2 tbsp olive oil Arugula to garnish Preheat oven to 320°F.

Directions

In a baking dish, combine the sausages with swerve, olive oil, black pepper, onion, bell peppers, salt, and mushrooms. Pour in 1 cup of water and toss to ensure everything is coated. Bake for 1 hour. Remove and let sit for 5 minutes. Serve scattered with arugula.

60. Hot Pork with Dill Pickles

Ready in about: 20 minutes + marinating time | Serves: 4 Per serving: Kcal 315, Fat 18g, Net Carbs 2.3g, Protein 36g

Ingredients

¼ cup lime juice 4 pork chops 2 tbsp coconut oil, melted 2 garlic cloves, minced ½ tsp chili powder 1 tsp ground cinnamon Salt and black pepper to taste ½ tsp hot pepper sauce 4 dill pickles, cut into spears

Directions

In a bowl, combine the lime juice with coconut oil, salt, hot pepper sauce, black pepper, cinnamon, garlic, and chili powder. Place in the pork chops, toss to coat, and refrigerate for 4 hours. Arrange the pork on the preheated grill over medium heat and cook for 7 minutes. Turn, add in the dill pickles, and cook for another 7 minutes. Split among serving plates and serve.

61. Mustardy Pork Chops

Ready in about: 15 minutes | Serves: 4 Per serving: Kcal 382, Fat 21.5g, Net Carbs 1.2g, Protein 38g

Ingredients

4 pork loin chops 1 tsp Dijon mustard 1 tbsp soy sauce 1 tsp lemon juice 1 tbsp water Salt and black pepper to taste 2 tbsp butter A bunch of scallions, chopped

Directions

In a bowl, combine the water with lemon juice, mustard, and soy sauce. Set aside. Set a pan over medium heat and melt the butter. Add in the pork chops and season with salt and black pepper. Cook for 4 minutes, turn, and cook for an additional 4 minutes. Remove to a plate. In the same pan, pour mustard sauce and simmer for 5 minutes. Drizzle the sauce over the pork, top with scallions, and serve.

62. Stuffed Pork with Red Cabbage Salad

Ready in about: 40 minutes + marinating time | Serves: 4 Per serving: Kcal 413, Fat 37g, Net Carbs 3g, Protein 26g

Ingredients

Zest and juice from 2 limes 2 garlic cloves, minced ¾ cup + 3 tbsp olive oil 1 cup fresh cilantro, chopped 1 tsp dried oregano Salt and black pepper to taste 1 tsp cumin 4 pork loin steaks 2 pickles, chopped 4 ham slices 6 Swiss cheese slices 2 tbsp mustard 1 head red cabbage, shredded 2 tbsp vinegar Salt to taste

Directions

In a food processor, blitz lime zest, ¾ cup oil, oregano, cumin, cilantro, lime juice, garlic, salt, and pepper. Rub the steaks with the mixture and toss to coat. Place in the fridge for 2 hours. Arrange the steaks on a working surface. Split the pickles, mustard, cheese, and ham on them, roll, and secure with toothpicks. Heat a pan over medium heat. Add in the pork rolls, cook each side for 2 minutes and remove to a baking sheet. Bake in the oven at 350°F for 25 minutes. In a bowl, mix the cabbage with the remaining olive oil, vinegar, and salt. Serve with the meat.

63. Bavarian-Style Ham and Cabbage

(Ready in about 45 minutes | Servings 4) Per serving: 123 Calories; 4.4g Fat; 6.8g Carbs; 9.8g Protein; 2.8g

Ingredients

6 ounces smoked ham, chopped 1 yellow onion, diced 2 cloves garlic, pressed 1 pound red cabbage, shredded 2 cups vegetable stock Sea salt and ground black pepper, to taste 1/4 teaspoon paprika 1 bay leaf

Directions

In a heavy-bottomed pot, cook the ham in over medium-high heat for 7 to 8 minutes. Then, sauté the onion and garlic for about 6 minutes or until tender and aromatic. Add in the cabbage and continue cooking for 10 minutes more. Add in the other ingredients and reduce the heat to simmer. Cover and continue to simmer for 20 to 25 minutes or until cooked through. Bon appétit!

64. Warm Pork Salad with Blue Cheese

(Ready in about 20 minutes | Servings 2) Per serving: 431 Calories; 22.9g Fat; 5.2g Carbs; 42.2g Protein; 5.2g

Ingredients

1/2 pound ground pork 1/2 cup Greek yogurt 1/2 cup blue cheese, crumbled 1 tablespoon lard 1/4 teaspoon thyme 1 bell pepper, deveined and chopped 1/4 cup beef bone broth 1/2 cup radicchio, trimmed and sliced 2 teaspoons fresh lemon juice Kosher salt and black pepper, to your liking 1 small head of Iceberg lettuce, leaves separated

Directions

In a frying pan, melt the lard over medium flame; cook the ground pork until browned, crumbling with a fork. Add the peppers and cook until they have softened. Pour in the bone broth to deglaze the pan; season with salt, pepper, and thyme; cook for a further 5 minutes and set aside. Drizzle fresh lemon juice over everything and serve.

65. Pork Stuffed Zucchini Boats

(Ready in about 50 minutes | Servings 8) Per serving: 302 Calories; 21.2g Fat; 5.2g Carbs; 18.2g Protein; 1.1g

Ingredients

1 pound ground pork 1 yellow onion, chopped 1 garlic clove, pressed 4 medium-sized zucchinis, cut into halves 1/2 cup chicken broth 2 tablespoons olive oil Salt and ground black pepper, to taste 1 cup tomato puree 1 cup cheddar cheese, freshly grated 1 cup Cremini mushrooms, chopped

Directions

Start by preheating your oven to 365 degrees F. Use a spoon to carefully scoop the flesh out of the zucchinis to create indentations. In a sauté pan, heat the oil in over medium-high flame. Cook the onion for about 3 minutes until tender and translucent. Stir in the garlic, pork and mushrooms; continue to sauté for 4 to 5 minutes more. Add in the salt, pepper, tomato puree and chicken broth. Continue simmer for 10 to 12 minutes or until thoroughly cooked. Spoon the filling into the zucchini boats and bake in the preheated oven approximately 20 minutes. Top with grated cheese and place under the preheated broiler for 5 minutes more until hot and bubbly. Bon appétit!

66. Easy Pork Sausage Frittata

(Ready in about 35 minutes | Servings 4) Per serving: 423 Calories; 35.4g Fat; 4.1g Carbs; 22.6g Protein; 0.8g

Ingredients

1/2 pound pork sausages, thinly sliced 8 eggs, whisked 1 teaspoon Serrano pepper, finely minced 2 garlic cloves, minced 1 teaspoon salt 1/2 teaspoon ground black pepper 1/4 teaspoon cayenne pepper 1 teaspoon dried thyme, crushed 3 tablespoons olive oil 1 cup onion, chopped

Directions

Start by preheating your oven to 410 degrees F. In a frying pan, heat the oil over a medium-high flame. Sauté the onions, Serrano pepper and garlic for about 5 minutes until they have softened. Sprinkle with salt, black pepper, and cayenne pepper. Then, cook the sausage until no longer pink, crumbling with a fork. Transfer the sautéed mixture to a lightly greased baking pan. Pour the whisked eggs over the top and sprinkle with dried thyme. Bake in the preheated oven for 22 to 25 minutes.

67. Pork Spare Ribs with Peppers

(Ready in about 2 hours | Servings 4) Per serving: 370 Calories; 21.3g Fat; 4.3g Carbs; 33.7g Protein; 1.6g

Ingredients

1 tablespoon lard, melted 1 tablespoon crushed sage 1 red onion, chopped 1 garlic clove, minced 1 tablespoon tamarind paste 1 cup beef broth 1/2 cup dry sherry Salt and pepper, to your liking 1 rosemary sprig 1 thyme sprig 1/2 cup coconut aminos 1 pound pork spare ribs 2 Italian peppers, deveined and chopped

Directions

Melt the lard in an oven-proof skillet over medium-high heat. Cook the meat on all sides until just browned; sprinkle with seasonings. Add in the remaining ingredients. Roast in the preheated oven at 330 degrees F for 1 hour 40 minutes. Storing Divide the ribs into four portions. Place each portion of ribs in an airtight container; keep in your refrigerator for 3 to 5 days. For freezing, place the ribs in airtight containers or heavy-duty freezer bags. Freeze up to 4 to 6 months. Defrost in your refrigerator. Bon appétit!

68. Chinese-Style Pork Tenderloin

Tenderloin (Ready in about 20 minutes | Servings 6) Per serving: 356 Calories; 19.5g Fat; 6.4g Carbs; 33.1g Protein; 1.8g

Ingredients

1 ½ pounds pork tenderloin, boneless 1 (8-ounce) can bamboo shoots 1 ½ tablespoons olive oil 1 shallot, chopped 1 head cauliflower, broken into florets Kosher salt and ground black pepper, to taste 1/4 teaspoon dried thyme 1/2 teaspoon dried rosemary 1/2 teaspoon granulated garlic 2 tablespoons fish sauce 1/4 cup vodka

Directions

Place the pork, salt, black pepper, thyme, rosemary, granulated garlic, fish sauce, vodka and 1/2 tablespoon of olive oil in Ziploc bag; shake to coat on all sides. Now, heat the remaining tablespoon of the olive oil in a frying pan over medium-high flame; sauté the onions until translucent. Add the shallot and cauliflower for about 6 minutes or until they have softened; reserve. In the same frying pan, brown the pork for 3 to 4 minutes per side. Add in the reserved marinade along with the shallot/cauliflower mixture and bamboo shoots. Continue to cook for a further 5 minutes or until cooked through. Bon appétit!

69. Classic Pork Stew

(Ready in about 45 minutes | Servings 8) Per serving: 390 Calories; 27.8g Fat; 4.7g Carbs; 28.3g Protein; 5g

Ingredients

1 cup fresh brown mushrooms, sliced 1/2 cup fresh cilantro, chopped 1 habanero pepper, minced 3 cups beef bone broth, no sugar added 2 ripe tomatoes, chopped 1 teaspoon garlic, pressed 2 carrots, peeled and chopped 1 celery stalk, chopped 2 tablespoons dry red wine 1/2 teaspoon dried oregano 2 tablespoons lard, at room temperature 2 pounds Boston butt, cut into 3/4-inch cubes 1 teaspoon sea salt 1/2 teaspoon black pepper 1 medium leek, chopped 1 teaspoon dried marjoram

Directions

In a heavy-bottomed pot, melt the lard until sizzling. Once hot, brown the pork for 4 to 5 minutes; season with salt and pepper and reserve. Then, cook the leeks, habanero pepper, garlic, carrots and celery until they have softened. Pour in the wine to deglaze the bottom of your pot. Add in the broth, tomatoes, oregano, marjoram, and mushrooms. Partially cover and continue to cook for 35 to 40 minutes. Serve with fresh cilantro. Bon appétit!

70. Authentic Greek Souvlaki

(Ready in about 20 minutes + marinating time | Servings 6) Per serving: 216 Calories; 4.1g Fat; 1.7g Carbs; 30g Protein; 0.2g

Ingredients

2 ½ pounds pork tenderloin, trimmed of silver skin and excess fat, cut into 1-inch cubes 1 teaspoon Greek oregano 3 cloves garlic, smashed Sea salt and ground black pepper, to taste 1/3 cup wine vinegar 2 tablespoons coriander, chopped 2 tablespoons fresh lime juice

Directions

Thoroughly combine all ingredients in a ceramic dish. Cover tightly and let it marinate in your refrigerator for 2 to 3 hours. Thread the pork cubes onto the skewers. Prepare the outdoor grill and brush the grates with a nonstick cooking spray. Grill your skewers until well browned and internal temperature registers 160 degrees F on an instant read thermometer. Bon appétit!

71. Mediterranean-Style Pork Medallions

(Ready in about 30 minutes | Servings 4) Per serving: 335 Calories; 26.3g Fat; 1.5g Carbs; 18.3g Protein; 0.2g Fiber

Ingredients

4 pork medallions 2 tablespoons coconut aminos 1/4 cup dry white wine 2 tablespoons olive oil 1 red onion, thinly sliced 2 cloves garlic, minced 1 teaspoon dried marjoram 1/2 teaspoon fresh ginger root, grated

Directions

In a saucepan, heat the olive oil over a moderate heat. Once hot, sauté the onions and garlic until browned. Cook the pork for about 20 minutes. Add the dry white wine to scrape up any browned bits from the bottom of your pot; add in the coconut aminos, marjoram, and ginger root. Continue to cook for 8 to 10 minutes or until cooked through. Bon appétit!

72. Mississippi Pulled Pork

(Ready in about 6 hours + marinating time | Servings 4) Per serving: 350 Calories; 11g Fat; 5g Carbs; 53.6g Protein; 2.2g Fiber

Ingredients

1 ½ pounds pork shoulder 1 tablespoon liquid smoke sauce 1 teaspoon chipotle powder Au Jus gravy seasoning packet 2 onions, cut into wedges Kosher salt and freshly ground black pepper, taste

Directions Mix the liquid smoke sauce, chipotle powder, Au Jus gravy seasoning packet, salt and pepper. Rub the spice mixture into the pork on all sides. Wrap in plastic wrap and let it marinate in your refrigerator for 3 hours. Prepare your grill for indirect heat. Place the pork butt roast on the grate over a drip pan and top with onions; cover the grill and cook for about 6 hours. Transfer the pork to a cutting board. Now, shred the meat into bite-sized pieces using two forks.Bon appétit!

73. Ground Pork Skillet

(Ready in about 25 minutes | Servings 4) Per serving: 349 Calories; 13g Fat; 4.4g Carbs; 45.3g Protein; 1.2g Fiber

Ingredients

1 ½ pounds ground pork 2 tablespoons olive oil 1 bunch kale, trimmed and roughly chopped 1 cup onions, sliced 1/4 teaspoon black pepper, or more to taste 1/4 cup tomato puree 1 bell pepper, chopped 1 teaspoon sea salt 1 cup chicken bone broth 1/4 cup port wine 2 cloves garlic, pressed 1 chili pepper, sliced

Directions Heat 1 tablespoon of the olive oil in a cast-iron skillet over a moderately high heat. Now, sauté the onion, garlic, and peppers until they are tender and fragrant; reserve. Heat the remaining tablespoon of olive oil; once hot, cook the ground pork and approximately 5 minutes until no longer pink. Add in the other ingredients and continue to cook for 15 to 17 minutes or until cooked through.Bon appétit!

74. Pork Chops with Herbs

(Ready in about 20 minutes | Servings 4) Per serving: 192 Calories; 6.9g Fat; 0.9g Carbs; 29.8g Protein; 0.4g Fiber

Ingredients

1 tablespoon butter 1 pound pork chops 2 rosemary sprigs, minced 1 teaspoon dried marjoram 1 teaspoon dried parsley A bunch of spring onions, roughly chopped 1 thyme sprig, minced 1/2 teaspoon granulated garlic 1/2 teaspoon paprika, crushed Coarse salt and ground black pepper, to taste

Directions

 Season the pork chops with the granulated garlic, paprika, salt, and black pepper. Melt the butter in a frying pan over a moderate flame. Cook the pork chops for 6 to 8 minutes, turning them occasionally to ensure even cooking. Add in the remaining ingredients and cook an additional 4 minutes.Bon appétit!

75. Old-Fashioned Goulash

(Ready in about 9 hours 10 minutes | Servings 4) Per serving: 456 Calories; 28.7g Fat; 6.7g Carbs; 32g Protein; 3.4g Fiber

Ingredients

1 ½ pounds pork butt, chopped 1 teaspoon sweet Hungarian paprika 2 Hungarian hot peppers, deveined and minced 1 cup leeks, chopped 1 ½ tablespoons lard 1 teaspoon caraway seeds, ground 4 cups vegetable broth 2 garlic cloves, crushed 1 teaspoons cayenne pepper 2 cups tomato sauce with herbs

Directions

Melt the lard in a heavy-bottomed pot over medium-high heat. Sear the pork for 5 to 6 minutes until just browned on all sides; set aside. Add in the leeks and garlic; continue to cook until they have softened. Place the reserved pork along with the sautéed mixture in your crock pot. Add in the other ingredients and stir to combine. Cover with the lid and slow cook for 9 hours on the lowest setting. Enjoy!

76. Mexican-Style Pork Chops

Chops (Ready in about 30 minutes | Servings 6) Per serving: 356 Calories; 20.3g Fat; 0.3g Carbs; 45.2g Protein; 0g

Ingredients

2 Mexican chilies, chopped 1 teaspoon dried Mexican oregano 1/2 teaspoon red pepper flakes, crushed Salt and ground black pepper, to taste 6 pork chops 1/2 cup chicken stock 2 garlic cloves, minced 2 tablespoons vegetable oil

Directions

Heat 1 tablespoon of the olive oil in a frying pan over a moderately high heat. Brow the pork chops for 5 to 6 minutes per side. Then, bring the Mexican chilies and chicken stock to a boil; remove from the heat and let it sit for about 20 minutes. Puree the chilies along with the liquid and the remaining ingredients in your food processor. Add in the remaining tablespoon of the oil. Bon appétit!

77. Mediterranean Meatballs in Tomato Sauce

(Ready in about 50 minutes | Servings 6) Per serving: 237 Calories; 12g Fat; 5.6g Carbs; 26.4g Protein; 1.6g

Ingredients

For the Meatballs: 3/4 cup grated parmesan cheese 1 teaspoon garlic paste 1 pound beef, ground 1 egg, beaten Salt and ground black pepper, to taste 1 white onion, finely chopped 1/2 tablespoon chili powder 1 teaspoon onion flakes 2 tablespoons fresh parsley, chopped 1/4 cup almond flour 2 ounces full-fat milk For the Sauce: 2 tablespoons olive oil 1 cup marinara sauce 1 tablespoon Mediterranean herb mix Salt and ground black pepper, to taste

Directions

Mix all ingredients for the meatballs. Then, roll the mixture into bite-sized balls and arrange them in a single layer on a lightly greased baking sheet. Mix all ingredients for the sauce. Pour the sauce over the meatballs. Bake in the preheated oven at 365 degrees F for 40 to 45 minutes or until they are golden brown on the top.Bon appétit!

78. Milk-Braised Pork

(Ready in about 1 hour 35 minutes | Servings 8) Per serving: 293 Calories; 15.4g Fat; 5.4g Carbs; 31.4g Protein; 0.4g

Ingredients

2 pounds pork sirloin roast 2 cup full-fat milk Salt and pepper, to taste 1 teaspoon dried marjoram 1/2 cup onion, sliced 3 teaspoons butter, room temperature 2 bell peppers, deveined and thinly sliced

Directions Melt the butter in a saucepan over medium-high flame. Sear the pork for about 7 minutes until just browned. Lower the pork sirloin roast into a baking dish. Season with salt, pepper, and marjoram. Scatter the onion and peppers around the pork. Pour in the milk and cover the dish with a piece of aluminum foil. Roast in the preheated oven at 330 degrees F for 1 hour 20 minutes, turning the pork halfway through the cooking time. Let it sit for 10 minutes before slicing. Bon appétit!

79. Hungarian-Style Pork Goulash

(Ready in about 25 minutes | Servings 6) Per serving: 228 Calories; 11.7g Fat; 6g Carbs; 23.1g Protein; 1.7g

Ingredients

1 tablespoon olive oil, room temperature 2 teaspoons paprika 2 bay laurels 1/2 cup loosely packed fresh parsley, roughly chopped 2 slices bacon, chopped Salt and red pepper, to taste 1 cup tomato sauce, no sugar added 1 cup onions, chopped 2 garlic cloves, minced 1 ¼ pounds pork stew meat, cubed 2 cups beef bone broth 1/2 teaspoon celery seeds

Directions Heat the olive oil in a stockpot over a moderately high flame. Sauté the onions and garlic until they've softened. Add in the pork and continue to cook for 7 to 8 minutes. Add in the bacon, salt, red pepper, and continue to cook for about 3 minutes. Add in the tomato sauce, beef bone broth, celery seeds, paprika, bay laurels, and parsley. Turn the heat to simmer. Continue to simmer for about 12 minutes until cooked through. Enjoy!

80. 3Keto Pork Wraps

(Ready in about 15 minutes | Servings 4) Per serving: 281 Calories; 19.4g Fat; 5.1g Carbs; 22.1g Protein; 1.3g Fiber

Ingredients

1 pound ground pork 2 garlic cloves, finely minced 1 chili pepper, deveined and finely minced 1 teaspoon mustard powder 1 tablespoon sunflower seeds 2 tablespoons champagne vinegar 1 tablespoon coconut aminos Celery salt and ground black pepper, to taste 2 scallion stalks, sliced 1 head lettuce

Directions Sear the ground pork in the preheated pan for about 8 minutes. Stir in the garlic, chili pepper, mustard seeds, and sunflower seeds; continue to sauté for 1 minute longer or until aromatic. Add in the vinegar, coconut aminos, salt, black pepper, and scallions. Stir to combine well.

81. Smoked Pork Sausage Keto Bombs

(Ready in about 15 minutes + chilling time | Servings 6) Per serving: 383 Calories; 32.7g Fat; 5.1g Carbs; 16.7g Protein; 1.7g Fiber

Ingredients

3/4 pound smoked pork sausage, ground 1 teaspoon ginger-garlic paste 2 tablespoons scallions, minced 1 tablespoon butter, room temperature 1 tomato, pureed 4 ounces mozzarella cheese, crumbled 2 tablespoons flaxseed meal 8 ounces cream cheese, room temperature Sea salt and ground black pepper, to taste

Directions

Melt the butter in a frying pan over medium-high heat. Cook the sausage for about 4 minutes, crumbling with a spatula. Add in the ginger-garlic paste, scallions, and tomato; continue to cook over medium-low heat for a further 6 minutes. Stir in the remaining ingredients. Place the mixture in your refrigerator for 1 to 2 hours until firm. Roll the mixture into bite-sized balls.Enjoy!

82. Easy Fall-Off-The-Bone Ribs

(Ready in about 8 hours | Servings 4) Per serving: 192 Calories; 6.9g Fat; 0.9g Carbs; 29.8g Protein; 0.5g Fiber

Ingredients

1 pound baby back ribs 4 tablespoons coconut aminos 1/4 cup dry red wine 1/2 teaspoon cayenne pepper 1 garlic clove, crushed 1 teaspoon Italian herb mix 1 tablespoon butter 1 teaspoon Serrano pepper, minced 1 Italian pepper, thinly sliced 1 teaspoon grated lemon zest

Directions

Butter the sides and bottom of your Crock pot. Place the pork and peppers on the bottom. Add in the remaining ingredients. Slow cook for 9 hours on Low heat setting.

83. Kansas-Style Meatloaf

(Ready in about 1 hour 10 minutes | Servings 8) Per serving: 318 Calories; 14.7g Fat; 6.2g Carbs; 39.3g Protein; 0.3g Fiber

Ingredients

2 pounds ground pork 2 eggs, beaten 1/2 cup onions, chopped 1/2 cup marinara sauce, bottled 8 ounces Colby cheese, shredded 1 teaspoon granulated garlic Sea salt and freshly ground black pepper, to taste 1 teaspoon lime zest 1 teaspoon mustard seeds 1/2 cup tomato puree 1 tablespoon Erythritol

Directions

Mix the ground pork with the eggs, onions, marinara salsa, cheese, granulated garlic, salt, pepper, lime zest, and mustard seeds; mix to combine. Press the mixture into a lightly-greased loaf pan. Mix the tomato paste with the Erythritol and spread the mixture over the top of your meatloaf. Bake in the preheated oven at 365 degrees F for about 1 hour 10 minutes, rotating the pan halfway through the cook time. Bon appétit!

84. Pork Casserole

Ready in about: 35 minutes | Serves: 4 Per serving: Kcal 495, Fat 29g, Net Carbs 2.7g, Protein 36.5g

Ingredients

1 lb ground pork 1 large yellow squash, thinly sliced Salt and black pepper to taste 1 clove garlic, minced 4 green onions, chopped 1 cup chopped cremini mushrooms 1 (15 oz) can diced tomatoes ½ cup pork rinds, crushed 2 tbsp fresh parsley, chopped 1 cup cottage cheese, crumbled 1 cup Mexican cheese blend 3 tbsp olive oil Preheat oven to 370°F.

Directions

Heat the olive oil in a skillet over medium heat. Add in the pork, season with salt and black pepper, and cook for 3 minutes or until no longer pink. Stir occasionally while breaking any lumps apart. Add the garlic, half of the green onions, mushrooms, and 2 tablespoons of pork rinds. Cook for 3 minutes. Stir in the tomatoes and ⅓ cup water. Cook for 3 minutes. Remove the pan. Mix the parsley, cottage cheese, and Mexican cheese blend in a bowl. Sprinkle the bottom of a baking dish with some pork rinds, top with half of the squash, and season with salt. Top with 2/3 of the pork mixture and 2/3 of the cheese mixture. Repeat the layering process a second time to exhaust the ingredients. Cover the baking dish with foil and bake for 20 minutes. After, remove the foil and brown the top of the casserole with the oven's broiler side for 2 minutes. Remove the dish when ready and serve warm.

85. Pork Sausage Bake

Ready in about: 50 minutes | Serves: 4 Per serving: Kcal 465, Fat 41.6g, Net Carbs 4.4g, Protein 15.1g

Ingredients

1 lb pork sausages 4 large tomatoes, cut in rings 1 red bell pepper, sliced 1 yellow bell pepper, sliced 1 green bell pepper, sliced 1 sprig thyme, chopped 1 sprig rosemary, chopped 2 cloves garlic, minced 2 bay leaves 2 tbsp olive oil 2 tbsp balsamic vinegar Preheat oven to 350°F.

Directions

In a greased baking pan, arrange the tomatoes and bell peppers. Sprinkle with thyme, rosemary, garlic, olive oil, and balsamic vinegar. Top with the sausages. Put the pan in the oven and bake for 20 minutes. After, remove the pan, shake it a bit, and turn the sausages over with a spoon. Continue cooking for 25 minutes or until the sausages have browned to your desired

color. Serve with the veggie and cooking sauce with cauli rice.

86. Spiced Pork Roast with Collard Greens

Ready in about: 60 minutes | Serves: 4 Per serving: Kcal 430, Fat 23g, Net Carbs 3g, Protein 45g

Ingredients

2 tbsp olive oil Salt and black pepper to taste 1 ½ lb pork loin A pinch of dry mustard 1 tsp red pepper flakes ½ tsp ginger, minced 1 cup collard greens, chopped 2 garlic cloves, minced ½ lemon, sliced

DirectionsIn a bowl, combine the ginger with mustard, salt, and pepper. Add in the meat and toss to coat. Heat the oil in a saucepan over medium heat. Brown the pork on all sides, about 5 minutes. Transfer to the oven. Pour in ¼ cup water and roast for 40 minutes at 390°F. To the saucepan, add collard greens, lemon slices, garlic, and ¼ cup water. Simmer for 10 minutes. Slice the loin and top with the sauce to serve.

87. Zoodle & Bacon Halloumi Gratin with Spinach

Ready in about: 35 minutes | Serves: 4 Per serving: Kcal 350, Fat 27g, Net Carbs 5.3g, Protein 16g

Ingredients

2 large zucchinis, spiralized 4 slices bacon, chopped 2 cups baby spinach 4 oz halloumi cheese, cut into cubes 2 cloves garlic, minced 1 cup heavy cream ½ cup sugar-free tomato sauce 1 cup mozzarella cheese, grated ½ tsp dried Italian herbs Preheat oven to 350°F.

Directions Place a pan over medium heat and fry the bacon for 4 minutes. Add in the garlic and cook for 1 minute. In a bowl, mix heavy cream, tomato sauce, and 1/6 cup of water and add it to the pan. Stir in zucchini, spinach, halloumi, Italian herbs, salt, and pepper. Sprinkle the mozzarella cheese on top and transfer the pan to the oven. Bake for 20 minutes or until the cheese is golden. Serve warm.

88. Creamy Pork Chops

Ready in about: 50 minutes | Serves: 4 Per serving: Kcal 612, Fat 40g, Net Carbs 6.8g, Protein 42g

Ingredients

8 oz mushrooms, sliced 1 tsp garlic powder 1 onion, chopped 1 cup heavy cream 4 pork chops, boneless ¼ cup coconut oil

Directions

Set a pan over medium heat and warm the oil. Add in the onion and mushrooms and cook for 4 minutes. Stir in the pork chops, season with garlic powder, and sear until browned. Put the pan in the oven. Bake for 30 minutes at 350°F. Remove the pork chops. Place the pan over medium heat, pour the heavy cream over the mushroom mixture, and cook for 5 minutes. Top the pork chops with the sauce to serve.

89. Herby Pork Chops with Berry Sauce

Ready in about: 17 minutes | Serves: 4 Per serving: Kcal 413, Fat 32.5g, Net Carbs 1.1g, Protein 26.3g

Ingredients

1 tbsp olive oil + extra for brushing 2 lb pork chops Pink salt and black pepper to taste 2 cups raspberries ¼ cup water 1 ½ tbsp Italian Herb mix 3 tbsp balsamic vinegar 2 tsp sugar-free Worcestershire sauce

Directions

Heat the olive oil in a skillet over medium heat, season the pork with salt and black pepper, and cook for 5 minutes on each side. Put on serving plates and reserve the pork drippings. Mash the raspberries with a fork in a bowl until jam-like. Pour into a saucepan, add the water, and herb mix. Bring to boil on low heat for 4 minutes. Stir in pork drippings, vinegar, and Worcestershire sauce. Simmer for 1 minute. Spoon sauce over the pork chops and serve with braised rapini.

90. Paprika Pork Chops

Ready in about: 25 minutes | Serves: 4 Per serving: Kcal 349, Fat 18.5g, Net Carbs 4g, Protein 41.8g

Ingredients

4 pork chops Salt and black pepper to taste 3 tbsp paprika ¾ cup cumin powder 1 tsp chili powder

Directions

In a bowl, combine the paprika with black pepper, cumin, salt, and chili. Place in the pork chops and toss to coat. Heat a grill to medium heat. Add in the pork chops and cook for 5 minutes. Flip and cook for 5 minutes. Serve with steamed vegetables.

91. Garlicky Pork with Bell Peppers

Ready in about: 40 minutes | Serves: 4 Per serving: Kcal 456, Fat 25g, Net Carbs 6g, Protein 40g

Ingredients

1 tbsp butter 4 pork steaks, bone-in 1 cup chicken stock Salt and black pepper to taste ½ tsp lemon pepper 2 tbsp olive oil 6 garlic cloves, minced 4 bell peppers, sliced 1 lemon, sliced

DirectionsHeat a pan with the olive oil and butter over medium heat. Add in the pork steaks, season with black pepper and salt, and cook until browned; remove to a plate. In the same pan, add garlic and bell peppers. Cook for 4 minutes. Pour in the chicken stock, lemon slices, salt, lemon pepper, and pepper and stir for 5 minutes. Return the pork steaks and cook for 10 minutes. Pour the sauce over the steaks and serve.

92. Pork Chops with Cranberry Sauce

Ready in about: 2 hours 40 minutes | Serves: 4 Per serving: Kcal 450, Fat 34g, Net Carbs 6g, Protein 26g

Ingredients

4 pork chops 1 tsp garlic powder Salt and black pepper to taste 3 tsp fresh basil, chopped 2 tbsp olive oil 1 shallot, chopped 1 cup white wine 1 bay leaf 2 cups vegetable stock 1 cup dried cranberries, soaked ½ tsp fresh rosemary, chopped ½ cup swerve sugar Juice of 1 lemon 1 cup water 1 tsp harissa paste

Directions

In a bowl, combine the pork chops with basil, salt, garlic powder, and black pepper. Heat the olive oil in a pan over medium heat. Add in the pork and cook until browned, about 6 minutes; set aside. Stir the shallot in the same pan and cook for 2 minutes. Pour in the wine and bay leaf and cook for 4 more minutes. Stir in juice from ½ lemon and vegetable stock and simmer for 5 minutes. Return the pork and simmer for 10 minutes. Cover the pan with foil and place it in the oven. Bake at 350°F for 2 hours. Set a pan over medium heat. Add in the cranberries, rosemary, harissa paste, water, swerve sugar, and remaining lemon juice and simmer for 15 minutes. Take out the pork chops from the oven. Remove and discard the bay leaf. Pour the cranberry sauce over the chops. Sprinkle with parsley and serve.

93. Pork in White Wine Sauce

Ready in about: 1 hour 25 minutes | Serves: 6 Per serving: Kcal 514, Fat 32.5g, Net Carbs 6g, Protein 43g

Ingredients

2 tbsp olive oil 2 lb pork stew meat, cubed Salt and black pepper to taste 2 tbsp butter 4 garlic cloves, minced ¾ cup vegetable stock ½ cup white wine 3 carrots, chopped 1 cabbage head, shredded ½ cup scallions, chopped 1 cup heavy cream

Directions

carrots and sauté for 5 minutes. Pour in the cabbage, vegetable stock, and wine. Stir and bring to a boil. Reduce the heat to low heat and cook for 1 hour covered. Add in heavy cream and stir for 1 minute. Adjust the seasoning with salt and pepper and serve.

94. Pork Burgers with Caramelized Onion Rings

Ready in about: 20 minutes | Serves: 6 Per serving: Kcal 445, Fat 32g, Net Carbs 7.6g, Protein 26g

Ingredients

2 lb ground pork Pink salt and chili pepper to taste 3 tbsp olive oil 1 tbsp butter 1 white onion, sliced into rings 1 tbsp balsamic vinegar 3 drops liquid stevia 6 zero carb burger buns, halved 2 firm tomatoes, sliced into rings

Directions

Combine the pork, salt, and chili pepper in a bowl and mold out 6 patties. Heat the olive oil in a skillet over medium heat. Fry the patties for 4-5 minutes on each side until golden brown. Remove to a plate. Melt butter in a skillet over medium heat, sauté onions for 2 minutes, and stir in the balsamic vinegar and liquid stevia. Cook for 30 seconds, stirring once or twice until caramelized. In each bun, place a patty, top with some onion rings and 2 tomato rings. Serve the burgers with cheddar cheese dip.

95. Sausage Links with Tomato & Spinach Salad

Ready in about: 15 minutes | Serves: 4 Per serving: Kcal 365, Fat 26g, Net Carbs 6.8g, Protein 18g

Ingredients

4 pork sausage links, sliced ½ lb mixed cherry tomatoes, halved 2 cups baby spinach 2 tbsp olive oil 4 oz Monterrey Jack cheese, cubed 1 tbsp lemon juice 1 cup basil pesto Salt and black pepper to taste

Directions

Warm the olive oil in a pan over medium heat. Cook the sausage links for 4 minutes per side. In a salad bowl, combine spinach, cheese, salt, pesto, pepper, cherry tomatoes, and lemon juice and toss to coat. Mix in the sausage. Serve.

96. Pork Sausage with Spinach

Ready in about: 35 minutes | Serves: 6 Per serving: Kcal 352, Fat 28g, Net Carbs 6.2g, Protein 29g

Ingredients

1 onion, chopped 2 tbsp olive oil 2 lb Italian pork sausage, sliced 1 red bell pepper, chopped Salt and black pepper to taste 4 lb spinach, chopped 1 garlic, minced ¼ cup green chili peppers, chopped 1 cup water

Directions

Warm the olive oil in a pan over medium heat. Add in the sausage and cook for 10 minutes. Stir in onion, garlic, and bell pepper and sauté for 4 minutes. Place in spinach, salt, water, pepper, chili pepper, and cook for 10 minutes until the liquid has reduced by half. Transfer to a plate and serve.

97. Easy Zucchini Beef Lasagna

Ready in about: 1 hour | Serves: 4 Per serving: Kcal 344, Fat 17.8g, Net Carbs 2.9g, Protein 40.4g

Ingredients

1 lb ground beef 2 large zucchinis, sliced lengthwise 3 cloves garlic 1 medium white onion, chopped 3 tomatoes, chopped Salt and black pepper to taste 2 tsp sweet paprika 1 tsp dried thyme 1 tsp dried basil 1 cup mozzarella cheese, shredded 1 tbsp olive oil Preheat the oven to 370°F.

Directions

Heat the olive oil in a skillet over medium heat. Cook the beef for 4 minutes while breaking any lumps as you stir. Top with onion, garlic, tomatoes, salt, paprika, and pepper. Stir and continue cooking for 5 minutes. Lay ⅓ of the zucchini slices in the baking dish. Top with ⅓ of the beef mixture and repeat the layering process two more times with the same quantities. Season with basil and thyme. Sprinkle the mozzarella cheese on top and tuck the baking dish in the oven. Bake for 35 minutes. Remove the lasagna and let it rest for 10 minutes before serving.

98. Grilled Sirloin Steak with Sauce Diane

Ready in about: 25 minutes | Serves: 6 Per serving: Kcal 434, Fat 17g, Net Carbs 2.9g, Protein 36g

Ingredients

Sirloin steak 1 ½ lb sirloin steak Salt and black pepper to taste 1 tsp olive oil Sauce Diane 1 tbsp olive oil 1 clove garlic, minced 1 cup sliced porcini mushrooms 1 small onion, finely diced 2 tbsp butter 1 tbsp Dijon mustard 2 tbsp Worcestershire sauce ¼ cup whiskey 2 cups heavy cream

Directions

Put a grill pan over high heat and as it heats, brush the steak with oil, sprinkle with salt and pepper, and rub the seasoning into the meat with your hands. Cook the steak in the pan for 4 minutes on each side for medium-rare and transfer to a chopping board to rest for 4 minutes before slicing. Reserve the juice. Heat the oil in a frying pan over medium heat and sauté the onion for 3 minutes. Add the butter, garlic, and mushrooms, and cook for 2 minutes. Add the Worcestershire sauce, the reserved juice, and mustard. Stir and cook for 1 minute. Pour in the whiskey and cook further 1 minute until the sauce reduces by half. Swirl the pan and add the cream. Let it simmer to thicken for about 3 minutes. Adjust the taste with salt and pepper. Spoon the sauce over the steaks slices and serve with celeriac mash.

99. Italian Beef Ragout

Ready in about: 1 hour 55 minutes | Serves: 4 Per serving: Kcal 328, Fat 21.6g, Net Carbs 4.2g, Protein 36.6g

Ingredients

1 lb chuck steak, cubed 2 tbsp olive oil Salt and black pepper to taste 2 tbsp almond flour 1 onion, diced ½ cup dry white wine 1 red bell pepper, seeded and diced 2 tsp Worcestershire sauce 4 oz tomato puree 3 tsp smoked paprika 1 cup beef broth 2 tbsp fresh thyme, chopped Lightly dredge the meat in the almond flour.

Directions

Place a large skillet over medium heat, add the olive oil to heat and then sauté the onion and bell pepper for 3 minutes. Stir in paprika. Add the beef and cook for 10 minutes in total while turning them halfway. Stir in white wine and let it reduce by half, about 3 minutes. Add in Worcestershire sauce, tomato puree, beef broth, salt, and pepper. Let the mixture boil for 2 minutes, reduce the heat, and let simmer for 1 ½ hours, stirring often. Serve garnished with thyme.

100. Rib Roast with Roasted Shallots & Garlic

Ready in about: 40 minutes | Serves: 6 Per serving: Kcal 556, Fat 38.6g, Net Carbs 2.5g, Protein 58.4g

Ingredients

5 lb beef rib roast, on the bone 3 heads garlic, cut in half 3 tbsp olive oil 6 shallots, peeled and halved 2 lemons, zested and juiced 3 tbsp mustard seeds 3 tbsp swerve Salt and black pepper to taste 3 tbsp thyme leaves Preheat oven to 400°F.

Directions

Place garlic heads and shallots in a roasting dish, toss with olive oil, and bake for 15 minutes. Pour lemon juice on them. Score shallow crisscrosses patterns on the meat and set aside. Mix swerve, mustard seeds, thyme, salt, pepper, and lemon zest to make a rub and apply it all over the beef. Place the beef on the shallots and garlic and cook in the oven for 20 minutes. Once ready, remove the dish, and let sit covered for 15 minutes before slicing. Serve.

101. Beef Cauliflower Curry

Ready in about: 26 minutes | Serves: 6 Per serving: Kcal 374, Fat 33g, Net Carbs 2g, Protein 22g

Ingredients

1 tbsp olive oil 1 ½ lb ground beef 1 tbsp ginger paste 1 tsp garam masala 1 (7 oz) can whole tomatoes 1 head cauliflower, cut into florets Salt to taste 2 garlic cloves, minced ½ tsp hot paprika

Directions

Heat oil in a saucepan over medium heat. Add the beef, ginger, garlic, garam masala, paprika, and salt and cook for 5 minutes while breaking any lumps. Stir in the tomatoes and cauliflower. Cook covered for 6 minutes. Add ½ cup water and bring to a boil. Simmer for 10 minutes or until the water has reduced by half. Spoon the curry into serving bowls and serve with shirataki rice.

102. Mustard-Lemon Beef

Ready in about: 25 minutes | Serves: 4 Per serving: Kcal 435, Fat 30g, Net Carbs 5g, Protein 32g

Ingredients

2 tbsp olive oil 1 tbsp fresh rosemary, chopped 2 garlic cloves, minced 1 ½ lb beef rump steak, thinly sliced Salt and black pepper to taste 1 shallot, chopped ½ cup heavy cream ½ cup beef stock 1 tbsp mustard 2 tsp Worcestershire sauce 2 tsp lemon juice 1 tsp erythritol 2 tbsp butter 1 tbsp fresh rosemary, chopped 1 tbsp fresh thyme, chopped

Directions

In a bowl, combine 1 tbsp of oil with black pepper, garlic, rosemary, and salt. Toss in the beef to coat and set aside for some minutes. Heat a pan with the rest of the oil over medium heat, place in the beef steak, cook for 6 minutes, flipping halfway through. Set aside and keep warm. Melt the butter in the pan. Add in the shallot and cook for 3 minutes. Stir in the stock, Worcestershire sauce, erythritol, thyme, cream, mustard, and rosemary and cook for 8 minutes. Mix in the lemon juice, pepper, and salt. Arrange the beef slices on serving plates, sprinkle over the sauce, and enjoy!

103. Parsley Beef Burgers

Ready in about: 25 minutes | Serves: 6 Per serving: Kcal 354, Fat: 28g, Net Carbs: 2.5g, Protein: 27g

Ingredients

2 lb ground beef 1 tbsp onion flakes ¾ cup almond flour ¼ cup beef broth 2 tbsp fresh parsley, chopped 1 tbsp Worcestershire sauce

Directions

Combine all ingredients in a bowl. Mix well with your hands and make 6 patties out of the mixture. Arrange on a lined baking sheet. Bake at 370°F for about 18 minutes, until nice and crispy. Serve.

104.   Spicy Spinach Pinwheel Steaks

Ready in about: 40 minutes | Serves: 6 Per serving: Kcal 490, Fat 41g, Net Carbs 2g, Protein 28g

Ingredients

1 ½ lb beef flank steak Salt and black pepper to taste 1 cup feta cheese, crumbled ½ loose cup baby spinach 1 jalapeño pepper, chopped ¼ cup chopped basil leaves Preheat oven to 400°F.

Directions

Wrap the steak in plastic wrap, place on a flat surface, and gently run a rolling pin over to flatten. Take off the wraps. Sprinkle with half of the feta cheese, top with spinach, jalapeno, basil leaves, and the remaining cheese. Roll the steak over on the stuffing and secure with toothpicks. Place in the baking sheet and cook for 30 minutes, flipping once until nicely browned on the outside and the cheese melted within. Cool for 3 minutes, slice into pinwheels, and serve with sautéed veggies.

105.   Beef Sausage Casserole

Ready in about: 60 minutes | Serves: 4 Per serving: Kcal 456, Fat 35g, Net Carbs 4g, Protein 32g

Ingredients

¼ cup almond flour 1 egg 1 lb beef sausages, chopped Salt and black pepper to taste ¼ tsp red pepper flakes ¼ cup Parmesan cheese, grated ¼ tsp onion powder ½ tsp garlic powder ¼ tsp dried oregano ½ cup ricotta cheese, crumbled ½ cup sugar-free marinara sauce ½ cups cheddar cheese, shredded

DirectionsIn a bowl, combine the sausages, black pepper, pepper flakes, oregano, egg, Parmesan cheese, onion powder, almond flour, salt, and garlic powder and mix well. Form balls and lay them on a greased baking sheet. Place in the oven and bake for 15 minutes at 370°F. Remove the balls from the oven. Cover the meatballs with half of the marinara sauce. Pour ricotta cheese all over, followed by the rest of the marinara sauce, and scatter with the cheddar cheese. Bake for 10 minutes. Allow to cool and serve.

106.   Soy-Glazed Meatloaf

Ready in about: 60 minutes | Serves: 6 Per serving: Kcal 474, Fat 21.4g, Net Carbs 7.5g, Protein 46g

Ingredients

1 cup white mushrooms, chopped 2 lb ground beef 2 tbsp fresh parsley, chopped 2 garlic cloves, minced 1 onion, chopped 1 red bell pepper, chopped ½ cup almond flour ⅓ cup Parmesan cheese, grated 2 eggs Salt and black pepper to taste ½ tbsp swerve sugar 1 tbsp soy sauce 2 tbsp sugar-free ketchup 2 cups balsamic vinegar Preheat oven to 370°F.

DirectionsIn a bowl, mix the beef, salt, mushrooms, bell pepper, Parmesan cheese, parsley, garlic, pepper, onion, almond flour, salt, and eggs. Shape into a loaf pan and bake for 30 minutes. Meanwhile, heat a small pan over medium heat, add in the balsamic vinegar, swerve, soy sauce, and ketchup and cook for 20 minutes. Remove the meatloaf from the oven, spread the glaze over the meatloaf, and bake in the oven for 5 more minutes. Allow the meatloaf to cool, slice, and enjoy.

107.   Herby Beef & Veggie Stew

Ready in about: 50 minutes | Serves: 4 Per serving: Kcal 253, Fat 13g, Net Carbs 5.2g, Protein 30g

Ingredients

1 lb stewed beef, cubed 2 tbsp olive oil 1 onion, chopped 2 garlic cloves, minced 14 oz canned diced tomatoes ¼ tsp dried oregano ¼ tsp dried basil ¼ tsp dried marjoram Salt and black pepper to taste 2 carrots, sliced 2 celery stalks, chopped 1 cup vegetable broth

Directions

Warm the olive oil in a pan over medium heat. Add in the onion, celery, and garlic and sauté for 5 minutes. Place in the ground beef and stir-fry for 6 minutes. Mix in the tomatoes, carrots, vegetable broth, black pepper, oregano, marjoram, basil, and salt and simmer for 35 minutes. Serve and enjoy!

108.   Beef with Dilled Yogurt

Ready in about: 25 minutes | Serves: 6 Per serving: Kcal 408, Fat 22.4g, Net Carbs 8.3g, Protein 27g

Ingredients

¼ cup almond milk 2 lb ground beef 1 onion, grated 5 zero carb bread slices, torn 1 egg, whisked Salt and black pepper to taste 2 garlic cloves, minced ¼ cup fresh mint, chopped ½ tsp dried oregano ¼ cup olive oil 1 cup cherry tomatoes, halved 1 cucumber, sliced 1 cup baby spinach 1 ½ tbsp lemon juice 1 cup dilled Greek yogurt Place the torn zero carb bread

Directions

In a bowl, add in the milk, and let it soak for 3 minutes. Squeeze the bread and place it into a bowl. Stir in the beef, salt, mint, onion, parsley, pepper, egg, oregano, and garlic. Form balls out of this mixture and place them on a working surface. Set a pan over medium heat and warm half of the oil. Fry the meatballs for 8 minutes on all sides. Remove to a tray. On a salad plate, combine the spinach with the cherry tomatoes and cucumber. Mix in the remaining oil, lemon juice, pepper, and salt. Spread dilled yogurt over. Top with meatballs to serve.

109.   Broccoli & Beef Slow Cooker Casserole

Ready in about: 4 hours 15 minutes | Serves: 6 Per serving: Kcal 434, Fat 21g, Net Carbs 5.6g, Protein 51g

Ingredients

2 tbsp olive oil 2 lb ground beef 1 head broccoli, cut into florets Salt and black pepper to taste 1 tsp mustard 2 tsp Worcestershire sauce 28 oz canned diced tomatoes 2 cups mozzarella cheese, grated 16 oz tomato sauce 2 tbsp fresh parsley, chopped 1 tsp dried oregano

DirectionsSeason the broccoli florets with pepper and salt to and drizzle over the olive oil. Toss to coat. In a separate bowl, combine the beef with Worcestershire sauce, salt, mustard, and black pepper, and stir well. Press on the slow cooker's bottom. Scatter with the broccoli and stir in the tomatoes, parsley, mozzarella, oregano, and tomato sauce. Cook for 4 hours on High. Split the casserole among bowls and serve hot.

110.   Beef & Cauliflower Rice Bowls

Ready in about: 25 minutes | Serves: 4 Per serving: Kcal 320, Fat 26g, Net Carbs 4g, Protein 15g

Ingredients

2 cups cauli rice 3 cups frozen mixed vegetables 3 tbsp ghee 1 lb skirt steaks Salt and black pepper to taste 4 eggs

DirectionsMix the cauli rice and vegetables in a bowl. Sprinkle with a little water and steam them in the microwave for 1 minute until tender. Share into 4 serving bowls. Melt the ghee in a skillet over medium heat. Season the beef with salt and pepper and brown for 5 minutes on each side. Remove onto the vegetables. Wipe out the skillet and return to medium heat. Crack in an egg, season with salt and pepper, and cook until the egg white has set, but the yolk is still runny 3 minutes. Remove egg onto the vegetable bowl and fry the remaining 3 eggs. Add to the other bowls and serve.

111. Beef Meatballs with Onion Sauce

Ready in about: 35 minutes | Serves: 4 Per serving: Kcal 435, Fat 23g, Net Carbs 6g, Protein 32g

Ingredients

1 lb ground beef Salt and black pepper to taste ½ tsp garlic powder 1 ¼ tbsp coconut aminos 1 cup beef stock ¾ cup almond flour 1 tbsp fresh parsley, chopped 1 tbsp dried onion flakes 1 onion, sliced 2 tbsp butter ¼ cup sour cream

Directions

In a bowl, mix the beef, salt, garlic powder, almond flour, onion flakes, parsley, 1 tbsp coconut aminos, and pepper. Form balls. Place them on a greased baking sheet. Bake in the oven for 20 minutes at 370ºF. Warm the butter in a pan over medium heat. Stir in the onion and cook for 3 minutes. Pour in the beef stock, sour cream, and remaining coconut aminos and bring to a simmer. Season with salt and pepper and cook for 3-4 minutes until the sauce thickens. Pour the sauce over the meatballs and serve.

112. Chuck Roast Beef

Ready in about: 3 hours 15 minutes | Serves: 6 Per serving: Kcal 325, Fat 18g, Net Carbs 7g, Protein 28g

Ingredients

2 lb beef chuck roast, cubed 2 tbsp olive oil 14.5 oz canned diced tomatoes 2 carrots, chopped Salt and black pepper to taste ½ lb mushrooms, sliced 1 celery stalk, chopped 1 onion, chopped 2 cups beef stock 1 tbsp fresh thyme, chopped ½ tsp dry mustard 1 tbsp almond flour

Directions

Set an ovenproof pot over medium heat, warm olive oil, and brown the beef on all sides for 5-6 minutes; Set aside. Add onions, carrots, mushrooms, and celery to the pot and sauté for 5 minutes. Pour in the stock and tomatoes and return the beef. Bring to a boil and simmer for 30 minutes. In a bowl, combine 1 cup of the cooking liquid with almond flour and dry mustard. Pour in the pot, sprinkle with thyme, salt, and black pepper, and cook for 3-4 minutes. Serve warm.

113. Beef Bourguignon

Ready in about: 60 minutes + marinated time | Serves: 4 Per serving: Kcal 435, Fat 26g, Net Carbs 7g, Protein 45g

Ingredients

3 tbsp coconut oil 1 tbsp dried parsley flakes 1 cup red wine 1 tsp dried thyme Salt and black pepper to taste 1 bay leaf ⅓ cup coconut flour 2 lb beef, cubed 12 small white onions 4 pancetta slices, chopped 2 garlic cloves, minced ½ lb mushrooms, chopped

Directions

In a bowl, combine the wine with bay leaf, olive oil, thyme, pepper, parsley, salt, and the beef cubes and toss to coat. Marinate for 3 hours. Drain the meat and reserve the marinade. Coat the meat with the flour. Heat a pan over medium heat, stir in the pancetta, and cook until slightly browned. Place in the onions and garlic, and cook for 3 minutes. Stir-fry in the meat and mushrooms for 4-5 minutes. Pour in the marinade and 1 cup of water; cover and cook for 50 minutes. Season to taste and serve.

114. Classic Italian Bolognese Sauce

Ready in about: 35 minutes | Serves: 4 Per serving: Kcal 318, Fat: 20g, Net Carbs: 5.9g, Protein: 26g

Ingredients

1 lb ground beef 2 garlic cloves, minced 1 onion, chopped ½ tsp dried oregano ½ tsp dried sage ½ tsp dried rosemary 14 oz canned diced tomatoes 2 tbsp olive oil

Directions

Heat the olive oil in a saucepan. Add onion and garlic and cook for 3 minutes. Add beef and cook until browned, about 4-5 minutes. Stir in the herbs and tomatoes. Cook for 15 minutes. Serve with zoodles.

115. Russian-Style Beef Gratin

Ready in about: 45 minutes | Serves: 4 Per serving: Kcal 584, Fat 48g, Net Carbs 5g, Protein 41g

Ingredients

1 onion, chopped 1 ½ lb ground beef 2 garlic cloves, minced Salt and black pepper to taste 1 cup mozzarella cheese, shredded 2 cups fontina cheese, shredded 1 cup crème fraîche 20 dill pickle slices 1 iceberg lettuce head, torn

Directions

Set a pan over medium heat, place in beef, garlic, salt, onion, and pepper and cook for 5 minutes. Remove to a baking dish, stir in crème fraîche, mozzarella cheese, and spread 1 cup of the fontina cheese. Lay the pickle slices on top and spread over the remaining fontina cheese. Place in the oven at 350ºF and bake for 20 minutes. Arrange the lettuce on a serving platter and top with the gratin.

116. Adobo Beef Fajitas

Ready in about: 35 minutes + marinating time | Serves: 4 Per serving: Kcal 348, Fat 25g, Net Carbs 5g, Protein 18g

Ingredients

1 ½ lb skirt steak 2 tbsp adobo seasoning 2 tbsp olive oil 2 large white onion, chopped 1 cup mixed bell peppers, chopped 8 zero carb tortillas Brush the steak with adobo seasoning and put in the fridge for 1 hour.

Directions

Preheat grill to high heat. Cook the steak for 12 minutes, flipping once until lightly browned. Remove, wrap in foil, and let sit for 10 minutes. Heat olive oil in a skillet over medium heat and sauté onion and bell peppers for 5 minutes until soft. Cut steak against the grain into strips and share on the tortillas. Top with the veggies and serve.

117. Beef Cotija Cheeseburger

Ready in about: 15 minutes | Serves: 4 Per serving: Kcal 386, Fat 32g, Net Carbs 2g, Protein 21g

Ingredients

1 ½ lb ground beef 1 tsp dried parsley ½ tsp Worcestershire sauce Salt and black pepper to taste 1 cup cotija cheese, shredded 4 zero carb buns, halved Preheat grill to 400°F.

Directions

Mix the beef, parsley, Worcestershire sauce, salt, and black pepper with your hands until evenly combined. Make medium-sized patties out of the mixture. Cook on the grill for 5 minutes. Flip and top with cheese. Cook for 5 more minutes until the cheese melts. Remove and sandwich into two halves of a bun each. Serve with a tomato sauce and zucchini fries.

118. Beef Reuben Soup

Ready in about: 20 minutes | Serves: 6 Per serving: Kcal 450, Fat: 37g, Net Carbs: 8g, Protein: 23g

Ingredients

1 onion, diced 6 cups beef stock 1 tsp caraway seeds 2 celery stalks, diced 2 garlic cloves, minced 2 cups heavy cream 1 cup sauerkraut, shredded 1 lb corned beef, chopped 3 tbsp butter 1 ½ cup swiss cheese, shredded Salt and black pepper to taste

Directions

Melt the butter in a large pot. Add onion, garlic, and celery and fry for 3 minutes until tender. Pour the beef stock over and stir in sauerkraut, salt, caraway seeds, and add a pinch of black pepper. Bring to a boil. Reduce the heat to low, and add the corned beef. Cook for about 15 minutes, adjust the seasoning. Stir in heavy cream and cheese and cook for 1 minute.

119. Winter Veal with Sauerkraut

Ready in about: 60 minutes | Serves: 4 Per serving: Kcal 430, Fat 27g, Net Carbs 6g, Protein 29g

Ingredients

1 lb veal, cut into cubes 18 oz sauerkraut, drained Salt and black pepper to taste ½ cup ham, chopped 1 keek, chopped 2 garlic cloves, minced 3 tbsp butter 1 cup canned tomatoes, chopped 1 cup beef broth

Directions

Heat a pot with the butter over medium heat. Add in the leek and garlic cook for 3 minutes, stirring occasionally. Place in the veal and ham and cook until slightly browned, about 5-6 minutes. Pour in the broth, tomatoes, and sauerkraut and cook until the meat becomes tender, about 30 minutes. Season with pepper and salt. Transfer to a baking dish. Bake in the oven for 10 minutes at 350°F. Serve.

120. Veal Stew

Ready in about: 2 hours | Serves: 6 Per serving: Kcal 415, Fat 21g, Net Carbs 5.2g, Protein 44g

Ingredients

3 tbsp olive oil 3 lb veal shoulder, cubed 1 onion, chopped 1 garlic clove, minced Salt and black pepper to taste 1 cup water 1 ½ cups red wine 12 oz canned tomato sauce 1 carrot, chopped 1 cup mushrooms, chopped ½ cup green beans 2 tsp dried oregano

Directions

Set a pot over medium heat and Warm the olive oil. Brown the veal for 5-6 minutes. Stir in the onion and garlic and cook for 3 minutes. Place in the wine, oregano, carrot, black pepper, salt, tomato sauce, water, and mushrooms. Bring to a boil and reduce the heat to low. Cook for 1 hour and 45 minutes, then add in the green beans, and cook for 5 minutes. Adjust the seasoning and split among bowls to serve.

121. Rolled Lamb Shoulder with Basil & Pine Nuts

Ready in about: 1 hour | Serves: 4 Per serving: Kcal 547, Fat 37.7g, Net Carbs 2.2g, Protein 42.7g

Ingredients

½ cup green olives, pitted and chopped 1 ½ lb lamb shoulder, boneless 1 ½ cups basil leaves, chopped 2 tbsp pine nuts, chopped 2 cloves garlic, minced Salt and black pepper to taste 1 cup chicken broth Preheat oven to 450°F.

Directions In a bowl, combine basil, pine nuts, olives, and garlic. Season with salt and pepper. Untie the lamb flat onto a chopping board, spread the basil mixture all over, and rub the spices onto the meat. Roll the lamb over the spice mixture and tie it together using 3 to 4 strings of butcher's twine. Place the lamb onto a baking dish, pour in the chicken broth, and cook in the oven for 10 minutes. Reduce the heat to 350°F and continue cooking for 40 minutes. When ready, transfer the meat to a cleaned chopping board. Let it rest for 10 minutes before slicing. Serve with roasted root vegetables.

122. Lamb Stew with Veggies

Ready in about: 1 hour 50 minutes | Serves: 2 Per serving: Kcal 584, Fat 42g, Net Carbs 8.1g, Protein 38g

Ingredients

1 garlic clove, minced 1 parsnip, chopped 1 onion, chopped 1 tbsp olive oil 1 celery stalk, chopped 10 oz lamb fillet, cut into pieces Salt and black pepper to taste 1 ¼ cups vegetable stock 1 carrot, chopped ½ tbsp fresh rosemary, chopped 1 leek, chopped 1 tbsp mint sauce 1 tsp stevia 1 tbsp tomato puree ½ head cauliflower, cut into florets ½ head celeriac, chopped 2 tbsp butter

Directions Set a pot over medium heat and warm the oil. Add in the celery, onion, and garlic and cook for 5 minutes. Stir in the lamb pieces and cook for 3 minutes. Add in the stevia, carrot, parsnip, rosemary, mint sauce, stock, leek, and tomato puree. Bring to a boil, reduce the heat, and cook for 1 hour and 30 minutes. Heat a pot with water over medium heat and place in the celeriac. Cover and simmer for 10 minutes. Add in the cauliflower florets and cook for 15 minutes. Drain everything and combine with butter, pepper, and salt. Mash using a potato masher. Top with vegetable mixture and lamb and serve.

123. White Wine Lamb Chops

Ready in about: 1 hour 10 minutes | Serves: 6 Per serving: Kcal 397, Fat: 30g, Net Carbs: 4.3g, Protein: 16g

Ingredients

6 lamb chops ½ tsp sage ½ tsp thyme 1 onion, sliced 3 garlic cloves, minced 2 tbsp olive oil ½ cup white wine Salt and black pepper to taste

Directions

Heat the olive oil in a pan. Add onion and garlic and cook for 3 minutes until soft. Rub the sage and thyme over the lamb chops. Cook it in the pan for about 3 minutes per side. Set aside. Pour the white wine and 1 cup of water into the pan and bring the mixture to a boil. Cook until the liquid is reduced by half, about 5 minutes. Add in the chops, reduce the heat, and let simmer for 1 hour. Serve.

124.   Sweet Chipotle Grilled Beef Ribs

Ready in about: 35 minutes + marinating time | Serves: 4 Per serving: Kcal 395, Fat 33g, Net Carbs 3g, Protein 21g

Ingredients

4 tbsp sugar-free BBQ sauce + extra for serving 2 tbsp erythritol Pink salt and black pepper to taste 2 tbsp olive oil 2 tsp chipotle powder 1 tsp garlic powder 1 lb beef spare ribs

Directions

Mix the erythritol, salt, pepper, oil, chipotle, and garlic powder. Brush on the meaty sides of the ribs and wrap in foil. Sit for 30 minutes to marinate. Preheat oven to 400°F. Place wrapped ribs on a baking sheet and cook for 40 minutes until cooked through. Remove ribs and aluminium foil, brush with BBQ sauce, and brown under the broiler for 10 minutes on both sides. Slice and serve with extra BBQ sauce and lettuce tomato salad.

125.   Habanero & Beef Balls

Ready in about: 45 minutes | Serves: 6 Per serving: Kcal 455, Fat 31g, Net Carbs 8.3g, Protein 27g

Ingredients

3 garlic cloves, minced 2 lb ground beef 1 onion, chopped 2 habanero peppers, chopped 1 tsp dried thyme 2 tsp fresh cilantro, chopped ½ tsp allspice 1 tsp cumin ½ tsp ground cloves Salt and black pepper to taste 2 tbsp butter 3 tbsp butter, melted 6 oz cream cheese 1 tsp turmeric ¼ tsp stevia ½ tsp baking powder 1½ cups flax meal ½ cup coconut flour In a blender, mix the onion with garlic, habaneros, and ½ cup water.

Directions

Set a pan over medium heat, add 2 tbsp butter, and cook the beef for 3 minutes. Stir in the onion mixture, and cook for 2 minutes. Stir in cilantro, cloves, salt, cumin, turmeric, thyme, allspice, and pepper and cook for 3 minutes. In a bowl, combine the coconut flour, stevia, flax meal, and baking powder and stir well. In a separate bowl, whisk the melted butter with the cream cheese. Mix the 2 mixtures to obtain a dough. Form 12 balls from the mixture and roll them into circles. Split the beef mix on one-half of the dough circles, cover with the other half, seal edges, and lay on a lined sheet. Bake for 25 minutes in the oven at 350°F.

126.   Warm Rump Steak Salad

Ready in about: 40 minutes | Serves: 4 Per serving: Kcal 325, Fat 19g, Net Carbs 4g, Protein 28g

Ingredients

1 lb rump steak, excess fat trimmed 3 green onions, sliced 3 tomatoes, sliced 1 cup cooked green beans, sliced 2 kohlrabi, peeled and chopped 1 tbsp butter, softened 2 cups mixed salad greens Salt and black pepper to taste Salad dressing 2 tsp Dijon mustard 1 tbsp erythritol Salt and black pepper to taste 3 tbsp olive oil 1 tbsp red wine vinegar Preheat oven to 400°F.

Directions

Place the kohlrabi on a baking sheet, drizzle with olive oil and bake in the oven for 25 minutes. Let it cool. In a bowl, mix the mustard, erythritol, salt, pepper, vinegar, and oil; reserve. Melt the butter in a pan over high heat. Season the meat with salt and pepper. Place the steak in the pan and brown on both sides for 4 minutes each. Remove and let it rest for 4 more minutes before slicing. In a salad bowl, add green onions, tomatoes, green beans, kohlrabi, salad greens, and steak slices. Drizzle the dressing over and toss with two spoons. Serve the steak salad warm with chunks of low carb bread.

127.Ribeye Steak with Shitake Mushrooms

Ready in about: 25 minutes | Serves: 4 Per serving: Kcal 478, Fat: 31g, Net Carbs: 3g, Protein: 33g

Ingredients

1 lb ribeye steaks 1 tbsp butter 2 tbsp olive oil 1 cup shitake mushrooms, sliced Salt and black pepper to taste 2 tbsp fresh parsley, chopped

Directions

Heat the olive oil in a pan over medium heat. Rub the steaks with salt and black pepper and cook about 4 minutes per side; reserve. Melt the butter in the pan and cook the shitakes for 4 minutes. Scatter the parsley over and pour the mixture over the steaks to serve.

128.   Beef & Ale Pot Roast

Ready in about: 2 hours 20 minutes | Serves: 6 Per serving: Kcal 513, Fat 34g, Net Carbs 6g, Protein 26g

Ingredients

1 ½ lb brisket 2 tbsp olive oil 8 baby carrots, peeled 2 medium red onions, quartered 1 celery stalk, cut into chunks Salt and black pepper to taste 2 bay leaves 1 ½ cups low carb beer (ale) Preheat oven to 370ºF.

Directions

Heat the olive oil in a large skillet over medium heat. Season the brisket with salt and pepper. Brown the meat on both sides for 8 minutes. After, transfer to a deep casserole dish. In the dish, arrange the carrots, onions, celery, and bay leaves around the brisket and pour the beer all over it. Cover the pot and cook in the oven for 2 hours. When ready, remove the casserole. Transfer the beef to a chopping board and cut it into thick slices. Serve the beef and vegetables with a drizzle of the sauce.

129.   Beef Cheeseburger Casserole

Ready in about: 30 minutes | Serves: 6 Per serving: Kcal 385, Fat 25g, Net Carbs 5g, Protein 20g

Ingredients

3 tbsp olive oil 2 lb ground beef 1 cup cauli rice 2 cups cabbage, chopped 14 oz can diced tomatoes 1 cup Colby jack cheese, shredded Preheat oven to 370ºF.

Directions

Warm the olive oil in a pan over medium heat. Add in the ground beef and cook for 6 minutes until no longer pink. Stir in the cauli rice, cabbage, tomatoes, and ¼ cup water. Bring to boil and cook covered for 5 minutes until the sauce thickens. Spoon the beef mixture into a baking dish and spread evenly. Sprinkle with cheese; bake for 15 minutes until the cheese has melted. Remove and cool for 4 minutes. Serve with zero carbs crusted bread.

130.   Beef Meatballs

Ready in about: 35 minutes | Serves: 4 Per serving: Kcal 332, Fat 18g, Net Carbs 7g, Protein 25g

Ingredients

½ cup pork rinds, crushed 1 egg Salt and black pepper to taste 1 ½ lb ground beef 10 oz canned onion soup 1 tbsp almond flour ¼ cup free-sugar ketchup 3 tsp Worcestershire sauce ½ tsp dry mustard In a bowl, combine ⅓ cup of the onion soup with the beef, pepper, pork rinds, egg, and salt.

Directions

Shape the mixture into 12 meatballs. Heat a greased pan over medium heat. Brown the meatballs for 12 minutes. In a separate bowl, combine the rest of the soup with almond flour, dry mustard, ketchup, Worcestershire sauce, and ¼ cup water. Pour this over the beef meatballs, cover the pan, and cook for 10 minutes as you stir occasionally. Split among bowls and serve.

131. Beef Stovies

Ready in about: 45 minutes | Serves: 4 Per serving: Kcal 316, Fat 18g, Net Carbs 3g, Protein 14g

Ingredients

1 lb ground beef 1 large onion, chopped 2 parsnips, peeled and chopped 1 large carrot, chopped 2 tbsp olive oil 2 garlic cloves, minced Salt and black pepper to taste 1 cup chicken broth ¼ tsp allspice 2 tsp fresh rosemary, chopped 1 tbsp Worcestershire sauce ½ small cabbage, shredded

Directions

Heat the olive oil in a skillet over medium heat and cook the beef for 4 minutes. Season with salt and pepper, stirring occasionally while breaking the lumps in it. Add in onion, garlic, carrot, rosemary, and parsnips. Stir and cook for a minute, and pour in the chicken broth, allspice, and Worcestershire sauce. Reduce the heat to low and cook for 20 minutes. Stir in the cabbage, season with salt and black pepper, and cook further for 15 minutes. Turn the heat off, plate the stovies, and serve warm.

132. Homemade Classic Beef Burgers

Ready in about: 15 minutes | Serves: 4 Per serving: Kcal 664, Fat: 55g, Net Carbs: 7.9g, Protein: 39g

Ingredients

1 lb ground beef ½ tsp onion powder 2 tbsp ghee 1 tsp Dijon mustard 4 zero carb buns, halved ¼ cup mayonnaise 1 tsp sriracha sauce 4 tbsp cabbage slaw Salt and black pepper to taste

Directions

Mix well the beef, onion powder, mustard, salt, and pepper in a bowl. Create 4 burgers. Melt the ghee in a skillet over medium heat and cook the burgers for about 3 minutes per side. Place in buns, top with mayonnaise, sriracha sauce, and cabbage slaw. Serve.

133. Beef Stuffed Roasted Squash

Ready in about: 1 hour 15 minutes | Serves: 4 Per serving: Kcal 406, Fat 14.7g, Net Carbs 12.4g, Protein 34g

Ingredients

2 lb butternut squash, pricked with a fork Salt and black pepper to taste 2 garlic cloves, minced 1 onion, chopped 1 cup button mushrooms, sliced 28 oz canned diced tomatoes 1 tsp dried oregano ¼ tsp cayenne pepper 1 lb ground beef 1 green bell pepper, chopped Lay the butternut squash on a lined baking sheet, set in the oven at 400°F, and bake for 40 minutes.

DirectionsAfter, cut in half and set aside to cool. Deseed, scoop out most of the flesh, and let sit. Heat a greased pan over medium heat. Add in the garlic, mushrooms, onion, and beef and cook until the meat browns. Stir in the green pepper, salt, tomatoes, oregano, pepper, butternut flesh, and cayenne and cook for 10 minutes. Stuff the squash halves with the beef mixture and bake in the oven for 10 minutes. Serve.

134. Beef with Grilled Vegetables

Ready in about: 30 minutes | Serves: 4 Per serving: Kcal 515, Fat 32.1g, Net Carbs 5.6g, Protein 66g

Ingredients

4 sirloin steaks 2 tbsp olive oil 3 tbsp balsamic vinegar Vegetables ½ lb asparagus, trimmed 1 cup green beans 1 cup snow peas 1 red bell peppers, cut into strips 1 orange bell peppers, cut into strips 1 medium red onion, quartered

Directions

Set a grill pan over high heat. Grab 2 separate bowls and put the beef in one and the vegetables in another. Mix salt, pepper, olive oil, and balsamic vinegar in a small bowl and pour half of the mixture over the beef and the other half over the vegetables. Coat the ingredients in both bowls with the sauce. Place the steaks in the grill pan and sear both sides for 2-3 minutes each. When done, remove the beef onto a plate; Set aside. Pour the vegetables and marinade in the pan and cook for 5 minutes, turning once. Share the vegetables into plates. Top with beef, drizzle the sauce from the pan all over, and serve.

135. Beef Zucchini Boats

Ready in about: 45 minutes | Serves: 4 Per serving: Kcal 422, Fat 33g, Net Carbs 7.8g, Protein 39g

Ingredients

2 garlic cloves, minced 1 tsp cumin 2 tbsp olive oil 1 lb ground beef ½ cup onions, chopped 1 tsp smoked paprika Salt and black pepper to taste 4 zucchinis ¼ cup fresh cilantro, chopped ½ cup Monterey Jack cheese, grated 1 ½ cups enchilada sauce 1 avocado, chopped, for serving

Directions

Green onions, chopped, for serving Tomatoes, chopped, for serving Set a pan over high heat and warm the oil. Add the onions, and cook for 2 minutes. Stir in the beef and brown for 4-5 minutes. Stir in the paprika, pepper, garlic, cumin, and salt; cook for 2 minutes. Slice the zucchini in half lengthwise and scoop out the seeds. Set the zucchini in a greased baking pan, stuff each with the beef, scatter enchilada sauce on top, and spread with the Monterey cheese. Bake in the oven at 350°F for 20 minutes while covered. Uncover, spread with cilantro, and bake for 5 minutes. Top with tomatoes, green onions, and avocado and place on serving plates. Enjoy!

136. Beef Provençal

Ready in about: 50 minutes | Serves: 4 Per serving: Kcal 230, Fat 11.3g, Net Carbs 5.2g, Protein 19g

Ingredients

12 oz beef steak racks 1 fennel bulb, sliced Salt and black pepper to taste 3 tbsp olive oil ½ cup apple cider vinegar 1 tsp herbs de Provence

Directions

In a bowl, mix the fennel with 2 tbsp of the olive oil and vinegar. Toss to coat and transfer to a baking dish. Season with herbs de Provence, pepper, and salt and cook in the oven at 400°F for 15 minutes. Sprinkle the beef with pepper and salt. Place into an oiled pan over medium heat and cook for 2 minutes. Place the beef in the baking dish with the fennel and bake for 20 minutes. Split among plates and serve.

137.Mexican Beef Chili

Ready in about: 40 minutes | Serves: 4 Per serving: Kcal 437, Fat 26g, Net Carbs 5g, Protein 17g

Ingredients

15 oz canned tomatoes with green chilies, chopped 1 onion, chopped 2 tbsp olive oil 1 ½ lb ground beef 1 cup beef broth 1 tbsp tomato paste ½ cup pickled jalapeños, chopped 1 tsp chipotle chili paste 2 garlic cloves, minced 3 celery stalks, chopped 2 tbsp coconut aminos Salt and black pepper to taste ½ tsp cayenne pepper 1 tsp cumin 1 bay leaf 1 tbsp fresh cilantro, chopped

Directions

Heat the olive oil in a pan over medium heat. Add in the onion, celery, garlic, ground beef, black pepper, and salt and cook until the meat browns, about 6-8 minutes. Stir in jalapeños, tomato paste, canned tomatoes with green chilies, salt, bay leaf, cayenne pepper, coconut aminos, chipotle chili paste, beef broth, and cumin. Cook for 30 minutes. Remove and discard the bay leaf. Serve sprinkled with cilantro.

138.   Beef Stew with Bacon

Ready in about: 1 hour 15 minutes | Serves: 6 Per serving: Kcal 592, Fat 36g, Net Carbs 5.7g, Protein 63g

Ingredients

4 oz bacon, chopped 4 lb beef meat for stew, cubed 2 garlic cloves, minced 1 onion, chopped 2 tbsp olive oil 2 tbsp red vinegar 2 cups beef stock 2 tbsp tomato puree 1 cinnamon stick 3 lemon peel strips ½ cup fresh parsley, chopped 4 thyme sprigs 2 tbsp butter Salt and black pepper to taste

Directions

Set a saucepan over medium heat and warm oil. Add in the garlic, bacon, and onion and cook for 5 minutes. Stir in the beef and cook until slightly brown, about 4-5 minutes. Pour in the vinegar, black pepper, butter, lemon peel strips, stock, salt, tomato puree, cinnamon, and thyme and stir for 3 minutes. Cook for 1 hour while covered. Get rid of the thyme, lemon peel, and cinnamon. Top with parsley to serve.

139.   Caribbean Beef

Ready in about: 1 hour 10 minutes | Serves: 4 Per serving: Kcal 305, Fat 14g, Net Carbs 8g, Protein 25g

Ingredients

1 onion, chopped 2 tbsp avocado oil 2 lb beef stew meat, cubed 1 red bell pepper, chopped 1 habanero pepper, chopped 2 green chilies, chopped 14.5 oz canned diced tomatoes 2 tbsp fresh cilantro, chopped 2 garlic cloves, minced 1 ½ cups vegetable broth Salt and black pepper to taste ½ tsp cumin ½ cup black olives, chopped ½tsp dried oregano

DirectionsSet a pan over medium heat and warm the avocado oil. Brown the beef on all sides for 5-6 minutes. Set aside. Stir-fry the bell pepper, green chilies, oregano, garlic, habanero pepper, onions, and cumin in the pan for about 5-6 minutes. Pour in the tomatoes and vegetable broth and return the beef. Cook for 1 hour. Stir in the olives, adjust the seasonings, and serve in bowls sprinkled with fresh cilantro.

140.   Beef & Feta Salad

Ready in about: 20 minutes | Serves: 4 Per serving: Kcal 434, Fat 43g, Net Carbs 3.5g, Protein 17g

Ingredients

3 tbsp olive oil ½ lb beef rump steak, cut into strips Salt and black pepper to taste 1 tsp cumin ½ tsp dried thyme 2 garlic cloves, minced 4 oz feta cheese, crumbled ½ cup pecans 2 cups spinach 1 ½ tbsp lemon juice ¼ cup fresh mint, chopped

DirectionsSeason the beef with salt, some olive oil, garlic, thyme, pepper, and cumin. Place on a preheated to medium heat grill and cook for 10 minutes, flipping once. Remove to a cutting board, leave to cool, and slice into strips. Toast the pecans in a dry pan over medium heat for 2 minutes, shaking often. In a salad bowl, combine the spinach with the remaining olive oil, mint, salt, black pepper, and lemon juice and toss well to coat. Sprinkle with feta cheese and pecans. Top with the beef slices and serve.

141. Italian Sausage Stew

Ready in about: 35 minutes | Serves: 6 Per serving: Kcal 314, Fat 25g, Net Carbs 7g, Protein 16g

Ingredients

1 lb Italian sausage, sliced 1 red bell pepper, chopped 2 onions, chopped Salt and black pepper to taste 1 cup fresh parsley, chopped 6 green onions, chopped ¼ cup avocado oil 1 cup beef stock 4 garlic cloves 24 oz canned diced tomatoes 16 oz okra, trimmed and sliced 6 oz tomato sauce 2 tbsp coconut aminos 1 tbsp hot sauce

Directions

Set a pot over medium heat and warm oil, place in the sausages, and cook for 2 minutes. Stir in the onions, green onions, garlic, black pepper, bell pepper, and salt and cook for 5 minutes. Add in the hot sauce, beef stock, tomatoes, coconut aminos, okra, and tomato sauce, bring to a simmer. Cook for 15 minutes. Share into serving bowls and sprinkle with fresh parsley to serve.

142. Roasted Spicy Beef

Ready in about: 70 minutes | Serves: 4 Per serving: Kcal 480, Fat 23.5g, Net Carbs 3.5g, Protein 55g

Ingredients

2 lb beef brisket ½ tsp celery salt 1 tsp chili powder 2 tbsp avocado oil ½ tsp cayenne pepper ½ tsp garlic powder ½ cup beef stock 1 tbsp garlic, minced ¼ tsp dry mustard Preheat oven to 340°F.

Directions

In a bowl, combine the dry mustard, chili powder, salt, garlic powder, cayenne pepper, and celery salt and mix well. Rub the meat with the mixture. Set a pan over medium heat. Warm the avocado oil in the pan. Place in the beef and sear until brown. Remove to a baking dish. Pour in the stock, add garlic, and bake for 60 minutes. Set the beef to a cutting board, leaving to cool before slicing. Take the juices from the baking dish and strain. Sprinkle over the meat and serve.

143. Beef Skewers with Ranch Dressing

Ready in about: 25 minutes | Serves: 4 Per serving: Kcal 230, Fat 14g, Net Carbs 3g, Protein 21g

Ingredients

1 lb sirloin steak, boneless, cubed ¼ cup ranch dressing Chopped scallions to garnish Preheat the grill to 400°F.

Directions

Thread the beef cubes on skewers. Brush half of the ranch dressing on the skewers (all around) and place them on the grill grate to cook for 12 minutes, turning once. Brush the remaining ranch dressing on the meat and cook them for 1 more minute on each side. Plate, garnish with the scallions, and serve with a mixed veggie salad and extra ranch dressing.

144. Thai Beef with Shiitake Mushrooms

Ready in about: 30 minutes | Serves: 6 Per serving: Kcal 224, Fat 15g, Net Carbs 3g, Protein 19g

Ingredients

1 cup beef stock 4 tbsp butter ¼ tsp garlic powder ¼ tsp onion powder 1 tbsp coconut aminos 1 ½ tsp lemon pepper 1 lb beef steak, cut into strips Salt and black pepper to taste 1 cup shiitake mushrooms, sliced 3 green onions, chopped 1 tbsp Thai red curry paste

Directions

Melt butter in a pan over medium heat. Add in the beef, garlic powder, pepper, salt, and onion powder, stir, and cook for 4 minutes. Mix in the mushrooms and stir-fry for 5 minutes. Pour in the stock, coconut aminos, lemon pepper, and Thai curry paste and cook for 15 minutes. Top with green onions and serve.

145. Beef & Butternut Squash Stew

Ready in about: 40 minutes | Serves: 4 Per serving: Kcal 343, Fat 17g, Net Carbs 7.3g, Protein 32g

Ingredients

2 tsp olive oil 1 ½ lb ground beef 1 cup beef stock 14 oz canned tomatoes with juice 1 tbsp stevia 1 lb butternut squash, chopped 1 tbsp Worcestershire sauce 2 bay leaves Salt and black pepper to taste 1 onion, chopped ½ tsp dried sage 1 tbsp garlic, minced

Directions

Set a pan over medium heat and heat olive oil. Stir in the onion, garlic, and beef and cook for 10 minutes. Add in butternut squash, Worcestershire sauce, bay leaves, stevia, stock, canned tomatoes, sage, salt, and pepper and bring to a boil. Simmer for 30 minutes. Remove and discard the bay leaves. Serve warm.

146. Pecorino Veal Cutlets

Ready in about: 55 minutes | Serves: 6 Per serving: Kcal 362, Fat 21g, Net Carbs 6g, Protein 26g

Ingredients

6 veal cutlets ½ cup Pecorino cheese, grated 6 provolone cheese slices Black pepper to taste 4 cups tomato sauce A pinch of garlic salt 2 tbsp butter 2 tbsp coconut oil, melted 1 tsp Italian seasoning Season the veal cutlets with garlic salt and pepper.

Directions

Set a pan over medium heat and warm coconut oil and butter. Add in the veal and cook until browned on all sides. Spread half of the tomato sauce on a greased baking dish. Place in the veal cutlets, then sprinkle with Italian seasoning and remaining sauce. Set in the oven at 360° F and bake for 40 minutes. Scatter with the provolone cheese, then sprinkle with Pecorino cheese, and bake for another 5 minutes until the cheese is golden and melted. Serve warm.

147. Venison Tenderloin with Cheese Stuffing

Ready in about: 30 minutes | Serves: 8 Per serving: Kcal 194, Fat: 12g, Net Carbs: 1.7g, Protein: 25g

Ingredients

2 lb venison tenderloin 2 garlic cloves, minced 2 tbsp almonds, chopped ½ cup gorgonzola cheese, crumbled ½ cup feta cheese, crumbled 1 tsp chopped onion

Directions

Preheat the grill to medium heat. Slice the tenderloin lengthwise to make a pocket for the filling. Combine the rest of the ingredients in a bowl. Stuff the tenderloin with the filling. Shut the meat with skewers and grill for as long as it takes to reach your desired density. Serve warm with sautéed vegetables.

148. Rack of Lamb in Red Bell Pepper Sauce

Ready in about: 65 minutes + marinating time | Serves: 4 Per serving: Kcal 415, Fat 25g, Carbs 2g, Protein 46g

Ingredients

1 lb rack of lamb Salt to taste 1 tbsp garlic powder ⅓ cup olive oil ⅓ cup white wine 6 sprigs fresh rosemary Sauce 2 tbsp olive oil 1 large red bell pepper, diced 2 cloves garlic, minced 1 cup chicken broth 2 oz butter Salt and white pepper to taste

Directions

cover the bowl with plastic wrap, and place in the refrigerator to marinate. Preheat the grill to high heat. Cook the lamb for 6 minutes on both sides. Remove and let rest for 4 minutes. Heat the olive oil in a frying pan and sauté the garlic and bell pepper for 5 minutes. Pour in the chicken broth and continue cooking the ingredients until the liquid reduces by half, about 10 minutes. Add the butter, salt, and white pepper. Stir to Melt the butter and turn the heat off. Use a stick blender to puree the ingredients until very smooth and strain the sauce through a fine-mesh into a bowl. Slice the lamb and serve drizzled with the sauce.

149. Grilled Lamb in Lemony Sauce

Ready in about: 25 minutes | Serves: 4 Per serving: Kcal 392, Fat: 31g, Net Carbs: 1g, Protein: 29g

Ingredients

1 ½ lb lamb chops Sal and black pepper to taste 2 tbsp olive oil Sauce ¼ cup olive oil 1 tsp red pepper flakes 2 tbsp lemon juice 2 tbsp fresh mint 3 garlic cloves, pressed 2 tbsp lemon zest ¼ cup parsley ½ tsp smoked paprika Rub lamb with olive oil, salt, and pepper.

Directions

Preheat the grill to medium heat. Grill the lamb chops for about 3 minutes per side. Whisk together the sauce ingredients in a bowl. Serve the lamb topped with sauce.

150.   Lamb Shashlyk

Ready in about: 20 minutes | Serves: 4 Per serving: Kcal 467, Fat: 37g, Net Carbs: 3.2g, Protein: 27g

Ingredients

1 lb ground lamb ¼ tsp cinnamon 1 egg 1 grated onion Salt and black pepper to taste Place all ingredients in a bowl.

Directions

Mix with your hands to combine well. Divide the meat into 4 pieces. Shape all meat portions around previously-soaked skewers. Preheat grill to medium heat and grill the kebabs for about 5 minutes per side. Serve

151. Beef Tripe Pot

Ready in about: 1 hour 30 minutes + cooling time | Serves: 6 Per serving: Kcal 248, Fat 12.8g, Net Carbs 4g, Protein 8g

Ingredients

1 ½ lb beef tripe, cleaned 4 cups buttermilk Salt and black pepper to taste 3 tbsp olive oil 2 onions, sliced 4 garlic cloves, minced 3 tomatoes, diced 1 tsp paprika 2 chili peppers, minced

Directions Put the tripe in a bowl and cover with buttermilk. Refrigerate for 3 hours to extract bitterness and a gamey taste. Remove from buttermilk, drain and rinse well under cold running water. Place in a pot over medium heat and cover with water. Bring to a boil and cook for about 1 hour until tender. Remove the tripe with a perforated spoon and let cool. Strain the broth and reserve. Chop the cooled tripe. Heat the oil in a skillet over medium heat. Sauté the onions, garlic, and chili peppers for 3 minutes until soft. Stir in the paprika and add in the tripe. Cook for 5-6 minutes. Include the tomatoes and 4 cups of the reserved tripe broth and cook for 10 minutes. Adjust the seasoning with salt and pepper. Serve.

152.   Jalapeno Beef Pot Roast

Ready in about: 1 hour 25 minutes | Serves: 4 Per serving: Kcal 745, Fat 46g, Net Carbs 3.2g, Protein 87g

Ingredients

1 ½ lb beef roast 4 oz mushrooms, sliced 12 oz beef stock 1 oz onion soup mix ½ cup Italian dressing 2 jalapeño peppers, shredded

Directions In a bowl, combine the stock with the Italian dressing and onion soup mixture. Place the beef roast in a baking pan, add in the stock mixture, mushrooms, and jalapeños, and cover with aluminum foil. Set in the oven and bake for 1 hour at 360°F. Take out the foil and continue baking for 15 minutes. Allow the roast to cool slightly. Slice and serve alongside a topping of the gravy.

153.   North African Lamb

Ready in about: 25 minutes | Serves: 4 Per serving: Kcal 445, Fat 32g, Net Carbs 4g, Protein 34g

Ingredients

1 tsp paprika 2 garlic cloves, minced ½ tsp dried oregano ½ tbsp sumac 12 lamb cutlets ¼ cup sesame oil 1 tsp cumin 2 carrots, sliced 2 tbsp fresh parsley, chopped 1 tsp harissa paste 1 tbsp red wine vinegar Salt and black pepper to taste 2 tbsp black olives, sliced 2 cucumbers, sliced

Directions

In a bowl, combine the cutlets with paprika, oregano, pepper, 2 tbsp water, half of the sesame oil, sumac, garlic, and salt and mix well. Place the carrots in a pot over medium heat and cover with water. Bring to a boil. Cook for 2 minutes. Drain, put in a salad bowl, and let them cool. Mix in cucumbers and olives. In another bowl, combine the harissa paste with the rest of the oil, a splash of water, parsley, vinegar, and cumin. Drizzle over the carrots mixture, season with pepper and salt, and toss to coat. Preheat the grill to medium heat. Arrange the lamb cutlets on it, grill each side for 3 minutes, and split among separate plates. Serve alongside the carrot salad.

154.   Easy and Spicy Sloppy Joes

(Ready in about 30 minutes | Servings 6) Per serving: 313 Calories; 20.6g Fat; 3.5g Carbs; 26.6g Protein; 2.1g Fiber

Ingredients

1 ½ pounds ground beef 2 teaspoons lard, room temperature 1 large onion, chopped 2 garlic cloves, minced Salt and ground pepper, to taste 1 teaspoon paprika 1 teaspoon mustard 1 tablespoon red wine vinegar 1/2 cup tomato sauce 1/2 teaspoon hot sauce

Directions

Melt 1 teaspoon of the lard in a saucepan over a moderately high heat. Once hot, sauté the onion and garlic until tender and translucent; reserve. In the same skillet, melt another teaspoon of the lard. Cook the ground beef, breaking apart with a fork, until well browned. Add the sautéed vegetables back to the saucepan; stir in the spices, vinegar, tomato sauce, and hot sauce. Reduce the heat to simmer and continue to cook for 17 to 20 minutes. Bon appétit!

155.   Restaurant-Style Soup with Lime-Chili Drizzle

(Ready in about 1 hour 10 minutes | Servings 6) Per serving: 375 Calories; 14.4g Fat; 4.8g Carbs; 47.6g Protein; 2.8g Fiber

Ingredients

2 pounds beef chuck-eye roast, cubed 1 medium leek, chopped 1/2 cup green peas, frozen 1 tablespoon ghee 1/2 cup bell peppers, chopped 1 cup tomato sauce 6 cups beef bone broth 1 parsnip, chopped 1 celery with leaves, chopped 1 bay laurel For the Lime-Chili Drizzle: 2 red chilies 2 tablespoons lime juice 1 tablespoon extra-virgin olive oil

Directions

In a heavy-bottomed pot, melt the ghee over a moderately high heat. Sear the beef for about 5 minutes, stirring continuously, until well browned on all sides; set aside. In the same pot, cook the leek, parsnip, celery, and peppers until they've softened. Add in the tomato sauce, beef bone broth and bay laurel; bring to a boil. Turn the heat to simmer; partially cover and continue to cook for 45 to 50 minutes. Add in the green peas and continue to cook for about 12 minutes longer. Make the lime-chili drizzle by whisking the ingredients.Garnish with the lime-chili drizzle and serve hot!

156.   Autumn Ground Chuck Casserole

(Ready in about 55 minutes | Servings 6) Per serving: 467 Calories; 37g Fat; 4.9g Carbs; 27.1g Protein; 3.1g Fiber

Ingredients

1 pound ground chuck 1 head of cabbage, cut into quarters 1 yellow onion, chopped 1/2 teaspoon mustard seeds 1 ½ cups Ricotta cheese, crumbled 8 slices Colby cheese 2 eggs 1/2 teaspoon fennel seeds Salt and black pepper, to taste 1 cup tomato sauce 2 slices bacon, chopped 1 teaspoon dried rosemary

Directions

Parboil the cabbage in a pot of a lightly salted water for 4 to 5 minutes; drain and reserve. Then, cook the ground chuck for about 5 minutes until it is no longer pink. Add in the onion and bacon and continue to sauté for 4 minutes more. Stir in the spices and tomato sauce; bring it to a boil. Turn the heat to simmer; partially cover, and continue to cook an additional 7 minutes. Spoon 1/2 of the mixture into the bottom of a lightly oiled casserole dish. Top with a layer of the boiled cabbage leaves. Repeat the layers one more time. Then, thoroughly combine the eggs, Ricotta cheese, and Colby cheese. Top your casserole with the cheese mixture; bake at 390 degrees F for 25 to 30 minutes or until cooked through.Bon appétit!

157. Saucy Flank Steak with Leeks

(Ready in about 2 hours 15 minutes | Servings 4) Per serving: 238 Calories; 9.2g Fat; 6.3g Carbs; 27.4g Protein; 0.6g Fiber

Ingredients

1 tablespoon lard, room temperature 1 pound flank steak, thinly sliced 1 cup leeks, sliced 1 parsnip, chopped 1 heaping teaspoon garlic, thinly sliced 1/2 teaspoon cardamom 1 teaspoon fresh ginger root, minced 1/2 teaspoon paprika 1/3 cup port wine 1 ½ cups beef stock

Directions

Melt the lard in a heavy-bottomed skillet over a moderately high heat. Cook the beef for about 12 minutes until no longer pink; reserve. In the pan drippings, cook the leeks, parsnip and garlic approximately 3 minutes until they are tender and fragrant. Add in the other ingredients and bring to a boil. Immediately reduce the heat to a simmer. Partially cover and continue to cook about 2 hours.Enjoy!

158.   Winter Beef and Beer Stew

(Ready in about 1 hour | Servings 6) Per serving: 444 Calories; 14.2g Fat; 6.1g Carbs; 66.3g Protein; 2g Fiber

Ingredients

1 ½ pounds chuck roast, cut into small chunks 1 ½ cups tomato puree 3 cups beef bone broth 1 parsnip, chopped 1 cup ale beer 1 bay leaf 1 ½ tablespoons olive oil 1/2 teaspoon mustard seeds 1/4 cup basil leaves, snipped 1 cup red onions, chopped 1 celery with leaves, chopped

Directions

Heat the olive oil in a heavy-bottomed pot or Dutch oven over medium-high flame. Cook the chuck roast for about 6 minutes or until it is browned; set aside. Sauté the vegetables in the same pot for about 8 minutes or until tender and fragrant, stirring occasionally. Add in the remaining ingredients and bring to a boil. Turn the heat to a simmer and continue to cook, partially covered, for about 45 minutes.Bon appétit!

159.   Breakfast Beef Sausage Quiche

(Ready in about 45 minutes | Servings 4) Per serving: 289 Calories; 19.7g Fat; 6.3g Carbs; 19.8g Protein; 1.4g Fiber

Ingredients

1 cup cauliflower, broken into florets 1 pound beef sausages, sliced 2 Italian pepper, thinly sliced 1 onion, chopped 2 garlic cloves, minced 6 eggs 2 tablespoons Greek-style yogurt Salt and black pepper, to taste 1 teaspoon rosemary 1/2 teaspoon caraway seeds

Directions

In a preheated saucepan, cook the beef sausage over a moderately high flame. Add in the peppers, onion, cauliflower, garlic, and spices; continue to sauté for 10 minutes more or until the cauliflower is crisp-tender. Spoon the sautéed mixture into a lightly oiled casserole dish. Whisk the eggs until pale and frothy; add in yogurt and whisk to combine well. Pour the eggs/yogurt mixture over the top and bake at 365 degrees F for 30 to 35 minutes.Enjoy!

160.   Grilled Flank Steak

(Ready in about 20 minutes + marinating time | Servings 6) Per serving: 314 Calories; 11.4g Fat; 1g Carbs; 48.2g Protein; 0.7g Fiber

Ingredients

2 pounds flank steak 2 garlic cloves, smashed 1 teaspoon Mediterranean spice mix Celery salt and ground black pepper, to taste 2 tablespoons dry sherry 2 tablespoons olive oil 1 tablespoon fish sauce 1 tablespoon coconut aminos 2 tablespoons BBQ sauce

Directions

In a ceramic bowl, thoroughly combine the fish sauce, coconut aminos, BBQ sauce, garlic, Mediterranean spice mix, salt, pepper, dry sherry, and olive oil. Add in the flank steaks and let it marinate for 2 hours in your refrigerator. Grill the flank steaks over direct heat for about 5 minutes per side (a meat thermometer should read 135 degrees F).Bon appétit!

161.Thai Steak Salad

(Ready in about 15 minutes | Servings 4) Per serving: 288 Calories; 21.5g Fat; 8.6g Carbs; 15.8g Protein; 5g Fiber

Ingredients

1/2 pound flank steak, trimmed 1 bunch fresh Thai basil 2 tablespoons white wine 1 garlic clove, minced 1 avocado, pitted, peeled and sliced 1 bell pepper, sliced 1 teaspoon coconut aminos 2 tablespoons olive oil 1 cup scallions, chopped 1 Bird's eye chili, minced 1/4 cup sunflower seeds Salt and black pepper, to season

Directions

Toss the flank steak with the salt, pepper and coconut aminos. In a frying pan, heat 1 tablespoon of olive oil over a moderate heat. Cook the scallions and garlic until tender for 3 to 4 minutes; reserve. In the same pan, heat another tablespoon of olive oil. Once hot, cook the flank steak for about 5 minutes per side; add in the sautéed mixture. Toss the remaining ingredients in a nice salad bowl; toss to combine well.Serve the flank steak on top of the salad and enjoy!

162.   Beef and Tomato Casserole

(Ready in about 25 minutes | Servings 4) Per serving: 509 Calories; 29.6g Fat; 6.1g Carbs; 45.2g Protein; 1.6g Fiber

Ingredients

2 tablespoons sun-dried tomatoes, chopped 1 cup Colby cheese, grated 1 tablespoon lard, room temperature 1 pound ground chuck 2 garlic cloves, minced 1/2 cup onions, finely chopped 2 tomatoes, chopped 1/2 tablespoon dill relish Sea salt and ground black pepper to taste 1/2 teaspoon mustard powder 3/4 cup Ricotta cream

Directions

Start by preheating your oven to 395 degrees F. Melt the lard in a saucepan over medium-high flame. Once hot, brown the ground chuck, breaking apart with a spatula. Add in the garlic and onions and cook until they are tender and aromatic. Stir in the tomatoes, dill relish and seasonings. Spoon the sautéed mixture into a lightly-oiled baking dish. Top with the cheese. Bake in the preheated oven for about 20 minutes.Enjoy!

163.   Old-Fashioned Beef Mélange

(Ready in about 1 hour 35 minutes | Servings 6) Per serving: 375 Calories; 13.3g Fat; 5.6g Carbs; 55.1g Protein; 1.2g Fiber

Ingredients

2 pounds beef rib-eye steak, cubed 1 bay laurel Salt and pepper, to taste 1 cup leeks, chopped 3 teaspoons lard, room temperature 1 teaspoon ginger-garlic paste 1 teaspoon dried parsley flakes 6 cups roasted vegetable broth 1 tablespoon oyster sauce 2 vine-ripened tomatoes, pureed 1 tablespoon paprika 1 teaspoon celery seeds, crushed 1/2 teaspoon mustard seeds

Directions

Melt 1 teaspoon of lard in a large stock pot over a moderately high heat. Now, brown the rib-eye steak until it is no longer pink or about 6 minutes. Season with salt and pepper to taste; reserve. Heat the remaining 2 teaspoons of lard and sauté the leeks until tender and fragrant. Now, add in the remaining ingredients. Continue to cook, partially covered, for 1 hour 20 minutes.Bon appétit!

164.   Authentic Hungarian Beef Paprikash

(Ready in about 1 hour 25 minutes | Servings 4) Per serving: 357 Calories; 15.8g Fat; 5g Carbs; 40.2g Protein; 2.2g Fiber

Ingredients

1 ¼ pounds beef roast, diced 1 tablespoon Hungarian paprika 4 cups beef broth 1 celery with leaves, chopped 2 bell pepper, deveined and chopped 1 tablespoon flaxseed meal 1 cup leeks, peeled and chopped Salt and pepper, to taste 2 tablespoons lard, room temperature 1/2 cup dry white wine

Directions

In a heavy-bottomed pot, melt the lard over moderate heat. Cook the beef and leeks for about 5 minutes. Sprinkle with salt, pepper, and Hungarian paprika. Add in wine to deglaze the bottom of your pot. Add in the beef broth, celery, and peppers. Turn the heat to a simmer and continue to cook for a further 1 hour 10 minutes. Stir in the flaxseed meal; continue stirring for about 4 minutes to thicken the liquid.Bon appétit!

165.   The Best Keto Lasagna Ever

(Ready in about 1 hour 30 minutes | Servings 6) Per serving: 494 Calories; 41g Fat; 3.8g Carbs; 24.1g Protein; 1.1g Fiber

Ingredients

For the Lasagna Sheets:

1 1/2 cup Romano cheese, grated 1/2 teaspoon dried Mediterranean spice mix 3 eggs, whisked 6 ounces cream cheese, at room temperature

For the Filling:

1 ½ pounds ground beef 1 cup marinara sauce 2 cups cream cheese 1 cup Cheddar cheese 1 onion, chopped 1 tablespoon butter, room temperature 1 teaspoon fresh garlic, smashed 2 slices bacon, chopped

Directions Begin by preheating your oven to 365 degrees F. Line a baking sheet with parchment paper. Combine the eggs and 6 ounces of cream cheese with a hand mixer. Stir in the remaining ingredients for the lasagna sheets and continue to mix until everything is well combined. Spread the mixture onto a baking sheet and bake in the preheated oven for 17 to 20 minutes. Let it cool and then, place in your refrigerator for about 30 minutes. Slice into lasagna sheets and reserve. In a saucepan, melt the butter over a moderately high heat. Cook the ground beef for about 4 minutes or until no longer pink. Stir in the onion, garlic and bacon; continue to cook an additional 4 minutes. Add in the marinara sauce and continue to simmer an additional 12 minutes. Pour 1/4 cup of the beef sauce into the bottom of a lightly greased baking dish. Top with the first lasagna sheet. Repeat until you run out of ingredients, ending with the sauce layer. Bake for about 20 minutes or until heated through.Enjoy!

166.   Summer Cold Steak Salad

(Ready in about 20 minutes | Servings 6) Per serving: 315 Calories; 13.8g Fat; 6.4g Carbs; 37.5g Protein; 0.9g Fiber

Ingredients

1 ½ pounds rib-eye steak, 1-inch thick piece 1 head of butter lettuce, leaves separated and torn into pieces 1 Serrano pepper, thinly sliced 1 onion, peeled and thinly sliced 1 cup cherry tomatoes, halved 1 Lebanese cucumber, sliced 2 bell peppers, thinly sliced 2 tablespoons fresh lime juice 1/4 cup extra-virgin olive oil Salt and pepper, to taste 1/2 teaspoon dried Mediterranean spice mix

Directions

Brush a frying pan with a nonstick cooking spray. One hot, cook the steak for about 3 to 4 minutes on each side for medium rare. After that, thinly slice the steak across the grain. In a salad bowl, mix the remaining ingredients; toss to coat.Bon appétit!

167.   French Beef Soup with Ventrèche

(Ready in about 2 hours 10 minutes | Servings 4) Per serving: 340 Calories; 19.6g Fat; 6.5g Carbs; 30.2g Protein; 2g Fiber

Ingredients

1 pound beef stew meat, cubed 2 tablespoons butter 4 ounces ventrèche, chopped 4 cups vegetable broth 1 yellow onion, chopped 2 cloves garlic, minced 1 bell pepper, deveined and chopped 1 small-sized ripe tomato, crushed 2 tablespoons fresh chives, chopped 1 tablespoon cider vinegar 2 tablespoons dry red wine 1 celery rib, chopped 2 sprigs rosemary 1 tablespoon flaxseed meal, dissolved in 2 tablespoons of cold water

Directions In a heavy-bottomed pot, melt 1 tablespoon of butter over a moderate heat. Cook the ventrèche for about 4 minutes and reserve. Melt another tablespoon of butter. Once hot, sauté the onions, garlic, pepper, and celery for 3 to 4 minutes until they have softened. Add in the beef and continue to cook until browned. Stir in the rosemary, tomato, vinegar, red wine, and broth. Turn the heat to a simmer, cover and continue to cook for a further 2 hours. Add in the flaxseed slurry and continue to cook an additional 3 to 4 minutes or until thoroughly cooked. Add in the reserved ventrèche.Serve with fresh chives. Bon appétit!

168.   Spicy Beef Medley

(Ready in about 2 hours 10 minutes | Servings 4) Per serving: 467 Calories; 18.7g Fat; 3.7g Carbs; 58g Protein; 2.1g Fiber

Ingredients

1 ½ pounds chuck roast, cut into small chunks 1 teaspoon garlic, minced 2 tablespoons butter 1 Serrano pepper, finely minced 1 celery with leaves, chopped 4 cups vegetable broth 1 tablespoon flaxseed meal, dissolved in 2 tablespoons of water 1 large onion, chopped 2 bell peppers, chopped Salt and pepper, to taste 1 teaspoon mustard seeds 1/4 teaspoon cardamom, ground

Directions In a Dutch oven, melt 1 tablespoon of butter and brown the beef, breaking apart with a fork; set aside. Then, melt the remaining tablespoon of butter and sauté the vegetables until they've softened. Add the reserved beef to the Dutch oven along with the vegetable broth. Add the seasonings and bring to a boil. Reduce the heat to a simmer and continue to cook approximately 2 hours. Stir in the flaxseed slurry. Let it cook, stirring continuously, until the cooking liquid has thickened about 2 minutes.Bon appétit!

169.   Easy Pan-Fried Skirt Steak

(Ready in about 20 minutes + marinating time | Servings 6) Per serving: 350 Calories; 17.3g Fat; 2.1g Carbs; 42.7g Protein; 0.8g Fiber

Ingredients

2 pounds skirt steak 1/2 cup onions, chopped 1/4 cup Pinot Noir 2 tablespoons sesame oil 2 tablespoons coconut aminos 2 garlic cloves, minced 1 teaspoon dried parsley flakes 1 teaspoon dried marjoram Salt and pepper, to taste

Directions

Place the skirt steak along with other ingredients in a ceramic dish. Let it marinate in your refrigerator overnight. Preheat a lightly oiled frying pan over a moderately high heat. Cook your skirt steaks for 8 to 10 minutes per side. Bon appétit!

170.   Slow Cooker Beef Shoulder

(Ready in about 6 hours + marinating time | Servings 6) Per serving: 296 Calories; 12g Fat; 5g Carbs; 35.2g Protein; 0.6g Fiber

Ingredients

1 ½ pounds beef shoulder 2 tablespoons coconut aminos 2 tablespoons olive oil 1 large-sized leek, chopped 2 celery stalks, chopped 1 cup chicken stock 1 teaspoon garlic, smashed 1 teaspoon Dijon mustard Salt and black pepper, to taste 2 tablespoons Marsala wine

Directions

Rub the beef shoulder with the garlic, mustard, salt, and black pepper. Add in Marsala wine and coconut aminos. Let it marinate for 3 hours in your refrigerator. Heat the olive oil in your slow cooker and sauté the leeks until they've softened. Then, cook the beef shoulder until it is golden-brown on top. Add in the celery and stock and stir to combine. Cover with the lid and cook on Low heat setting for 5 to 6 hours.Bon appétit!

171. Beef Stuffed Avocado

(Ready in about 20 minutes | Servings 6) Per serving: 407 Calories; 28.8g Fat; 16.4g Carbs; 23.4g Protein; 6.1g Fiber

Ingredients

3 ripe avocados, pitted and halved 1 tablespoon butter, room temperature 1/2 cup onions, sliced 3/4 cup Swiss cheese, shredded 3 tablespoons green olives, pitted and sliced 3/4 pound ground chuck 1/3 cup vegetable broth 1/2 cup mayonnaise 1 large tomato, chopped Salt and pepper, to taste

Directions

Melt the butter in a nonstick skillet a moderate heat; cook the ground chuck for about 3 minutes, crumbling it with a fork. Add in the broth and onions. Continue to sauté until the onions are tender translucent. Season with salt and pepper to taste. Scoop out some of the middle of your avocados. Combine the avocado flash with the chopped tomatoes and green olives. Add in the reserved beef mixture and stuff your avocado. Place the stuffed avocado in a parchment-lined baking pan. Bake in the preheated oven at 350 degrees F for about 10 minutes.Serve with mayonnaise. Bon appétit!

172.Tender Chuck Short Ribs

(Ready in about 2 hours 35 minutes | Servings 8) Per serving: 231 Calories; 8.9g Fat; 1.3g Carbs; 34.7g Protein; 0.2g Fiber

Ingredients

2 pounds chuck short ribs 1 vine-ripened tomato 2 garlic cloves, minced 1/2 teaspoon red pepper flakes 1 tablespoon butter, at room temperature 1/2 cup dry red wine Sea salt and black pepper, to taste

Directions

Start by preheating your oven to 325 degrees F. Toss the beef ribs with salt, pepper and red pepper flakes until well coated. In a large frying pan, melt the butter over medium-high heat. Sear the short ribs until browned, about 9 minutes. Place the ribs in a lightly-oiled baking pan. Add in the remaining ingredients. Cover with foil and roast in the preheated oven at 330 degrees F for 2 hours. Remove the foil and roast an additional 30 minute.Bon appétit!

173.Italian-Style Herbed Meatloaf

(Ready in about 50 minutes | Servings 6) Per serving: 163 Calories; 8.4g Fat; 5.6g Carbs; 12.2g Protein; 1.9g Fiber

Ingredients

2 garlic cloves, minced 1/3 cup almond meal 2 tablespoons flaxseed meal 1 tablespoon yellow mustard 1 ½ teaspoons coconut aminos 1/3 cup heavy cream 2 pounds ground beef 1 egg, slightly beaten 1 large onions, chopped 1 teaspoon Italian seasoning mix For the Tomato Sauce: 2 vine-ripened tomatoes, pureed 1 tablespoon dried parsley flakes Salt and pepper, to taste

Directions

In a mixing bowl, combine all ingredients for the meatloaf. Press the meatloaf mixture into a lightly greased loaf pan. In a saucepan, over a moderate heat, cook all ingredients for the sauce until reduced slightly, about 4 minutes. Pour the sauce over the top of your meatloaf. Bake at 365 degrees F for 40 to 45 minutes.Bon appétit!

174.   Saucy Mediterranean Tenderloin

(Ready in about 30 minutes | Servings 4) Per serving: 451 Calories; 34.4g Fat; 3.6g Carbs; 29.7g Protein; 1.1g Fiber

Ingredients

1 ½ pounds tenderloin 1 teaspoon Mediterranean seasoning mix 2 tablespoons olive oil 1 cup red onions, chopped 1/2 cup dry red wine 2 garlic cloves, minced 1 tablespoon Dijon mustard Kosher salt and black pepper, to taste 1 Italian pepper, deveined and chopped

Directions

Rub the tenderloin steak with the mustard, salt, pepper, and Mediterranean seasoning mix. Heat the olive oil in a nonstick skillet over moderately high heat. Cook the tenderloin steak for 9 to 10 minutes per side. Sauté the onion, garlic, and Italian pepper for 3 to 4 minutes more until they've softened. Add in red wine to scrape up any browned bits from the bottom of the skillet. Continue to cook until the cooking liquid has thickened and reduced by half.Bon appétit!

175. Mini Meatloaf Muffins

(Ready in about 40 minutes | Servings 6) Per serving: 404 Calories; 22.8g Fat; 6.2g Carbs; 44g Protein; 1.3g Fiber

Ingredients

1 ¼ pounds ground chuck 1 shallot, chopped 3/4 cup mozzarella cheese, grated 1/2 cup pork rinds, crushed Salt and pepper, to taste 1 tablespoon lard, room temperature 2 garlic cloves, minced 2 eggs, lightly beaten 1/4 cup almond meal 1/2 pound button mushrooms, chopped 1/2 cup tomato puree

Directions

Melt the lard in a saucepan over a moderately high flame. Sauté the shallot and mushrooms until they are just tender and aromatic. Add in the remaining ingredients and mix to combine well. Press the mixture into a lightly greased muffin pan. Bake in the preheated oven at 380 degrees F for 25 to 30 minutes. Bon appétit!

176. Beef Brisket with Provolone Cheese

(Ready in about 6 hours | Servings 8) Per serving: 519 Calories; 39.6g Fat; 2.7g Carbs; 34.4g Protein; 0.6g Fiber

Ingredients

2 pounds beef brisket 2 tablespoons soy sauce 1/2 cup beef bone broth 2 tablespoons fresh coriander, chopped 2 garlic cloves, minced 1 rosemary springs 1 thyme sprig 2 tablespoons lard, room temperature 1 onion, cut into wedges 1/3 cup Marsala wine Salt and pepper, to season 1 cup Provolone cheese, sliced

Directions

Place all ingredients, except for the Provolone cheese, in your Slow Cooker. Cook on High settings about 6 hours. Cut the beef brisket into eight portions. Enjoy!

177. Omelet with New York Strip Steak

(Ready in about 30 minutes | Servings 6) Per serving: 429 Calories; 27.8g Fat; 3.2g Carbs; 39.1g Protein; 0.8g Fiber

Ingredients

2 tablespoons butter, at room temperature 1 ½ pounds New York strip, cut into cubes Flaky sea salt and pepper, to season 1/2 teaspoon smoked paprika 1/2 cup scallions, chopped 2 garlic cloves, pressed 2 Spanish peppers, deveined and chopped 6 eggs

Directions

Ina frying pan, melt the butter over a moderately high heat. Cook the beef until browned on all sided or for 10 to 12 minutes. Season with salt, pepper, and paprika; reserve. In the same pan, cook the scallions, garlic, and pepper until just tender and aromatic. Add in the eggs and gently stir to combine. Continue to cook, covered, for 10 minutes more or until the eggs are set. Bon appétit!

178. Porterhouse Steak with Sriracha Sauce

(Ready in about 15 minutes + marinating time | Servings 4) Per serving: 292 Calories; 14.3g Fat; 3.9g Carbs; 36.9g Protein; 0.6g Fiber

Ingredients

1 ½ pounds Porterhouse steak, cubed 1/2 tablespoon lard, melted Salt and pepper, to taste 1 teaspoon celery seeds 1/2 teaspoon dried rosemary 1/2 cup green onions, chopped 1 tablespoon fresh cilantro, chopped 2 tablespoons coconut aminos 1 teaspoon Sriracha sauce 1 tablespoon ginger-garlic paste

Directions

In a ceramic bowl, thoroughly combine the coconut aminos, Sriracha sauce, ginger-garlic paste, salt, pepper, celery seeds, rosemary, and green onions. Add in the cubed beef and allow it to marinate in your refrigerator for 1 hour. Melt the lard in a frying pan over medium-high heat. Cook the Porterhouse steak for 5 to 6 minutes until it is fall-apart-tender. Add in the cilantro and remove from the heat.Bon appétit!

179. Beef Tenderloin with Cabbage

(Ready in about 20 minutes + marinating time | Servings 4) Per serving: 321 Calories; 14g Fat; 5.3g Carbs; 36.7g Protein; 1.4g Fiber

Ingredients

1 pound beef tenderloin, cut into bite-sized strips 1 tablespoon fish sauce Sea salt and pepper, to taste 1/2 teaspoon dried marjoram 1/2 teaspoon dried rosemary 1/2 teaspoon dried basil 2 tablespoons olive oil 1 red onion, chopped 1 teaspoon garlic, minced 1 cup cabbage, shredded 1 Spanish pepper, deseeded and chopped

Directions Toss the beef tenderloin with the fish sauce and spices. Allow it to marinate in your refrigerator for at least 2 hours. In a Dutch oven, heat the olive oil over a moderately high heat. Cook the marinated beef for about 5 minutes, stirring periodically to ensure even cooking. Add in the onions and garlic and cook for 2 minutes more. Now, stir in the cabbage and pepper; turn the heat to a simmer. Continue to simmer, partially covered, for 10 to 12 minutes more.Bon appétit!

180. Mexican-Style Stuffed Tomatoes

(Ready in about 35 minutes | Servings 4) Per serving: 244 Calories; 9.6g Fat; 6g Carbs; 28.9g Protein; 3.2g Fiber

Ingredients

8 tomatoes, scoop out the pulp and chop it 3/4 cup Mexican cheese blend, crumbled 1 pound ground chuck 2 tablespoons tomato sauce Flaky salt and pepper, to taste 1 teaspoon ancho chili powder 1/2 teaspoon caraway seeds 1 tablespoon butter 1 cup onions, chopped 2 cloves garlic, minced 1 teaspoon dried parsley flakes 1/2 cup vegetable broth

Directions Start by preheating your oven to 350 degrees F. Lightly grease a casserole dish with cooking spray. In a sauté pan, melt the butter over a moderately high flame. Now, cook the onion and garlic until tender and fragrant. Add in the ground chuck and continue to cook for 5 to 6 minutes, breaking apart with a wide spatula. Add in the tomato sauce, salt, and pepper. Divide the filling between the prepared tomatoes. Place the stuffed tomatoes in a lightly oiled baking dish. Mix the scooped tomato pulp with the ancho chili powder and caraway seeds; salt to taste and pour it into the baking dish. Bake in the preheated oven at 360 degrees F for about 25 minutes until the tomatoes have softened and everything is thoroughly cooked.Enjoy!

181. Zoodles with Bolognese Sauce

(Ready in about 1 hour 35 minutes | Servings 4) Per serving: 477 Calories; 25.6g Fat; 6.3g Carbs; 41.8g Protein; 1.4g Fiber

Ingredients

For Bolognese: 2 tablespoons sesame oil 1 shallot, finely chopped 1 teaspoon garlic, thinly sliced 1 cup celery with leaves, finely chopped 2 slices bacon, chopped 1 pound ground chuck 1 cup tomato puree 1/2 cup Sauvignon blanc wine 1/2 cup water 1 tablespoons Greek spice mix Salt and ground black pepper, to taste

For Zucchini Spaghetti: 4 zucchinis, peeled and jullianed (tagliatelle shape)

Directions In a saucepan, heat the sesame oil over a moderately high flame. Sweat the shallot until just tender and translucent; add in the garlic and celery and continue to cook until they are just tender and fragrant. Stir in the bacon and ground chuck; continue to cook for 6 to 7 more minutes, breaking up lumps with a fork. Stir in the tomato puree, wine, water, and spices and continue to simmer, partially covered, for 1 hour 10 minutes. Meanwhile, cook your zucchini in a lightly buttered wok for about 2 minutes or until they've softened. Fold in the prepared Bolognese sauce and stir to combine well. Enjoy!

182. Beef Kabobs with Mustard Relish

(Ready in about 20 minutes | Servings 6) Per serving: 413 Calories; 21.1g Fat; 5.8g Carbs; 45.3g Protein; 1g Fiber

Ingredients

2 pounds beef shoulder, cut into cubes 2 teaspoons stone-ground mustard 3 tablespoons olive oil 2 ½ tablespoons apple cider vinegar 1 cup shallots, cut into wedges 1 large zucchini, sliced 2 garlic cloves, minced 1 jalapeno pepper, minced 2 bell peppers, sliced Salt and ground black pepper, to taste

Directions Season the meat and vegetables with the salt and pepper to taste. Brush them with a nonstick cooking spray. Thread the meat cubes and vegetables onto bamboo skewers. Grill the beef kabobs for about 10 minutes, flipping them occasionally to ensure even cooking. Make the relish by whisking the mustard, garlic, jalapeno pepper, olive oil and apple cider vinegar. Bon appétit!

183. Beef Sausage with Aioli Sauce

(Ready in about 15 minutes | Servings 4) Per serving: 549 Calories; 49.3g Fat; 4.7g Carbs; 16.2g Protein; 0.8g Fiber

Ingredients

1 pound beef sausage, crumbled Kosher salt and pepper, to taste 2 tablespoons coriander 1 tablespoon olive oil 1/2 cup onion, chopped 1 teaspoon garlic, finely minced For the Sauce: 1/4 cup aioli 1 teaspoon paprika 1 ½ teaspoon mustard

Directions

In a frying pan, heat the olive oil over a moderate heat. Stir in the onion and garlic and continue to cook for 2 to 3 minutes or until they've softened. Stir in the beef sausage; continue to cook for 3 to 4 minutes or until no longer pink. Add in the salt, pepper, and coriander and stir to combine well. Make the sauce by whisking all the sauce ingredients. Enjoy!

184.   Hearty Winter Beef Stew

(Ready in about 40 minutes | Servings 6) Per serving: 259 Calories; 10.1g Fat; 4.1g Carbs; 35.7g Protein; 0.5g Fiber

Ingredients

1 ½ pounds beef shoulder, cubed 1 tablespoon olive oil 1 tablespoon white mushrooms, thinly sliced 1 teaspoon dried caraway seeds 1/4 teaspoon hot paprika 1 bay leaf 4 cups beef bone broth 1 egg, lightly whisked 1 cup onions, thinly sliced 1 teaspoon garlic, chopped Salt and pepper, to taste

Directions

In a heavy-bottomed pot, heat the olive oil over a moderately high flame. Sear the beef for about 7 minutes until it's just browned; reserve. In the same pot, cook the onions for about 3 minutes or until fragrant. Stir in the garlic and mushrooms and continue to cook for a minute or so. Stir in the remaining ingredients, cover, and cook for 35 minutes more. Add in the egg, remove from the heat, and stir to combine.Bon appétit!

185.   Family Sausage and Vegetable Casserole

(Ready in about 30 minutes | Servings 4) Per serving: 424 Calories; 32.4g Fat; 6g Carbs; 23.7g Protein; 1.6g Fiber

Ingredients

4 beef sausages, sliced 2 Spanish peppers, sliced 1 tablespoon butter 2 garlic cloves, finely chopped 1 teaspoon dry chili pepper, crushed Salt and pepper, to taste 1 teaspoon paprika 1 ½ cups vegetable broth 1 yellow onion, sliced 1 cup cauliflower, broken into small florets 1 celery stalk, chopped

Directions

In a frying pan, melt the butter over a moderately high heat. Brown the sausage until browned on all sides or about 5 minutes; reserve. Sauté the onion, cauliflower, peppers, celery, and garlic for about 8 minutes or until the vegetables have softened. Place the sautéed vegetables in a lightly buttered baking dish. Season with salt, pepper, and paprika. Nestle the reserved sausages within the vegetables. Pour in the vegetable broth and bake in the preheated oven at 360 degrees F for 10 to 12 minutes.Enjoy!

186.   Beef and Broccoli Skillet

(Ready in about 20 minutes | Servings 4) Per serving: 241 Calories; 7.6g Fat; 6g Carbs; 36g Protein; 3.9g Fiber

Ingredients

1 pound ground beef 1 head broccoli, cut into small florets 2 garlic cloves, minced 1/2 teaspoon red pepper flakes, crushed 1/2 cup vegetable broth 2 teaspoons olive oil 1/2 teaspoon curry paste 1 large onion, sliced Kosher salt and black pepper, to season

Directions

In a cast-iron skillet, heat 1 teaspoon of the olive oil over a moderately high flame. Cook the broccoli for 3 to 4 minutes until crisp-tender. Stir in the garlic and onion and continue to cook for 2 to 3 minutes more until tender and aromatic. Reserve. In the same skillet, heat another teaspoon of the oil and cook the beef until it is well browned, crumbling with a fork. Add in the sauteed broccoli mixture, turn the heat to a simmer, and stir in the other ingredients. Cover and continue to cook for 12 minutes more.Bon appétit!

187. Finger-Lickin' Good Filet Mignon

(Ready in about 3 hours 30 minutes | Servings 8) Per serving: 219 Calories; 7.2g Fat; 0.6g Carbs; 34.6g Protein; 0.3g Fiber

Ingredients

2 pounds filet mignon 1 teaspoon porcini powder 1 teaspoon dried thyme 1/4 cup Marsala wine 1 tablespoon brown mustard 1 heaping teaspoon garlic, sliced Sea salt and pepper, to taste

Directions

Rub the filet mignon with mustard and garlic. Toss with spices and place on a lightly oiled baking pan. Pour in Marsala wine. Roast in the preheated oven at 370 degrees F for 1 hour 30 minutes. Turn the oven temperature to 310 degrees F and roast an additional 2 hours.Bon appétit!

188. Winter Sausage and Vegetable Bowl

(Ready in about 40 minutes | Servings 4) Per serving: 250 Calories; 17.5g Fat; 5.4g Carbs; 6.8g Protein; 2.8g Fiber

Ingredients

4 beef sausages, sliced 2 Italian peppers, deveined and chopped 1 large onion, chopped 2 tablespoons olive oil 1 celery rib, chopped Salt and pepper, to taste 1 teaspoon fresh garlic, smashed 1 cup tomato sauce 1 teaspoon dried parsley flakes 1 ½ cups vegetable broth 1/4 cup dry red wine 2 rosemary sprigs

Directions

In a saucepan, heat the oil over a moderately high heat. Brown the sausage for about 3 minutes, stirring periodically to ensure even cooking. Stir in the onion, garlic, peppers, and celery rib; season with salt and pepper to taste. Continue to cook for 6 to 7 minutes or until they've softened. Add in the other ingredients, bringing it to a rolling boil. Turn the heat to a simmer and continue to cook for 20 to 25 minutes or until heated through.Enjoy!

189. Beef Brisket with Provolone Cheese

(Ready in about 6 hours | Servings 8) Per serving: 519 Calories; 39.6g Fat; 2.7g Carbs; 34.4g Protein; 0.6g Fiber

Ingredients

2 pounds beef brisket   2 tablespoons soy sauce 1/2 cup beef bone broth 2 tablespoons fresh coriander, chopped 2 garlic cloves, minced 1 rosemary springs 1 thyme sprig 2 tablespoons lard, room temperature 1 onion, cut into wedges 1/3 cup Marsala wine Salt and pepper, to season 1 cup Provolone cheese, sliced

Directions

Place all ingredients, except for the Provolone cheese, in your Slow Cooker. Cook on High settings about 6 hours. Cut the beef brisket into eight portions.Enjoy!

190.   Omelet with New York Strip Steak

(Ready in about 30 minutes | Servings 6) Per serving: 429 Calories; 27.8g Fat; 3.2g Carbs; 39.1g Protein; 0.8g Fiber

Ingredients

2 tablespoons butter, at room temperature 1 ½ pounds New York strip, cut into cubes Flaky sea salt and pepper, to season 1/2 teaspoon smoked paprika 1/2 cup scallions, chopped 2 garlic cloves, pressed 2 Spanish peppers, deveined and chopped 6 eggs

Directions

Ina frying pan, melt the butter over a moderately high heat. Cook the beef until browned on all sided or for 10 to 12 minutes. Season with salt, pepper, and paprika; reserve. In the same pan, cook the scallions, garlic, and pepper until just tender and aromatic. Add in the eggs and gently stir to combine. Continue to cook, covered, for 10 minutes more or until the eggs are set. Bon appétit!

191. Porterhouse Steak with Sriracha Sauce

(Ready in about 15 minutes + marinating time | Servings 4) Per serving: 292 Calories; 14.3g Fat; 3.9g Carbs; 36.9g Protein; 0.6g Fiber

Ingredients

1 ½ pounds Porterhouse steak, cubed 1/2 tablespoon lard, melted Salt and pepper, to taste 1 teaspoon celery seeds 1/2 teaspoon dried rosemary 1/2 cup green onions, chopped 1 tablespoon fresh cilantro, chopped 2 tablespoons coconut aminos 1 teaspoon Sriracha sauce 1 tablespoon ginger-garlic paste

Directions

In a ceramic bowl, thoroughly combine the coconut aminos, Sriracha sauce, ginger-garlic paste, salt, pepper, celery seeds, rosemary, and green onions. Add in the cubed beef and allow it to marinate in your refrigerator for 1 hour. Melt the lard in a frying pan over medium-high heat. Cook the Porterhouse steak for 5 to 6 minutes until it is fall-apart-tender. Add in the cilantro and remove from the heat.Bon appétit!

192.   Beef Tenderloin with Cabbage

(Ready in about 20 minutes + marinating time | Servings 4) Per serving: 321 Calories; 14g Fat; 5.3g Carbs; 36.7g Protein; 1.4g Fiber

Ingredients

1 pound beef tenderloin, cut into bite-sized strips 1 tablespoon fish sauce Sea salt and pepper, to taste 1/2 teaspoon dried marjoram 1/2 teaspoon dried rosemary 1/2 teaspoon dried basil 2 tablespoons olive oil 1 red onion, chopped 1 teaspoon garlic, minced 1 cup cabbage, shredded 1 Spanish pepper, deseeded and chopped

Directions

Toss the beef tenderloin with the fish sauce and spices. Allow it to marinate in your refrigerator for at least 2 hours. In a Dutch oven, heat the olive oil over a moderately high heat. Cook the marinated beef for about 5 minutes, stirring periodically to ensure even cooking. Add in the onions and garlic and cook for 2 minutes more. Now, stir in the cabbage and pepper; turn the heat to a simmer. Continue to simmer, partially covered, for 10 to 12 minutes more.Bon appétit!

193.   Mexican-Style Stuffed Tomatoes

(Ready in about 35 minutes | Servings 4) Per serving: 244 Calories; 9.6g Fat; 6g Carbs; 28.9g Protein; 3.2g Fiber

Ingredients

8 tomatoes, scoop out the pulp and chop it 3/4 cup Mexican cheese blend, crumbled 1 pound ground chuck 2 tablespoons tomato sauce Flaky salt and pepper, to taste 1 teaspoon ancho chili powder 1/2 teaspoon caraway seeds 1 tablespoon butter 1 cup onions, chopped 2 cloves garlic, minced 1 teaspoon dried parsley flakes 1/2 cup vegetable broth

Directions

Start by preheating your oven to 350 degrees F. Lightly grease a casserole dish with cooking spray. In a sauté pan, melt the butter over a moderately high flame. Now, cook the onion and garlic until tender and fragrant. Add in the ground chuck and continue to cook for 5 to 6 minutes, breaking apart with a wide spatula. Add in the tomato sauce, salt, and pepper. Divide the filling between the prepared tomatoes. Place the stuffed tomatoes in a lightly oiled baking dish. Mix the scooped tomato pulp with the ancho chili powder and caraway seeds; salt to taste and pour it into the baking dish. Bake in the preheated oven at 360 degrees F for about 25 minutes until the tomatoes have softened and everything is thoroughly cooked.Enjoy!

194.   Beef Kabobs with Mustard Relish

(Ready in about 20 minutes | Servings 6) Per serving: 413 Calories; 21.1g Fat; 5.8g Carbs; 45.3g Protein; 1g Fiber

Ingredients

2 pounds beef shoulder, cut into cubes 2 teaspoons stone-ground mustard 3 tablespoons olive oil 2 ½ tablespoons apple cider vinegar 1 cup shallots, cut into wedges 1 large zucchini, sliced 2 garlic cloves, minced 1 jalapeno pepper, minced 2 bell peppers, sliced Salt and ground black pepper, to taste

Directions

Season the meat and vegetables with the salt and pepper to taste. Brush them with a nonstick cooking spray. Thread the meat cubes and vegetables onto bamboo skewers. Grill the beef kabobs for about 10 minutes, flipping them occasionally to ensure even cooking. Make the relish by whisking the mustard, garlic, jalapeno pepper, olive oil and apple cider vinegar.Bon appétit!

195.   Beef Sausage with Aioli Sauce

(Ready in about 15 minutes | Servings 4) Per serving: 549 Calories; 49.3g Fat; 4.7g Carbs; 16.2g Protein; 0.8g Fiber

Ingredients

1 pound beef sausage, crumbled Kosher salt and pepper, to taste 2 tablespoons coriander 1 tablespoon olive oil 1/2 cup onion, chopped 1 teaspoon garlic, finely minced For the Sauce: 1/4 cup aioli 1 teaspoon paprika 1 ½ teaspoon mustard

Directions

 In a frying pan, heat the olive oil over a moderate heat. Stir in the onion and garlic and continue to cook for 2 to 3 minutes or until they've softened. Stir in the beef sausage; continue to cook for 3 to 4 minutes or until no longer pink. Add in the salt, pepper, and coriander and stir to combine well. Make the sauce by whisking all the sauce ingredients.Enjoy!

196. Hearty Winter Beef Stew

(Ready in about 40 minutes | Servings 6) Per serving: 259 Calories; 10.1g Fat; 4.1g Carbs; 35.7g Protein; 0.5g Fiber

Ingredients

1 ½ pounds beef shoulder, cubed 1 tablespoon olive oil 1 tablespoon white mushrooms, thinly sliced 1 teaspoon dried caraway seeds 1/4 teaspoon hot paprika 1 bay leaf 4 cups beef bone broth 1 egg, lightly whisked 1 cup onions, thinly sliced 1 teaspoon garlic, chopped Salt and pepper, to taste

Directions

In a heavy-bottomed pot, heat the olive oil over a moderately high flame. Sear the beef for about 7 minutes until it's just browned; reserve. In the same pot, cook the onions for about 3 minutes or until fragrant. Stir in the garlic and mushrooms and continue to cook for a minute or so. Stir in the remaining ingredients, cover, and cook for 35 minutes more. Add in the egg, remove from the heat, and stir to combine.Bon appétit!

197. Family Sausage and Vegetable Casserole

(Ready in about 30 minutes | Servings 4) Per serving: 424 Calories; 32.4g Fat; 6g Carbs; 23.7g Protein; 1.6g Fiber

Ingredients

4 beef sausages, sliced 2 Spanish peppers, sliced 1 tablespoon butter 2 garlic cloves, finely chopped 1 teaspoon dry chili pepper, crushed Salt and pepper, to taste 1 teaspoon paprika 1 ½ cups vegetable broth 1 yellow onion, sliced 1 cup cauliflower, broken into small florets 1 celery stalk, chopped

Directions

In a frying pan, melt the butter over a moderately high heat. Brown the sausage until browned on all sides or about 5 minutes; reserve. Sauté the onion, cauliflower, peppers, celery, and garlic for about 8 minutes or until the vegetables have softened. Place the sautéed vegetables in a lightly buttered baking dish. Season with salt, pepper, and paprika. Nestle the reserved sausages within the vegetables. Pour in the vegetable broth and bake in the preheated oven at 360 degrees F for 10 to 12 minutes.Enjoy!

198. Beef and Broccoli Skillet

(Ready in about 20 minutes | Servings 4) Per serving: 241 Calories; 7.6g Fat; 6g Carbs; 36g Protein; 3.9g Fiber

Ingredients

1 pound ground beef 1 head broccoli, cut into small florets 2 garlic cloves, minced 1/2 teaspoon red pepper flakes, crushed 1/2 cup vegetable broth 2 teaspoons olive oil 1/2 teaspoon curry paste 1 large onion, sliced Kosher salt and black pepper, to season

Directions

In a cast-iron skillet, heat 1 teaspoon of the olive oil over a moderately high flame. Cook the broccoli for 3 to 4 minutes until crisp-tender. Stir in the garlic and onion and continue to cook for 2 to 3 minutes more until tender and aromatic. Reserve. In the same skillet, heat another teaspoon of the oil and cook the beef until it is well browned, crumbling with a fork. Add in the sauteed broccoli mixture, turn the heat to a simmer, and stir in the other ingredients. Cover and continue to cook for 12 minutes more.Bon appétit!

199.   Finger-Lickin' Good Filet Mignon

(Ready in about 3 hours 30 minutes | Servings 8) Per serving: 219 Calories; 7.2g Fat; 0.6g Carbs; 34.6g Protein; 0.3g Fiber

Ingredients

2 pounds filet mignon 1 teaspoon porcini powder 1 teaspoon dried thyme 1/4 cup Marsala wine 1 tablespoon brown mustard 1 heaping teaspoon garlic, sliced Sea salt and pepper, to taste

Directions

Rub the filet mignon with mustard and garlic. Toss with spices and place on a lightly oiled baking pan. Pour in Marsala wine. Roast in the preheated oven at 370 degrees F for 1 hour 30 minutes. Turn the oven temperature to 310 degrees F and roast an additional 2 hours.Bon appétit!

200.   Winter Sausage and Vegetable Bowl

(Ready in about 40 minutes | Servings 4) Per serving: 250 Calories; 17.5g Fat; 5.4g Carbs; 6.8g Protein; 2.8g Fiber

Ingredients

4 beef sausages, sliced 2 Italian peppers, deveined and chopped 1 large onion, chopped 2 tablespoons olive oil 1 celery rib, chopped Salt and pepper, to taste 1 teaspoon fresh garlic, smashed 1 cup tomato sauce 1 teaspoon dried parsley flakes 1 ½ cups vegetable broth 1/4 cup dry red wine 2 rosemary sprigs

Directions

In a saucepan, heat the oil over a moderately high heat. Brown the sausage for about 3 minutes, stirring periodically to ensure even cooking. Stir in the onion, garlic, peppers, and celery rib; season with salt and pepper to taste. Continue to cook for 6 to 7 minutes or until they've softened. Add in the other ingredients, bringing it to a rolling boil. Turn the heat to a simmer and continue to cook for 20 to 25 minutes or until heated through.Enjoy!

201.   Cheeseburger Soup with Herbs

(Ready in about 25 minutes | Servings 4) Per serving: 326 Calories; 20.5g Fat; 4.5g Carbs; 26.8g Protein; 0.7g Fiber

Ingredients

1/2 pound ground chuck 1 cup cream cheese 1 cup scallions, chopped 2 tablespoons butter, softened 1 celery with leaves, chopped 4 cups chicken broth ½ cup sour cream 1 tablespoon fresh parsley, chopped 1 tablespoon fresh basil, chopped

Directions

Ina heavy-bottomed pot, melt the butter over a moderately high heat. Cook the ground chuck for about 5 minutes, crumbling with a fork; set aside. Add in the scallions and celery and continue to cook for a further 4 minutes, adding a splash of broth if needed. Add in parsley, basil, and broth; bring to a boil. Immediately reduce heat to a simmer. Add the cooked meat back to the pot, partially cover, and continue to cook for 8 to 10 minutes. Add in the sour cream and let it cook for 3 minutes more until cooked through.Bon appétit!

202.   Mexican-Style Keto Tacos

(Ready in about 30 minutes | Servings 4) Per serving: 258 Calories; 19.3g Fat; 5g Carbs; 16.3g Protein; 1.9g Fiber

Ingredients

1 ½ cups ground beef 6 slices bacon, chopped 2 teaspoon white vinegar 2 chili peppers, minced Salt and pepper, to taste 1/2 teaspoon shallot powder 1/2 teaspoon ground cumin 1 cup tomato puree 1/2 cup cream of onion soup 1 ½ cups Mexican cheese blend, shredded

Directions

Place 6 piles of the Mexican cheese on a parchment-lined baking pan; bake in the preheated oven at 385 degrees F for 13 to 15 minutes and let them cool slightly. Then, in a frying pan, cook the ground beef until no longer pink or about 5 minutes. Add in the tomato puree, salt, pepper, shallot powder, and ground cumin; continue to cook for 5 minutes more. In another pan, cook the bacon along with the remaining ingredients for about 3 minutes or until cooked through.Bon appétit! Assemble your tacos. Divide the meat mixture among the 6 taco shells; top with the bacon sauce. Enjoy!

203.   Rustic Hamburger and Cabbage Soup

(Ready in about 35 minutes | Servings 4) Per serving: 307 Calories; 23.6g Fat; 5.4g Carbs; 14.8g Protein; 2.9g Fiber

Ingredients

3/4 pound ground beef 1 cup tomato sauce 4 cups vegetable broth 1 sprig thyme 1/2 cup onions, chopped 1 bell pepper, diced 1 ½ tablespoons tallow, room temperature 1 cup green cabbage, shredded 1 celery with leaves, diced Salt and pepper, to taste 2 cloves garlic, minced 1 cup sour cream

Directions

In a large soup pot, melt the tallow until sizzling. Once hot, cook the ground beef for about 5 minutes, falling apart with a fork; reserve. Add in the onions, garlic, bell pepper, cabbage, and celery and continue to cook for 5 to 6 minutes more or until the vegetables have softened. Stir in the remaining ingredients along with the reserved ground beef; bring to a boil. Reduce the heat to a simmer and continue to cook an additional 20 minutes until everything is thoroughly cooked.Enjoy!

204.   German Szegediner Gulasch

(Beef with Sauerkraut) (Ready in about 20 minutes | Servings 4) Per serving: 342 Calories; 22g Fat; 7.7g Carbs; 29.4g Protein; 4.3g Fiber

Ingredients

18 ounces sauerkraut, rinsed and well drained 1 ¼ pounds ground chuck roast 1 teaspoon hot paprika 1 teaspoon celery powder 1 tablespoon lard, melted 1 medium leek, chopped 1 teaspoon fresh garlic, minced 1 bay laurel

Directions

In a saucepan, melt the lard over a moderately high heat. Sauté the leek and garlic until tender and fragrant. Add in the ground chuck and continue to cook until slightly browned or about 5 minutes. Add in the remaining ingredients. Reduce the heat to a simmer. Cover and continue to cook for a further 7 minutes until everything is cooked through.Bon appétit!

205.   Perfect Roast Beef with Horseradish Sauce

(Ready in about 2 hours + marinating time | Servings 6) Per serving: 493 Calories; 39.4g Fat; 2.9g Carbs; 27.9g Protein; 0.5g Fiber

Ingredients

1 ½ pounds top sirloin roast 1 ½ tablespoons Dijon mustard 1/2 teaspoon paprika 1/3 cup Merlot 1 sprig thyme 1 sprig rosemary 1 teaspoon dried marjoram 1/4 cup olive oil 1 garlic clove, minced

For the Sauce: 2 tablespoons prepared horseradish 2 tablespoons mayonnaise 1/4 cup cream cheese

Directions

Place all ingredients for the roast beef in a ceramic bowl; let it marinate in your refrigerator for 3 to 4 hours. Transfer the top sirloin roast along with the marinade to a lightly oiled baking pan. Wrap with the foil and bake in the preheated oven at 370 degrees F approximately 1 hour. Rotate the pan and continue to roast for 1 hour longer (a meat thermometer should register 125 degrees F). Whisk all ingredients for the horseradish sauce.Bon appétit!

206.   Cheeseburger Chowder with Tomatoes and Plum Vinegar

(Ready in about 30 minutes | Servings 6) Per serving: 238 Calories; 12.6g Fat; 5.6g Carbs; 25.1g Protein; 0.9g Fiber

Ingredients

1 ½ pounds ground beef 1 tablespoon butter, room temperature 2 Roma tomatoes, pureed 1 bay laurel 1 leek, chopped 2 garlic cloves, chopped 2 cups vegetable broth 1 cup Cheddar cheese, shredded 2 tablespoons plum vinegar Salt and pepper, to your liking

Directions

Melt the butter in a soup pot over a moderately-high flame. Cook the beef until it is no longer pink, breaking apart with a fork. Reserve. In the pan drippings, cook the leeks and garlic until they've softened, for 5 to 6 minutes. Add in the vegetable broth, tomatoes, salt, pepper, and bay laurel. Cover and continue to cook for 18 to 20 minutes more.Serve in individual bowls garnished with plum vinegar.Bon appétit!

207.   Greek-Style Meatloaf

(Ready in about 55 minutes | Servings 8) Per serving: 442 Calories; 20.6g Fat; 4.9g Carbs; 56.3g Protein; 0.7g Fiber

Ingredients

2 ½ pounds ground beef 8 slices of bacon 2 teaspoons Greek seasoning mix 1 tablespoon Dijon mustard 3 teaspoons olive oil 6 ounces Halloumi cheese, crumbled 2 eggs, beaten 1 tablespoon Greek red wine 1/2 cup Greek black olives, chopped 1 red onion, finely chopped 1/4 cup half-and-half

Directions In a frying pan, heat the oil over a moderate flame. Once hot, cook the onion and beef until the onion is tender and the beef is no longer pink or 5 to 6 minutes. Then, thoroughly combine half-and-half, cheese eggs, seasoning mix, mustard, wine and olives; add in sautéed mixture. Mix until everything is well combined. Press the mixture into a loaf pan. Top the meatloaf with the bacon slices and cover with a piece of foil. Bake in the preheated oven at 385 degrees F for 35 to 40 minutes. Remove the foil and bake for a further 13 minutes.Bon appétit!

208. Spicy Ground Beef Bowl

(Ready in about 40 minutes | Servings 6) Per serving: 361 Calories; 21.9g Fat; 6.4g Carbs; 29g Protein; 2g Fiber

Ingredients

1 ½ pounds ground beef 1 teaspoon Fresno pepper, minced 1/2 teaspoon dried rosemary 1/2 teaspoon dried thyme 1/2 teaspoon red pepper flakes 1/4 teaspoon mustard seeds, ground 2 tablespoons butter, room temperature 1 bay laurel 1 onion, chopped 1 teaspoon garlic, minced 1 cup tomato puree 1/2 cup port wine Sea salt and ground black pepper, to taste For Ketogenic Tortillas: 1 tablespoon flaxseed meal 1/3 teaspoon baking powder 6 tablespoons water 4 egg whites 1/4 cup almond meal 1/4 teaspoon granulated Swerve A pinch of salt

Directions Melt the butter in a large saucepan over a moderately high flame. Brown the ground beef for about 5 minutes, stirring and crumbling it with a wide spatula. Stir in all seasonings, onion, garlic, and Fresno pepper. Continue to cook for a further 10 minutes. Add in the tomato puree and port wine. Turn the heat to a simmer, partially cover, and continue to cook for 15 to 20 minutes. To make the tortillas, whisk the eggs, almond meal, flaxseed meal, and baking powder until well combined. Add in water, Swerve and salt and whisk until everything is well combined. Cook the tortillas in a lightly oiled skillet that is previously preheated over medium-high heat. Repeat until you run out of ingredients.Enjoy!

209. Cheesy Meatballs with Roasted Peppers

(Ready in about 1 hour | Servings 4) Per serving: 348 Calories; 13.7g Fat; 5.9g Carbs; 42.8g Protein; 2.7g Fiber

Ingredients

1 pound ground chuck 1 cup onions, chopped 2 garlic cloves 3 tablespoons Romano cheese, grated 1 cup tomato puree 1 egg 4 Spanish peppers, deveined and chopped 1 jalapeno pepper, deveined and minced Salt and ground black pepper, to taste 1/2 cup Cheddar cheese, crumbled 1 ½ cups chicken broth 1/2 teaspoon mustard seeds

Directions Place the Spanish peppers under the preheated broiler for about 15 minutes. Peel the peppers and discard the seeds. Thoroughly combine the jalapeno pepper, onion, garlic, Romano cheese, egg, salt, black pepper, and ground chuck; add in roasted peppers. Roll the mixture into balls. In a lightly oiled skillet, sear the meatballs until browned on all sides about 8 to 10 minutes. In a saucepan, heat the tomato puree, chicken broth, and mustard seeds; bring to a boil. Turn the heat to a simmer and continue to cook until cooked through. Fold in the prepared meatballs.Bon appétit!

210. Swiss Cheese and Beef Dipping Sauce

(Ready in about 20 minutes | Servings 8) Per serving: 333 Calories; 29.2g Fat; 2.9g Carbs; 14.7g Protein; 0.1g Fiber

Ingredients

1 ½ cups beef sausages, crumbled 1 tablespoon olive oil 1 shallot, chopped 2 garlic cloves, minced 2 tablespoons fresh Italian parsley, roughly chopped 1 ½ cups Swiss cheese, shredded 1 cup Ricotta cheese, at room temperature

Directions

In a saucepan, heat the olive oil over a moderately high flame. Cook the shallot until tender and translucent or about 4 minutes. Stir in the garlic and continue to cook for 30 seconds more until fragrant. Add in the sausage, cheese and parsley. Bake in the preheated oven at 320 degrees F for 15 to 18 minutes.Enjoy!

211. Tender and Spicy Flank Steak

(Ready in about 1 hour 20 minutes + marinating time | Servings 4) Per serving: 326 Calories; 11.1g Fat; 1.6g Carbs; 52g Protein; 0g Fiber

Ingredients

1 ½ pounds flank steak 1/2 teaspoon ancho chile powder 1 teaspoon fresh ginger root, minced Sea salt and black pepper, to taste 1 teaspoon celery seeds

Directions

Place all ingredients in a ceramic dish and let it marinate for 1 hour in your refrigerator. Preheat your grill to medium-high. Then, grill the flank steak for about 15 minutes, basting them with the reserved marinade.Bon appétit!

212. Easy Roasted Skirt Steak

(Ready in about 25 minutes + marinating time | Servings 6) Per serving: 343 Calories; 27.3g Fat; 3g Carbs; 20.1g Protein; 0.9g Fiber

Ingredients

1 ½ pounds skirt steak 1 tablespoon stone-ground mustard Sea salt and black pepper, to taste 2 tablespoons green garlic, chopped 1/2 cup dry red wine 1 tablespoon olive oil

Directions

Remove the connective tissue from one side of your steak using a knife. Place the skirt steak, mustard, salt, black pepper, green garlic, and red wine in a ceramic dish. Let it marinate in your refrigerator at least 1 hour. Brush the marinated steak with olive oil and place on a parchment-lined baking pan. Bake in the preheated oven at 360 degrees F for about 20 minutes, basting with the reserved marinade.Bon appétit!

213. Bacon-Wrapped Meatballs

(Ready in about 30 minutes | Servings 6) Per serving: 399 Calories; 27g Fat; 1.8g Carbs; 37.7g Protein; 0.9g Fiber

Ingredients

For the Meatballs:

1 ½ pounds ground chuck 6 slices bacon, cut into thirds lengthwise 1 egg, beaten Sea salt and ground black pepper, to your liking 1 ½ tablespoons sesame oil 1/2 cup crushed pork rinds 1/2 cup onion, chopped 2 cloves garlic, smashed

For the Parsley Sauce:

1 cup fresh Italian parsley Flaky salt, to taste 2 tablespoons sunflower seeds, soaked 1/2 tablespoon olive oil

Directions

Thoroughly combine all ingredients for the meatballs. Roll the mixture into 18 balls and wrap each of them with a slice of bacon; secure with a toothpick. Bake the meatballs in the preheated oven at 385 degrees F for about 30 minutes, rotating the pan once or twice. Pulse all ingredients for the parsley sauce in your blender or food processor until your desired consistency is reached.Bon appétit!

214. Porterhouse Steak in Red Wine Sauce

(Ready in about 1 hour 40 minutes | Servings 6) Per serving: 339 Calories; 21.7g Fat; 5.2g Carbs; 35g Protein; 1.5g Fiber

Ingredients

1 ½ pounds Porterhouse steak, cut into 6 serving-size pieces 1/2 teaspoon dried oregano 1 tablespoon dried marjoram 1 red onion, chopped 1/2 teaspoon fresh garlic, minced 1 ½ cups Brussels sprouts, quartered Kosher salt and black pepper, to taste 1 cup roasted vegetable broth 2 tablespoons olive oil For the Sauce: 1/2 cup dry red wine 3/4 teaspoon yellow mustard 1 cup heavy cream 1/2 cup roasted vegetable broth 1/4 teaspoon ground cardamom

Directions

Heat the olive oil in an oven-proof skillet over medium-high flame. Sear the steak until just browned, 4 to 5 minutes per side; reserve. In the same skillet, cook the onion and garlic until they've softened. Add in the Brussels sprouts and continue to cook until just tender. Add the Porterhouse steak back to the skillet. Add all spices along with 1 cup of vegetable broth. Cover with foil and roast at 350 degrees F for 1 hour 15 minutes. Reserve. Add the remaining ingredients to the pan and continue to simmer for about 15 minutes until the sauce has thickened and reduced.Bon appétit!

215. Grandma's Blead Roast with Goat Cheese

(Ready in about 8 hours | Servings 6) Per serving: 439 Calories; 33.4g Fat; 4.2g Carbs; 25.5g Protein; 0.6g Fiber

Ingredients

1 ½ pounds blade roast 1 ¼ cups water 2 tablespoons butter, room temperature 1 large onion, chopped 2 cloves garlic, minced 1 Italian pepper, deveined, and sliced 6 ounces goat cheese, crumbled 2 tablespoons coconut aminos 1 tablespoon red wine vinegar 1/3 teaspoon ground mustard seeds

Directions

Brush the sides and bottom of your Crock pot with a nonstick spray. Melt the butter in a large saucepan over a moderate heat. Now, sauté the onion, garlic, and pepper until they've softened. Transfer the sautéed mixture to your Crock pot. Add in the blade roast coconut aminos, vinegar, mustard seeds, and water. Cover with the lid; cook on Low heat setting for 7 hours.Enjoy!

216. Beef Sirloin with Tangy Mustard Sauce

(Ready in about 20 minutes | Servings 4) Per serving: 321 Calories; 13.7g Fat; 1g Carbs; 45g Protein; 0.4g Fiber

Ingredients

1 tablespoon olive oil 4 (1 ½-inch) thick sirloin steaks Seasoned salt and black pepper, to taste 1 tablespoon deli mustard 1 sprig rosemary, chopped 1/3 cup cream cheese, room temperature 1 tablespoon fresh basil, finely chopped

Directions

Season the sirloin steaks with salt, pepper, and rosemary. Heat olive oil in a large grill pan over medium-high flame. Sear the sirloin steaks in the grill pan for 5 minutes; flip them over and cook for 4 to 5 minutes on the other side. Combine together the cream cheese, mustard, and basil. Place in your refrigerator until ready to serve.Bon appétit!

Poultry

217. Autumn Chicken Soup with Root Vegetables

(Ready in about 25 minutes | Servings 4) Per serving: 342 Calories; 22.4g Fat; 6.3g Carbs; 25.2g Protein; 1.3g Fiber

Ingredients

4 cups chicken broth 1 cup full-fat milk 1 cup double cream 1/2 cup turnip, chopped 2 chicken drumsticks, boneless and cut into small pieces Salt and pepper, to taste 1 tablespoon butter 1 teaspoon garlic, finely minced 1 carrot, chopped 1/2 parsnip, chopped 1/2 celery 1 whole egg

Directions Melt the butter in a heavy-bottomed pot over medium-high heat; sauté the garlic until aromatic or about 1 minute. Add in the vegetables and continue to cook until they've softened. Add in the chicken and cook until it is no longer pink for about 4 minutes. Season with salt and pepper. Pour in the chicken broth, milk, and heavy cream and bring it to a boil. Reduce the heat to. Partially cover and continue to simmer for 20 to 25 minutes longer. Afterwards, fold the beaten egg and stir until it is well incorporated.Bon appétit!

218.   Breaded Chicken Fillets

(Ready in about 30 minutes | Servings 4) Per serving: 367 Calories; 16.9g Fat; 6g Carbs; 43g Protein; 0.7g Fiber

Ingredients

1 pound chicken fillets 3 bell peppers, quartered lengthwise 1/3 cup Romano cheese 2 teaspoons olive oil 1 garlic clove, minced Kosher salt and ground black pepper, to taste 1/3 cup crushed pork rinds

Directions Start by preheating your oven to 410 degrees F. Mix the crushed pork rinds, Romano cheese, olive oil and minced garlic. Dredge the chicken into this mixture. Place the chicken in a lightly greased baking dish. Season with salt and black pepper to taste. Scatter the peppers around the chicken and bake in the preheated oven for 20 to 25 minutes or until thoroughly cooked. Enjoy!

219.   Greek-Style Saucy Chicken Drumettes

(Ready in about 50 minutes | Servings 6) Per serving: 333 Calories; 20.2g Fat; 2g Carbs; 33.5g Protein; 0.2g Fiber

Ingredients

1 ½ pounds chicken drumettes 1/2 cup port wine 1/2 cup onions, chopped 2 garlic cloves, minced 1 teaspoon tzatziki spice mix 1 cup double cream 2 tablespoons butter Sea salt and crushed mixed peppercorns, to season

Directions

Melt the butter in an oven-proof skillet over a moderate heat; then, cook the chicken for about 8 minutes. Add in the onions, garlic, wine, tzatziki spice mix, double cream, salt, and pepper. Bake in the preheated oven at 390 degrees F for 35 to 40 minutes (a meat thermometer should register 165 degrees F).Enjoy!

220.   Herbed Chicken Breasts

(Ready in about 40 minutes | Servings 8) Per serving: 306 Calories; 17.8g Fat; 3.1g Carbs; 31.7g Protein; 0.2g Fiber

Ingredients

4 chicken breasts, skinless and boneless 1 Italian pepper, deveined and thinly sliced 10 black olives, pitted 1 ½ cups vegetable broth 2 garlic cloves, pressed 2 tablespoons olive oil 1 tablespoon Old Sub Sailor Salt, to taste

Directions

Rub the chicken with the garlic and Old Sub Sailor; salt to taste. Heat the oil in a frying pan over a moderately high heat. Sear the chicken until it is browned on all sides, about 5 minutes. Add in the pepper, olives, and vegetable broth and bring it to boil. Reduce the heat simmer and continue to cook, partially covered, for 30 to 35 minutes. Bon appétit!

221.   Festive Turkey Rouladen

(Ready in about 30 minutes | Servings 5) Per serving: 286 Calories; 9.7g Fat; 6.9g Carbs; 39.9g Protein; 0.3g Fiber

Ingredients

2 pounds turkey fillet, marinated and cut into 10 pieces 10 strips prosciutto 1/2 teaspoon chili powder 1 teaspoon marjoram 1 sprig rosemary, finely chopped 2 tablespoons dry white wine 1 teaspoon garlic, finely minced 1 ½ tablespoons butter, room temperature 1 tablespoon Dijon mustard Sea salt and freshly ground black pepper, to your liking

Directions

Start by preheating your oven to 430 degrees F. Pat the turkey dry and cook in hot butter for about 3 minutes per side. Add in the mustard, chili powder, marjoram, rosemary, wine, and garlic. Continue to cook for 2 minutes more. Wrap each turkey piece into one prosciutto strip and secure with toothpicks. Roast in the preheated oven for about 30 minutes.Bon appétit!

222.   Chinese Bok Choy and Turkey Soup

(Ready in about 40 minutes | Servings 8) Per serving: 211 Calories; 11.8g Fat; 3.1g Carbs; 23.7g Protein; 0.9g Fiber

Ingredients

1/2 pound baby Bok choy, sliced into quarters lengthwise 2 pounds turkey carcass 1 tablespoon olive oil 1/2 cup leeks, chopped 1 celery rib, chopped 2 carrots, sliced 6 cups turkey stock Himalayan salt and black pepper, to taste

Directions

In a heavy-bottomed pot, heat the olive oil until sizzling. Once hot, sauté the celery, carrots, leek and Bok choy for about 6 minutes. Add the salt, pepper, turkey, and stock; bring to a boil. Turn the heat to simmer. Continue to cook, partially covered, for about 35 minutes.Bon appétit!

223.   Spicy Breakfast Sausage

(Ready in about 15 minutes | Servings 4) Per serving: 156 Calories; 4.2g Fat; 4.1g Carbs; 16.2g Protein; 2.1g Fiber

Ingredients

4 chicken sausages, sliced 1 chili pepper, minced 1 cup shallots, diced 1/4 cup dry white wine 2 teaspoons lard, room temperature 1 teaspoon garlic, minced 2 Spanish peppers, deveined and chopped 2 tablespoons fresh coriander, minced 2 teaspoons balsamic vinegar 1 cup pureed tomatoes

Directions

In a frying pan, warm the lard over moderately high flame. Then, sear the sausage until well browned on all sides; add in the remaining ingredients and stir to combine. Allow it to simmer over low heat for 10 minutes or until thickened slightly.Enjoy!

224.   Chicken Fajitas with Peppers and Cheese

(Ready in about 15 minutes | Servings 4) Per serving: 301 Calories; 11.4g Fat; 5.2g Carbs; 37.9g Protein; 2.2g Fiber

Ingredients

1 Habanero pepper, deveined and chopped 4 banana peppers, deveined and chopped 1 teaspoon Mexican seasoning blend 1 tablespoon avocado oil 2 garlic cloves, minced 1 cup onions, chopped 1 pound chicken, ground 1/3 cup dry sherry Salt and black pepper, to taste 1/2 cup Cotija cheese, shredded

Directions

In a skillet, heat the avocado oil over a moderate flame. Sauté the garlic, onions, and peppers until they are tender and aromatic or about 5 minutes. Fold in the ground chicken and continue to cook until the juices run clear. Add in the dry sherry, Mexican seasonings, salt and pepper. Continue to cook for 5 to 6 minutes more or until cooked through.Enjoy!

225.   Chicken Breasts with Mustard Sauce

(Ready in about 25 minutes | Servings 4) Per serving: 415 Calories; 33.2g Fat; 4.5g Carbs; 24.6g Protein; 1.1g Fiber

Ingredients

1/4 cup vegetable broth 1/2 cup heavy whipped cream 1/2 cup onions, chopped 2 garlic cloves, minced 1/4 cup Marsala wine 2 tablespoons brown mustard 1/2 cup fresh parsley, roughly chopped 1 tablespoon olive oil 1 pound chicken breasts, butterflied Salt and pepper, to taste

Directions

Heat the oil in a frying pan over a moderate flame. Cook the chicken breasts until no longer pink or about 6 minutes; season with salt and pepper to taste and reserve. Cook the onion and garlic until it is fragrant or about 5 minutes. Add in the wine to scrape the bits that may be stuck to the bottom of your frying pan. Pour in the broth and bring to boil. Fold in the double cream, mustard, and parsley.Bon appétit!

226.   Easy Turkey Meatballs

(Ready in about 20 minutes | Servings 4) Per serving: 244 Calories; 13.7g Fat; 5g Carbs; 27.6g Protein; 2.2g Fiber

Ingredients

For the Meatballs: 1/3 cup Colby cheese, freshly grated 3/4 pound ground turkey 1/3 teaspoon Five-spice powder 1 egg For the Sauce: 1 1/3 cups water 1/3 cup champagne vinegar 2 tablespoons soy sauce 1/2 cup Swerve 1/2 cup tomato sauce, no sugar added 1/2 teaspoon paprika 1/3 teaspoon guar gum

Directions

Thoroughly combine all ingredients for the meatballs. Roll the mixture into balls and sear them until browned on all sides. In a saucepan, mix all of the sauce ingredients and cook until the sauce has thickened, whisking continuously. Fold the meatballs into the sauce and continue to cook, partially covered, for about 10 minutes.Bon appétit!

227.   Chicken Drumettes with Leeks and Herbs

(Ready in about 30 minutes | Servings 4) Per serving: 165 Calories; 9.8g Fat; 4.7g Carbs; 12.4g Protein; 1.3g Fiber

Ingredients

4 chicken drumettes 2 tomatoes, crushed 2 tablespoons lard, room temperature 1 tablespoon coconut aminos 1 teaspoon dried marjoram 2 thyme sprigs Salt and pepper, to taste 2 cloves garlic, minced 1/2 teaspoon fennel seeds 1 cup chicken bone broth 1/2 cup leeks, chopped 1 celery rib, sliced

Directions

Melt the lard in a frying pan over a moderate heat. Sprinkle the chicken with salt and pepper to taste. Then, fry the chicken until no longer pink or about 8 minutes; set aside. In the same frying pan, cook the leeks, celery rib, and garlic for about 5 minutes, stirring continuously. Reduce the heat to medium-low; add the remaining ingredients along with the reserved chicken drumettes. Let it simmer for about 20 minutes.Enjoy!

228.   Roasted Chicken with Cashew Pesto

(Ready in about 35 minutes | Servings 4) Per serving: 580 Calories; 44.8g Fat; 5g Carbs; 38.7g Protein; 1g Fiber

Ingredients

1 cup leeks, chopped 1 pound chicken legs, skinless Salt and ground black pepper, to taste 1/2 teaspoon red pepper flakes For the Cashew-Basil Pesto: 1/2 cup cashews 2 garlic cloves, minced 1/2 cup fresh basil leaves 1/2 cup Parmigiano-Reggiano cheese, preferably freshly grated 1/2 cup olive oil

Directions

Place the chicken legs in a parchnemt-lined baking pan. Season with salt and pepper, Then, scatter the leeks around the chicken legs. Roast in the preheated oven at 390 degrees F for 30 to 35 minutes, rotating the pan occasionally. Pulse the cashews, basil, garlic, and cheese in your blender until pieces are small. Continue blending while adding olive oil to the mixture. Mix until the desired consistency is reached.Bon appétit!

229. Turkey Chorizo with Bok Choy

(Ready in about 50 minutes | Servings 4) Per serving: 189 Calories; 12g Fat; 2.6g Carbs; 9.4g Protein; 1g Fiber

Ingredients

4 mild turkey Chorizo, sliced 1/2 cup full-fat milk 6 ounces Gruyère cheese, preferably freshly grated 1 yellow onion, chopped Coarse salt and ground black pepper, to taste 1 pound Bok choy, tough stem ends trimmed 1 cup cream of mushroom soup 1 tablespoon lard, room temperature

Directions

Melt the lard in a nonstick skillet over a moderate flame; cook the Chorizo sausage for about 5 minutes, stirring occasionally to ensure even cooking; reserve. Add in the onion, salt, pepper, Bok choy, and cream of mushroom soup. Continue to cook for 4 minutes longer or until the vegetables have softened. Spoon the mixture into a lightly oiled casserole dish. Top with the reserved Chorizo. In a mixing bowl, thoroughly combine the milk and cheese. Pour the cheese mixture over the sausage. Cover with foil and bake at 365 degrees F for about 35 minutes.Enjoy!

230. Taro Leaf and Chicken Soup

(Ready in about 45 minutes | Servings 4) Per serving: 256 Calories; 12.9g Fat; 3.2g Carbs; 35.1g Protein; 2.2g Fiber

Ingredients

1 pound whole chicken, boneless and chopped into small chunks 1/2 cup onions, chopped 1/2 cup rutabaga, cubed 2 carrots, peeled 2 celery stalks Salt and black pepper, to taste 1 cup chicken bone broth 1/2 teaspoon ginger-garlic paste 1/2 cup taro leaves, roughly chopped 1 tablespoon fresh coriander, chopped 3 cups water 1 teaspoon paprika

Directions Place all ingredients in a heavy-bottomed pot. Bring to a boil over the highest heat. Turn the heat to simmer. Continue to cook, partially covered, an additional 40 minutes. Storing Spoon the soup into four airtight containers or Ziploc bags; keep in your refrigerator for up to 3 to 4 days. For freezing, place the soup in airtight containers. It will maintain the best quality for about 5 to 6 months. Defrost in the refrigerator. Bon appétit!

231. Italian-Style Chicken Meatballs with Parmesan

(Ready in about 20 minutes | Servings 6) Per serving: 252 Calories; 9.7g Fat; 5.3g Carbs; 34.2g Protein; 1.4g Fiber

Ingredients

For the Meatballs: 1 ¼ pounds chicken, ground 1 tablespoon sage leaves, chopped 1 teaspoon shallot powder 1 teaspoon porcini powder 2 garlic cloves, finely minced 1/3 teaspoon dried basil 3/4 cup Parmesan cheese, grated 2 eggs, lightly beaten Salt and ground black pepper, to your liking 1/2 teaspoon cayenne pepper For the sauce: 2 tomatoes, pureed 1 cup chicken consommé 2 ½ tablespoons lard, room temperature 1 onion, peeled and finely chopped

Directions In a mixing bowl, combine all ingredients for the meatballs. Roll the mixture into bite-sized balls. Melt 1 tablespoon of lard in a skillet over a moderately high heat. Sear the meatballs for about 3 minutes or until they are thoroughly cooked; reserve. Melt the remaining lard and cook the onions until tender and translucent. Add in pureed tomatoes and chicken consommé and continue to cook for 4 minutes longer. Add in the reserved meatballs, turn the heat to simmer and continue to cook for 6 to 7 minutes. Bon appétit!

232.   Spicy Chicken Breasts

(Ready in about 30 minutes | Servings 6) Per serving: 239 Calories; 8.6g Fat; 5.5g Carbs; 34.3g Protein; 1g Fiber

Ingredients

1 ½ pounds chicken breasts 1 bell pepper, deveined and chopped 1 leek, chopped 1 tomato, pureed 2 tablespoons coriander 2 garlic cloves, minced 1 teaspoon cayenne pepper 1 teaspoon dry thyme 1/4 cup coconut aminos Sea salt and ground black pepper, to taste

Directions

Rub each chicken breasts with the garlic, cayenne pepper, thyme, salt and black pepper. Cook the chicken in a saucepan over medium-high heat. Sear for about 5 minutes until golden brown on all sides. Fold in the tomato puree and coconut aminos and bring it to a boil. Add in the pepper, leek, and coriander. Reduce the heat to simmer. Continue to cook, partially covered, for about 20 minutes.Bon appétit!

233.   Spicy and Cheesy Turkey Dip

(Ready in about 25 minutes | Servings 4) Per serving: 284 Calories; 19g Fat; 3.2g Carbs; 26.7g Protein; 1.6g Fiber

Ingredients

1 Fresno chili pepper, deveined and minced 1 ½ cups Ricotta cheese, creamed, 4% fat, softened 1/4 cup sour cream 1 tablespoon butter, room temperature 1 shallot, chopped 1 teaspoon garlic, pressed 1 pound ground turkey 1/2 cup goat cheese, shredded Salt and black pepper, to taste 1 ½ cups Gruyère, shredded

Directions

Melt the butter in a frying pan over a moderately high flame. Now, sauté the onion and garlic until they have softened. Stir in the ground turkey and continue to cook until it is no longer pink. Transfer the sautéed mixture to a lightly greased baking dish. Add in Ricotta, sour cream, goat cheese, salt, pepper, and chili pepper. Top with the shredded Gruyère cheese. Bake in the preheated oven at 350 degrees F for about 20 minutes or until hot and bubbly in top.Enjoy!

234.   Spicy and Tangy Chicken Drumsticks

(Ready in about 55 minutes | Servings 6) Per serving: 420 Calories; 28.2g Fat; 5g Carbs; 35.3g Protein; 0.8g Fiber

Ingredients

3 chicken drumsticks, cut into chunks 1/2 stick butter 2 eggs 1/4 cup hemp seeds, ground Salt and cayenne pepper, to taste 2 tablespoons coconut aminos 3 teaspoons red wine vinegar 2 tablespoons salsa 2 cloves garlic, minced

Directions

Rub the chicken with the butter, salt, and cayenne pepper. Drizzle the chicken with the coconut aminos, vinegar, salsa, and garlic. Allow it to stand for 30 minutes in your refrigerator. Whisk the eggs with the hemp seeds. Dip each chicken strip in the egg mixture. Place the chicken chunks in a parchment-lined baking pan. Roast in the preheated oven at 390 degrees F for 25 minutes.Enjoy!

235.   Mexican-Style Turkey Bacon Bites

(Ready in about 5 minutes | Servings 4) Per serving: 195 Calories; 16.7g Fat; 2.2g Carbs; 8.8g Protein; 0.3g Fiber

Ingredients

4 ounces turkey bacon, chopped 4 ounces Neufchatel cheese 1 tablespoon butter, cold 1 jalapeno pepper, deveined and minced 1 teaspoon Mexican oregano 2 tablespoons scallions, finely chopped

Directions

Thoroughly combine all ingredients in a mixing bowl. Roll the mixture into 8 balls.

236.   Bacon-Wrapped Chicken with Grilled Asparagus

Ready in about: 50 minutes | Serves: 4 Per serving: Kcal 468, Fat 38g, Net Carbs 2g, Protein 26g

Ingredients

4 chicken breasts Pink salt and black pepper to taste 8 bacon slices 2 tbsp olive oil 1 lb asparagus spears 3 tbsp olive oil 2 tbsp fresh lemon juice 2 oz Manchego cheese for topping Preheat oven to 400°F.

DirectionsSeason the chicken breasts with salt and pepper. Wrap 2 bacon slices around each chicken breast. Arrange them on a baking sheet, drizzle with olive oil, and bake for 25-30 minutes until the bacon is brown and crispy. Remove and cover with foil to keep warm. Preheat grill to high heat. Brush the asparagus with olive oil and season with salt. Grill for 8-10 minutes, frequently turning until slightly charred. Remove to a plate and drizzle with lemon juice. Grate over Manchego cheese to melts a little on contact with the hot asparagus and forms a cheesy dressing. Serve.

237.   Chicken Drumsticks in Tomato Sauce

Ready in about: 1 ½ hours | Serves: 4 Per serving: Kcal 515, Fat 34.2g, Net Carbs 7.3g, Protein 50.8g

Ingredients

8 chicken drumsticks 2 tbsp olive oil 1 medium white onion, chopped 2 medium turnips, peeled and diced 1 medium carrot, chopped 2 green bell peppers, cut into chunks 2 cloves garlic, minced ¼ cup coconut flour 1 cup chicken broth 1 (28 oz) can sugar-free tomato sauce 2 tbsp dried Italian herbs Salt and black pepper to taste Preheat oven to 400°F.

DirectionsHeat the olive oil in a skillet over medium heat. Season the drumsticks with salt and pepper and fry for 10 minutes on all sides until brown. Remove to a baking dish. Sauté the onion, turnips, bell peppers, carrot, and garlic in the same oil for 10 minutes with continuous stirring. In a bowl, combine the broth, coconut flour, tomato paste, and Italian herbs together and pour it over the vegetables in the skillet. Stir and cook for 4 minutes until thickened. Pour the mixture over the chicken in the baking dish. Bake for around 1 hour. Remove from the oven and serve with steamed cauli rice.

238.   Sweet Garlic Chicken Skewers

Ready in about: 20 minutes + time refrigeration | Serves: 4 Per serving: Kcal 225, Fat 17.4g, Net Carbs 2g, Protein 15g

Ingredients

Skewers 3 tbsp soy sauce 1 tbsp ginger-garlic paste 2 tbsp swerve brown sugar 1 tsp chili pepper 2 tbsp olive oil 1 lb chicken breasts, cut into cubes Dressing ½ cup tahini ½ tsp garlic powder Pink salt to taste

Directions

In a bowl, whisk soy sauce, ginger-garlic paste, swerve brown sugar, chili pepper, and olive oil. Put the chicken in a zipper bag. Pour in the marinade, seal, and shake to coat. Marinate in the fridge for 2 hours. Preheat grill to 400°F. Thread the chicken on skewers. Cook for 10 minutes in total with three to four turnings until golden brown; remove to a plate. Mix the tahini, garlic powder, salt, and ¼ cup of warm water in a bowl. Pour into serving jars. Serve the chicken skewers and tahini dressing with cauli rice.

239.   Parmesan Wings with Yogurt

Sauce Ready in about: 25 minutes | Serves: 6 Per serving: Kcal 452, Fat 36.4g, Net Carbs 4g, Protein 24g

Ingredients

1 cup Greek-style yogurt 2 tbsp extra-virgin olive oil 1 tbsp fresh dill, chopped 2 lb chicken wings Salt and black pepper to taste ½ cup butter, melted ½ cup hot sauce ¼ cup Parmesan cheese, grated Preheat oven to 400°F.

Directions

Mix yogurt, olive oil, dill, salt, and black pepper in a bowl. Chill while making the chicken. Season wings with salt and pepper. Line them on a baking sheet and grease with cooking spray. Bake for 20 minutes until golden brown. Mix butter, hot sauce, and Parmesan cheese in a bowl. Toss chicken in the sauce to evenly coat and plate. Serve with yogurt dipping sauce.

240.   Chicken Cauliflower Bake

Ready in about: 50 minutes | Serves: 6 Per serving: Kcal 390, Fat 27g, Net Carbs 3g, Protein 22g

Ingredients

3 cups cubed leftover chicken 3 cups spinach 2 cauliflower heads, cut into florets 3 eggs, lightly beaten 2 cups grated sharp cheddar cheese 1 cup pork rinds, crushed ½ cup unsweetened almond milk 3 tbsp olive oil 3 cloves garlic, minced Preheat oven to 350°F.

DirectionsPour the cauli florets and 3 cups water in a pot over medium heat and bring to a boil. Cover and steam the cauli florets for 8 minutes. Drain through a colander and set aside. Combine the cheddar cheese and pork rinds in a large bowl and mix in the chicken. Set aside. Heat the olive oil in a skillet and cook the garlic and spinach until the spinach has wilted, about 5 minutes. Add the spinach mixture and cauli florets to the chicken bowl. Add in the eggs and almond milk, mix, and transfer everything to a greased baking dish. Layer the top of the ingredients. Place the dish in the oven and bake for 30 minutes. By this time, the edges and top must have browned nicely. Remove the chicken from the oven, let rest for 5 minutes, and serve.

241.   Easy Chicken Chili

Ready in about: 30 minutes | Serves: 4 Per serving: Kcal: 421, Fat: 21g, Net Carbs: 5.6g, Protein: 45g

Ingredients

4 chicken breasts 2 tbsp butter 1 onion, chopped 8 oz diced tomatoes 2 tbsp tomato puree ½ tsp chili powder ½ tsp cumin ½ tsp garlic powder 1 serrano pepper, minced ½ cup cheddar cheese, shredded Salt and black pepper to taste

DirectionsPut a large saucepan over medium heat and add the chicken. Cover with water and bring to a boil. Cook for 10 minutes. Transfer the chicken to a flat surface and shred with forks. Reserve 2 cups of the broth. Melt the butter in a large pot over medium heat. Sauté onion until transparent for 3 minutes. Stir in the chicken, tomatoes, cumin, serrano pepper, garlic powder, tomato puree, broth, and chili powder. Adjust the seasoning and let the mixture boil. Simmer for 10 minutes. Top with shredded cheese and serve.

242.   Lemon-Garlic Chicken Skewers

Ready in about: 20 minutes + marinating time | Serves: 4 Per serving: Kcal 350, Fat 11g, Net Carbs 3.5g, Protein 34g

Ingredients

1 lb chicken breasts, cut into cubes 2 tbsp olive oil 2/3 jar preserved lemon, drained 2 garlic cloves, minced ½ cup lemon juice Salt and black pepper to taste 1 tsp fresh rosemary, chopped 4 lemon wedges

Directions

In a wide bowl, mix half of the oil, garlic, salt, pepper, and lemon juice and add the chicken cubes and lemon rind. Let marinate for 2 hours in the refrigerator. Remove the chicken and thread it onto skewers. Heat a grill pan over high heat. Add in the chicken skewers and sear them for 6 minutes per side. Remove to a plate and serve warm garnished with rosemary and lemons wedges.

243. Cheese & Spinach Stuffed Chicken Breasts

Ready in about: 50 minutes | Serves: 4 Per serving: Kcal 491, Fat: 36g, Net Carbs: 3.5g, Protein: 38g

Ingredients

4 chicken breasts ½ cup mozzarella cheese, grated ⅓ cup Parmesan cheese 6 oz cream cheese, softened 2 cups spinach, chopped ½ tsp ground nutmeg Breading 2 eggs ⅓ cup almond flour 2 tbsp olive oil ½ tsp parsley ⅓ cup Parmesan cheese 1 tsp onion powder

Directions

Pound the chicken until it doubles in size. Mix the cream cheese, spinach, mozzarella cheese, nutmeg, salt, black pepper, and Parmesan cheese in a bowl. Divide the mixture between the chicken breasts. Close the chicken around the filling. Wrap the breasts with cling film. Refrigerate for 15 minutes. Preheat oven to 370ºF. Beat the eggs in a shallow dish. Combine all other breading ingredients in a bowl. Dip the chicken in egg first, then in the breading mixture. Heat the olive oil in a pan over medium heat. Cook chicken for 3-5 minutes on all sides. Transfer to a baking sheet. Bake for 20 minutes. Serve.

244. Greek Chicken with Capers

Ready in about: 30 minutes | Serves: 4 Per serving: Kcal 387, Fat 21g, Net Carbs 2.2g, Protein 25g

Ingredients

½ cup Kalamata olives, pitted and chopped ¼ cup olive oil 1 onion, chopped 4 chicken breasts 2 garlic cloves, minced Salt and black pepper to taste 1 tbsp capers 1 lb tomatoes, chopped ½ tsp red chili flakes

DirectionsSprinkle black pepper and salt on the chicken and brush with some olive oil. Add it to a pan set over high heat and cook for 2 minutes. Flip to the other side and cook for 2 more minutes. Transfer the chicken breasts to the oven and bake for 8 minutes at 450ºF. Split the chicken into serving plates. Put the same pan over medium heat and warm the remaining oil. Place in the onion, olives, capers, garlic, and chili flakes and cook for 1 minute. Stir in the tomatoes, black pepper, and salt, and cook for 2 minutes. Sprinkle over the chicken breasts and serve.

245. Chicken in Creamy Tomato Sauce

Ready in about: 25 minutes | Serves: 6 Per serving: Kcal 456, Fat 38.2g, Net Carbs 2g, Protein 24g

Ingredients

3 tbsp butter 6 chicken thighs Salt and black pepper to taste 14 oz canned tomato sauce 2 tsp Italian seasoning ½ cup heavy cream 1 cup mozzarella cheese, shredded ½ cup Parmesan cheese, grated

DirectionsIn a saucepan, melt the butter over medium heat. Season the chicken with salt and black pepper and brown for 5 minutes on each side. Plate the chicken. Pour the tomato sauce and Italian seasoning in the pan and cook for 8 minutes. Adjust the taste with salt and black pepper. Stir in the heavy cream and mozzarella cheese. Once the cheese has melted, return the chicken to the pot and simmer for 4 minutes. Remove to a plate, garnish with Parmesan cheese, and serve.

246. Spicy Chicken Kebabs

Ready in about: 20 minutes + marinade time | Serves: 6 Per serving: Kcal 198, Fat: 13.5g, Net Carbs: 3.1g, Protein: 17.5g

Ingredients

2 lb chicken breasts, cubed 3 tbsp sesame oil 1 cup red bell peppers, chopped 2 tbsp five-spice powder 2 tbsp granulated sweetener 1 tbsp fish sauce

Directions

Combine the sesame oil, fish sauce, five-spice powder, and granulated sweetener in a bowl and mix well. Add in the chicken and toss to coat. Let marinate for 1 hour in the fridge. Preheat the grill. Thread the chicken and bell peppers onto skewers. Grill for 3 minutes per side. Serve warm with steamed broccoli.

247.   Roasted Chicken Kabobs with Celery Fries

Ready in about: 50 minutes | Serves: 4 Per serving: Kcal: 579, Fat: 43g, Net Carbs: 6g, Protein: 39g

Ingredients

1 lb chicken breasts, cubed 4 tbsp olive oil 1 cup chicken broth 1 head celery root, sliced 2 tbsp olive oil Salt and black pepper to taste Preheat oven to 400°F.

Directions

In a bowl, mix 2 tbsp of the olive oil, salt, and pepper. Add in the chicken and toss to coat. Cover with foil and place in the fridge. Arrange the celery slices in a baking tray in an even layer and coat with the remaining olive oil. Season with salt and black pepper and place in the oven. Bake for 10 minutes. Take out the chicken of the refrigerator and thread it onto skewers. Place over the celery, pour in the chicken broth, and roast in the oven for 30 minutes. Serve warm in plates.

248.   Chicken Garam Masala

Ready in about: 35 minutes | Serves: 4 Per serving: Kcal: 564, Fat: 50g, Net Carbs: 5g, Protein: 33g

Ingredients

1 lb chicken breasts, cut lengthwise 2 tbsp butter 1 tbsp olive oil 1 yellow bell pepper, finely chopped 1 ¼ cups heavy whipping cream 1 tbsp fresh cilantro, finely chopped Salt and pepper, to taste Garam masala 1 tsp ground cumin 2 tsp ground coriander 1 tsp ground cardamom 1 tsp turmeric 1 tsp ginger 1 tsp paprika 1 tsp cayenne, ground 1 pinch ground nutmeg Preheat oven to 400°F.

Directions

In a bowl, mix the garam masala spices. Coat the chicken with half of the mixture. Heat the olive oil and butter in a frying pan over medium heat. Brown the chicken for 3 minutes per side. Transfer to a baking dish. To the remaining masala, add heavy cream, bell pepper, salt, and pepper. Pour over the chicken. Bake for 20 minutes until the mixture starts to bubble. Garnish with cilantro to serve.

249.   Yummy Chicken Nuggets

Ready in about: 25 minutes | Serves: 2 Per serving: Kcal 417, Fat 37g, Net Carbs 4.3g, Protein 35g

Ingredients

½ cup almond flour 1 egg, beaten ½ tsp garlic powder 2 chicken breasts, cut into chunks Salt and black pepper to taste ½ cup butter

Directions

In a bowl, mix salt, garlic powder, flour, and pepper and stir. Dip the chicken chunks in egg, then in the flour mixture. Warm butter in a pan over medium heat. Add in the chicken nuggets and cook for 6 minutes on each side. Remove to paper towels, drain the excess grease, and serve with your favorite dip.

250.   Stuffed Avocados with Chicken

Ready in about: 10 minutes | Serves: 2 Per serving: Kcal 511, Fat 40, Net Carbs 5g, Protein 24g

Ingredients

2 avocados, cut in half and pitted ¼ cup pesto 2 tbsp cream cheese 1 ½ cups chicken, cooked, shredded ¼ tsp cayenne pepper ½ tsp onion powder ½ tsp garlic powder Salt and black pepper to taste 2 tbsp lemon juice

Directions

Scoop the insides of the avocado halves, and place the flesh in a bowl. Add in the chicken and stir in the remaining ingredients. Stuff the avocado cups with chicken mixture and enjoy.

251.   Homemade Chicken Pizza Calzone

Ready in about: 60 minutes | Serves: 4 Per serving: Kcal 425, Fat 15g, Net Carbs 4.6g, Protein 28g

Ingredients

2 eggs 1 low carb pizza crust ½ cup Pecorino cheese, grated ½ lb chicken breasts, halved ½ cup sugar-free marinara sauce 1 tsp Italian seasoning 1 tsp onion powder Salt and black pepper to taste ¼ cup flax seed, ground 1 cup provolone cheese, grated

Directions

In a bowl, combine the Italian seasoning with onion powder, salt, Pecorino cheese, pepper, and flaxseed. In a separate bowl, beat the eggs with pepper and salt. Dip the chicken pieces in eggs and then in cheese mixture. Lay them on a lined baking sheet and bake for 25 minutes in the oven at 390ºF. Remove the chicken from the oven and leave it to cool slightly before chopping. Place the pizza dough on a lined baking sheet. Spread ½ cup of the provolone cheese on 1 half of the crust, leaving a ⅓ inch edge around the trim. Scatter the chopped chicken over the cheese and top with marinara sauce. Sprinkle with the remaining cheese. Fold the other half of the dough over the filling. Seal the edges, set in the oven, and bake for 20 minutes. Allow the calzone to cool down before slicing. Serve.

252.   Easy Chicken Meatloaf

Ready in about: 50 minutes | Serves: 6 Per serving: Kcal 273, Fat 14g, Net Carbs 4g, Protein 28

Ingredients

1 cup sugar-free marinara sauce 2 lb ground chicken 2 garlic cloves, minced 2 tsp onion powder 1 tsp Italian seasoning Salt and black pepper to taste Filling ½ cup ricotta cheese 1 cup Grana Padano cheese, grated 1 cup Colby cheese, shredded 2 tsp fresh chives, chopped 2 tbsp fresh parsley, chopped

Directions

In a bowl, combine the ground chicken with half of the marinara sauce, pepper, onion powder, Italian seasoning, salt, and garlic. In a separate bowl, mix the ricotta cheese with half of the Grana Padano cheese, chives, pepper, half of the Colby cheese, salt, and parsley. Place half of the chicken mixture into a loaf pan and spread evenly. Top with the cheese filling. Cover with the rest of the chicken mixture and spread again. Set the meatloaf in the preheated to 380ºF oven. Bake for 25 minutes. Remove meatloaf and spread the rest of the marinara sauce, Grana Padano cheese, and Colby cheese. Bake for 18 minutes. Allow meatloaf cooling and serve in sliced.

253.   Thyme Chicken Thighs

Ready in about: 30 minutes | Serves: 4 Per serving: Kcal 528, Fat: 42g, Net Carbs: 4g, Protein: 33g

Ingredients

½ cup chicken stock 2 tbsp olive oil 1 onion, chopped 4 chicken thighs ¼ cup heavy cream 2 tbsp Dijon mustard 1 tsp thyme 1 tsp garlic powder

Directions

Heat the olive oil in a pan over medium heat. Cook the chicken for about 4 minutes per side. Set aside. Sauté the onion in the same pan for 3 minutes, add the stock, and simmer for 5 minutes. Stir in mustard, heavy cream, thyme, and garlic powder. Pour the sauce over the chicken and serve.

254. Grilled Paprika Chicken with Steamed Broccoli

Ready in about: 17 minutes | Serves: 6 Per serving: Kcal 422, Fat 35.3g, Net Carbs 2g, Protein 26g

Ingredients

1 tsp smoked paprika Salt and black pepper to taste 1 tsp garlic powder 3 tbsp olive oil 6 chicken breasts 1 head broccoli, cut into florets

Directions

Place broccoli florets onto the steamer basket over the boiling water and steam for 8 minutes or until crisp-tender. Set aside. Preheat grill to high and grease the grate with cooking spray Mix paprika, salt, pepper, and garlic powder in a bowl. Brush chicken with olive oil, sprinkle spice mixture over, and massage with hands. Grill chicken for 7 minutes per side until well-cooked. Serve warm.

255. Chicken Goujons with Tomato Sauce

Ready in about: 50 minutes | Serves: 6 Per serving: Kcal 415, Fat 36g, Net Carbs 5g, Protein 28g

Ingredients

1 ½ lb chicken breasts, cubed Salt and black pepper to taste 1 egg, beaten in a bowl 1 cup almond flour ¼ cup Parmesan cheese, grated ½ tsp garlic powder ½ tsp dried parsley ½ tsp dried basil 4 tbsp avocado oil 4 cups butternut squash spirals 6 oz Gruyere cheese, shredded 1½ cups tomato sauce

Directions

In a bowl, combine the almond flour, Parmesan cheese, pepper, and garlic powder. Dip the chicken in the egg first, and then in the almond flour mixture. Set a pan over medium heat and warm 3 tablespoons avocado oil. Add in the chicken and cook until golden, about 5-6 minutes. Remove to paper towels. In a bowl, combine the butternut squash spirals with salt, dried basil, remaining avocado oil, and black pepper. Transfer to a baking dish and top with the chicken pieces, followed by the tomato sauce. Scatter shredded Gruyere cheese on top and bake for 30 minutes at 360°F. Remove and serve.

256. Chicken with Anchovy Tapenade

Ready in about: 30 minutes | Serves: 2 Per serving: Kcal 155, Fat 13g, Net Carbs 3g, Protein 25g

Ingredients

1 chicken breast, cut into 4 pieces 1 tbsp coconut oil 2 garlic cloves, crushed Anchovy tapenade ½ cup black olives, pitted 1 oz anchovy fillets, rinsed 1 garlic clove, crushed Salt and black pepper to taste 1 tbsp olive oil 1 tbsp lemon juice

Directions

Blend the tapenade ingredients in a food processor until smooth and set aside. Warm the coconut oil in a pan over medium heat. Stir in the garlic and sauté for 1 minute. Add in the chicken pieces and cook each side for 4 minutes. Top the chicken with the anchovy tapenade and serve.

257.   Baked Chicken with Parmesan Topping

Ready in about: 45 minutes | Serves: 4 Per serving: Kcal 361, Fat 15g, Net Carbs 5g, Protein 25g

Ingredients

4 chicken breast halves Salt and black pepper to taste ¼ cup green chilies, chopped 4 bacon slices, chopped 4 oz cream cheese, softened 1 onion, chopped ½ cup mayonnaise ½ cup Grana Padano cheese, grated 1 cup cheddar cheese, grated 2 oz pork rinds, crushed 2 tbsp olive oil ½ cup Parmesan cheese, shredded Season the chicken with salt and pepper.

Directions

Heat the olive oil in a pan over medium heat and fry the chicken for about 4-6 minutes until cooked through with no pink showing. Remove to a baking dish. In the same pan, fry bacon until crispy and remove to a plate. Sauté the onion in the same fat for 3 minutes until soft. Remove from heat, add in the fried bacon, cream cheese, 1 cup of water, Grana Padano cheese, mayonnaise, chilies, and cheddar cheese and spread over the chicken. Bake in the oven for 10-15 minutes at 370°F. Remove and sprinkle with mixed Parmesan cheese and pork rinds and return to the oven. Bake for another 10-15 minutes until the cheese melts. Serve immediately.

258.   Cheddar Chicken Tenders

Ready in about: 35 minutes | Serves: 4 Per serving: Kcal 507, Fat 54g, Net Carbs 1.3g, Protein 42g

Ingredients

2 eggs 2 tbsp butter, melted 3 cups cheddar cheese, crushed ½ cup pork rinds, crushed 1 lb chicken tenders Pink salt to taste Preheat oven to 350°F. Line a baking sheet with parchment paper.

Directions

Whisk the eggs with butter in a bowl. Mix the cheese and pork rinds in another bowl. Season the chicken with salt. Dip it in the egg mixture. Coat with the cheddar mixture. Place on the baking sheet, cover with aluminium foil, and bake for 15 minutes. Remove foil and bake for 10 more minutes until golden brown. Serve chicken with mustard dip.

259.   Bacon & Cheese Chicken

Ready in about: 30 minutes | Serves: 4 Per serving: Kcal 423, Fat 21g, Net Carbs 3.3g, Protein 34g

Ingredients

4 bacon strips 4 chicken breasts 2 tbsp avocado jalapeño sauce 1 oz coconut aminos 2 tbsp coconut oil 4 oz Monterey Jack cheese, grated

DirectionsHeat a pan over medium heat and add in the bacon. Cook for 5 minutes until crispy. Remove to paper towels, drain the grease, and crumble. To the pan, add and warm the coconut oil. Place in the chicken breasts, cook for 4 minutes, flip, and cook for an additional 4 minutes. Transfer to a baking dish. Top with the coconut aminos, Monterey Jack cheese, and crumbled bacon. Insert in the oven, turn on the broiler, and cook for 5 minutes. Serve topped with avocado jalapeño sauce.

260.   Chicken with Tarragon

Ready in about: 50 minutes | Serves: 4 Per serving: Kcal: 415, Fat: 23g, Net Carbs: 5.5g, Protein: 42g

Ingredients

1 lb chicken thighs 1 lb radishes, sliced 2 oz butter, sliced 1 tbsp tarragon Salt and black pepper to taste 1 cup mayonnaise Preheat oven to 400°F.

Directions

Place the chicken on a greased baking dish. Add in radishes and season with tarragon, pepper, and salt. Top with butter and bake in the oven for 40 minutes. Serve with mayonnaise.

261. Pacific Chicken

Ready in about: 50 minutes | Serves: 6 Per serving: Kcal: 465, Fat: 31g, Net Carbs: 2.6g, Protein: 33g

Ingredients

4 chicken breasts Salt and black pepper to taste ½ cup mayonnaise 1 tbsp Dijon mustard 1 tsp xylitol ¾ cup pork rinds, crushed ¾ cup Grana Padano cheese, grated 1 tsp garlic powder 1 tsp onion powder Salt and black pepper to taste 8 pieces ham, sliced 4 Gruyere cheese slices

Directions

Preheat oven to 350°F. In a bowl, mix mustard, mayonnaise, and xylitol. Rub the mixture onto the chicken. In another bowl, combine the pork rinds, garlic and onion powders, salt, pepper, and Grana Padano cheese. Pour half of the mixture in a greased baking dish. Add the chicken to the top. Cover with the remaining pork rind mixture. Roast for 40 minutes until the chicken is cooked thoroughly. Take out from the oven and top with Gruyere cheese and ham. Place back in the oven and cook until golden brown. Serve warm.

262. Coconut Chicken Soup

Ready in about: 30 minutes | Serves: 4 Per serving: Kcal 387, Fat 23g, Net Carbs 5g, Protein 31g

Ingredients

2 tbsp coconut oil 1-inch piece peeled ginger, grated 2 chicken breasts, diced 4 cups chicken stock ½ cup coconut cream ¼ cup celery, chopped 1 cup mushrooms, sliced 1 tbsp lime juice ½ tsp red pepper flakes 2 tbsp fresh cilantro, chopped 2 tbsp fish sauce Salt and black pepper to taste

Directions

Warm the coconut oil in a large saucepan over medium heat. Add in the chicken, ginger, mushrooms, and celery and sauté for 3-4 minutes, stirring occasionally. Pour in the chicken stock, fish sauce, lime juice, and pepper flakes and bring to a boil. Reduce the heat and simmer for 18-20 minutes. Whisk in the coconut cream and season with salt and pepper. Continue cooking for about 5 minutes. Garnish with cilantro, spoon onto soup bowls, and serve.

263. Slow Cooker Chicken Stroganoff

Ready in about: 4 hours 15 minutes | Serves: 4 Per serving: Kcal 365, Fat 22g, Net Carbs 4g, Protein 26g

Ingredients

2 garlic cloves, minced 8 oz mushrooms, chopped ¼ tsp celery seeds, ground 1 cup chicken stock 1 cup sour cream 1 cup leeks, chopped 1 lb chicken breasts ½ tsp dried thyme 2 tbsp fresh parsley, chopped Salt and black pepper to taste 4 zucchinis, spiralized 2 tbsp olive oil

Directions

Place the chicken in the slow cooker. Season with salt and pepper and add in the leeks, sour cream, parsley, celery seeds, garlic, mushrooms, stock, and thyme. Cover and cook on high for 4 hours on High. Heat the olive oil in a pan over medium heat. Add in the zucchini pasta and cook for 1-2 minutes until tender. Divide the zucchini between serving plates, top with the chicken mixture, and serve.

264. One-Pot Chicken with Mushrooms & Spinach

Ready in about: 40 minutes | Serves: 4 Per serving: Kcal 453, Fat 23g, Net Carbs 1g, Protein 32g

Ingredients

1 lb chicken thighs 1 cup mushrooms, sliced 2 cups spinach, chopped ¼ cup butter Salt and black pepper to taste ½ tsp onion powder ½ tsp garlic powder 1 tsp Dijon mustard 1 tbsp fresh tarragon, chopped

Directions

Melt the butter in a pan over medium heat. Add in the thighs, onion powder, pepper, garlic powder, and salt. Cook each side for 3 minutes. Set aside. To the same pan, add the mushrooms and cook for 5 minutes. Place in ½ cup water and mustard, take the chicken pieces back to the pan, and cook for 15 minutes while covered. Stir in the tarragon and spinach and cook for 5 minutes. Serve warm.

265. Stuffed Mushrooms with Chicken

Ready in about: 40 minutes | Serves: 4 Per serving: Kcal 261, Fat 16g, Net Carbs 6g, Protein 14g

Ingredients

8 portobello mushrooms, stems removed 3 cups cauliflower florets Salt and black pepper to taste 1 onion, chopped 1 lb ground chicken 2 tbsp butter ½ cup vegetable broth

Directions

In a food processor, add the cauliflower florets, pepper, and salt and blend until it has a rice texture. Transfer to a plate. Warm the butter in a pan over medium heat. Stir in onion and cook for 3 minutes. Add in the cauliflower rice and ground chicken and cook for 5 minutes. Stir in the broth, salt, and pepper and cook for further 2 minutes. Arrange the mushrooms on a lined baking sheet, stuff each one with chicken mixture, put in the oven, and bake for 30 minutes at 350°F. Place on serving plates and enjoy!

266. Paprika Chicken with Cream Sauce

Ready in about: 50 minutes | Serves: 4 Per serving: Kcal 381, Fat 33g, Net Carbs 2.6g, Protein 31.3g

Ingredients

1 lb chicken thighs Salt and black pepper to taste 1 tsp onion powder ¼ cup heavy cream 2 tbsp butter 2 tbsp sweet paprika In a bowl, combine paprika with onion powder, pepper, and salt.

Directions

Rub the chicken with the mixture and lay on a lined baking sheet. Bake for 40 minutes in the oven at 400°F. Set aside. Add the cooking juices to a skillet over medium heat, and mix with the heavy cream and butter. Cook for 5-6 minutes until the sauce is thickened. Sprinkle the sauce over the chicken and serve.

267. Chicken Breasts with Spinach & Artichoke

Ready in about: 40 minutes | Serves: 4 Per serving: Kcal 431, Fat 21g, Net Carbs 3.5g, Protein 36g

Ingredients

4 oz cream cheese, softened 4 chicken breasts 8 oz canned artichoke hearts 1 cup spinach ½ cup Pecorino cheese, grated ½ tsp onion powder ½ tbsp garlic powder Salt and black pepper to taste 4 oz Monterrey Jack cheese, grated

Directions

Lay the chicken breasts on a lined baking sheet, season with pepper and salt, and set in the preheated oven at 350°F. Bake for 25 minutes. Chop the artichoke hearts and place them in a bowl. Add in onion powder, Pecorino cheese, salt, spinach, cream cheese, garlic powder, and pepper and toss to combine. Remove the chicken from the oven and cut each piece in half lengthwise. Divide the artichokes mixture on top, sprinkle with Monterrey cheese, and return in the oven. Bake for 10 minutes. Serve warm.

268. Country-Style Chicken Stew

(Ready in about 1 hour | Servings 6) Per serving: 280 Calories; 14.7g Fat; 2.5g Carbs; 25.6g Protein; 2.5g Fiber

Ingredients

1 pound chicken thighs 2 tablespoons butter, room temperature 1/2 pound carrots, chopped 1 bell pepper, chopped 1 chile pepper, deveined and minced 1 cup tomato puree Kosher salt and ground black pepper, to taste 1/2 teaspoon smoked paprika 1 onion, finely chopped 1 teaspoon garlic, sliced 4 cups vegetable broth 1 teaspoon dried basil 1 celery, chopped

Directions

Melt the butter in a stockpot over medium-high flame. Sweat the onion and garlic until just tender and fragrant. Reduce the heat to medium-low. Stir in the broth, chicken thighs, and basil; bring to a rolling boil. Add in the remaining ingredients. Partially cover and let it simmer for 45 to 50 minutes. Shred the meat, discarding the bones; add the chicken back to the pot.Bon appétit!

269. Panna Cotta with Chicken and Bleu d' Auvergne

(Ready in about 20 minutes + chilling time | Servings 4) Per serving: 306 Calories; 18.3g Fat; 4.7g Carbs; 29.5g Protein; 0g Fiber

Ingredients

2 chicken legs, boneless and skinless 1 tablespoon avocado oil 2 teaspoons granular erythritol 3 tablespoons water 1 cup Bleu d' Auvergne, crumbled 2 gelatin sheets 3/4 cup double cream Salt and cayenne pepper, to your liking

Directions

Heat the oil in a frying pan over medium-high heat; fry the chicken for about 10 minutes. Soak the gelatin sheets in cold water. Cook with the cream, erythritol, water, and Bleu d' Auvergne. Season with salt and pepper and let it simmer over the low heat, stirring for about 3 minutes. Spoon the mixture into four ramekins.Enjoy!

270. Chicken Drumsticks with Broccoli and Cheese

(Ready in about 1 hour 15 minutes | Servings 4) Per serving: 533 Calories; 40.2g Fat; 5.4g Carbs; 35.1g Protein; 3.5g Fiber

Ingredients

1 pound chicken drumsticks 1 pound broccoli, broken into florets 2 cups cheddar cheese, shredded 1/2 teaspoon dried oregano 1/2 teaspoon dried basil 3 tablespoons olive oil 1 celery, sliced 1 cup green onions, chopped 1 teaspoon minced green garlic

Directions

Roast the chicken drumsticks in the preheated oven at 380 degrees F for 30 to 35 minutes. Add in the broccoli, celery, green onions, and green garlic. Add in the oregano, basil and olive oil; roast an additional 15 minutes. Bon appétit!

271. Chicken with Avocado Sauce

(Ready in about 20 minutes | Servings 4) Per serving: 370 Calories; 25g Fat; 4.1g Carbs; 31.4g Protein; 2.6g Fiber

Ingredients

8 chicken wings, boneless, cut into bite-size chunks 2 tablespoons olive oil Sea salt and pepper, to your liking 2 eggs 1 teaspoon onion powder 1 teaspoon hot paprika 1/3 teaspoon mustard seeds 1/3 cup almond meal For the Sauce: 1/2 cup mayonnaise 1/2 medium avocado 1/2 teaspoon sea salt 1 teaspoon green garlic, minced

Directions

Pat dry the chicken wings with a paper towel. Thoroughly combine the almond meal, salt, pepper, onion powder, paprika, and mustard seeds. Whisk the eggs in a separate dish. Dredge the chicken chunks into the whisked eggs, then in the almond meal mixture. In a frying pan, heat the oil over a moderate heat; once hot, fry the chicken for about 10 minutes, stirring continuously to ensure even cooking. Make the sauce by whisking all of the sauce ingredients.

272. Cheese and Prosciutto Chicken Roulade

(Ready in about 35 minutes | Servings 2) Per serving: 499 Calories; 18.9g Fat; 5.7g Carbs; 41.6g Protein; 0.6g Fiber

Ingredients

1/2 cup Ricotta cheese 4 slices of prosciutto 1 pound chicken fillet 1 tablespoon fresh coriander, chopped Salt and ground black pepper, to taste pepper 1 teaspoon cayenne pepper

Directions

Season the chicken fillet with salt and pepper. Spread the Ricotta cheese over the chicken fillet; sprinkle with the fresh coriander. Roll up and cut into 4 pieces. Wrap each piece with one slice of prosciutto; secure with a kitchen twine. Place the wrapped chicken in a parchment-lined baking pan. Now, bake in the preheated oven at 385 degrees F for about 30 minutes. Enjoy!

273. Pan-Fried Chorizo Sausage

(Ready in about 20 minutes | Servings 4) Per serving: 330 Calories; 17.2g Fat; 4.5g Carbs; 34.4g Protein; 1.6g Fiber

Ingredients

16 ounces smoked turkey chorizo 1 ½ cups Asiago cheese, grated 1 teaspoon oregano 1 teaspoon basil 1 cup tomato puree 4 scallion stalks, chopped 1 teaspoon garlic paste Sea salt and ground black pepper, to taste 1 tablespoon dry sherry 1 tablespoon extra-virgin olive oil 2 tablespoons fresh coriander, roughly chopped

Directions

Heat the oil in a frying pan over moderately high heat. Now, brown the turkey chorizo, crumbling with a fork for about 5 minutes. Add in the other ingredients, except for cheese; continue to cook for 10 minutes more or until cooked through.Enjoy!

274.   Italian-Style Turkey Wings

(Ready in about 1 hour | Servings 2) Per serving: 488 Calories; 24.5g Fat; 2.1g Carbs; 33.6g Protein; 0.9g Fiber

Ingredients

2 tablespoons sesame oil 1 pound turkey wings 1/2 cup marinara sauce 1 tablespoon Italian herb mix 2 tablespoons balsamic vinegar 1 teaspoon garlic, minced Salt and black pepper, to taste

Directions

Place the turkey wings, Italian herb mix, balsamic vinegar, and garlic in a ceramic dish. Cover and let it marinate for 2 to 3 hours in your refrigerator. Rub the sesame oil over turkey wings. Grill the turkey wings on the preheated grill for about 1 hour, basting with the reserved marinade. Sprinkle with salt and black pepper to taste. Serve with marinara sauce.

275.   Creamed Sausage with Spaghetti Squash

(Ready in about 20 minutes | Servings 4) Per serving: 591 Calories; 32g Fat; 4.8g Carbs; 32g Protein; 1.5g Fiber

Ingredients

1 ½ pounds cheese & bacon chicken sausages, sliced 8 ounces spaghetti squash 1/2 cup green onions, finely chopped 2/3 cup double cream 1 Spanish pepper, deveined and finely minced 1 garlic clove, pressed 2 teaspoons butter, room temperature 1 ¼ cups cream of onion soup Sea salt and ground black pepper, to taste

Directions

Melt the butter in a saucepan over a moderate flame. Then, sear the sausages until no longer pink about 9 minutes. Reserve. In the same saucepan, cook the green onions, pepper and garlic until they've softened. Add in the spaghetti squash, salt, black pepper and cream of onion soup; bring to a boil. Reduce the heat to medium-low and fold in the cream; let it simmer until the sauce has reduced slightly or about 7 minutes. Add in the reserved sausage and gently stir to combine. Enjoy!

276.   Crispy Chicken Drumsticks

(Ready in about 50 minutes | Servings 4) Per serving: 345 Calories; 14.1g Fat; 0.4g Carbs; 50.8g Protein; 0.2g Fiber

Ingredients

4 chicken drumsticks 1/4 teaspoon ground black pepper, or more to the taste 1 teaspoon dried basil 1 teaspoon dried oregano 1 tablespoon olive oil 1 teaspoon paprika Salt, to your liking

Directions

Pat dry the chicken drumsticks and rub them with the olive oil, salt, black pepper, paprika, basil, and oregano. Preheat your oven to 410 degrees F. Coat a baking pan with a piece of parchment paper. Bake the chicken drumsticks until they are browned on all sides for 40 to 45 minutes. Enjoy!

277.   Chinese-Style Cabbage with Turkey

(Ready in about 45 minutes | Servings 4) Per serving: 293 Calories; 17.5g Fat; 9.1g Carbs; 26.2g Protein; 2.6g Fiber

Ingredients

1 pound turkey, ground 2 slices smoked bacon, chopped 1 pound Chinese cabbage, finely chopped 1 tablespoon sesame oil 1/2 cup onions, chopped 1 teaspoon ginger-garlic paste 2 ripe tomatoes, chopped 1 teaspoon Five-spice powder Coarse salt and ground black pepper, to taste

Directions

Heat the oil in a wok over a moderate flame. Cook the onions until tender and translucent. Now, add in the remaining ingredients and bring to a boil. Reduce the temperature to medium-low and partially cover. Reduce the heat to medium-low and cook an additional 30 minutes, crumbling the turkey and bacon with a fork.Bon appétit!

278.   Chicken with Mediterranean Sauce

(Ready in about 15 minutes | Servings 6) Per serving: 357 Calories; 26.2g Fat; 0.6g Carbs; 29.2g Protein; 0.2g Fiber

Ingredients

1 stick butter 1 ½ pounds chicken breasts 2 teaspoons red wine vinegar 1 ½ tablespoons olive oil 1/3 cup fresh Italian parsley, chopped 2 tablespoon green garlic, finely minced 2 tablespoons red onions, finely minced Flaky sea salt and ground black pepper, to taste Directions In a cast-iron skillet, heat the oil over a moderate flame. Sear the chicken for 10 to 12 minutes or until no longer pink. Season with salt and black pepper. Add in the melted butter and continue to cook until heated through. Stir in the green garlic, onion, and Italian parsley; let it cook for 3 to 4 minutes more. Stir in the red wine vinegar and remove from heat.Enjoy!

279.   Old-Fashioned Turkey Soup

(Ready in about 35 minutes | Servings 4) Per serving: 274 Calories; 14.4g Fat; 5.6g Carbs; 26.7g Protein; 3g Fiber

Ingredients

1 pound turkey drumettes 2 tablespoons olive oil 4 ½ cups vegetable broth Salt and ground black pepper, to your liking 1/2 teaspoon hot paprika 4 dollops of sour cream 1/2 head cauliflower, broken into florets 1 rosemary sprig 1 large onion, chopped 2 garlic cloves, chopped 1 celery, chopped 1 parsnip, chopped 2 bay leaves

Directions

Heat the oil in a heavy-bottomed pot over a moderate flame. Then, sauté the onion, garlic, celery and parsnip until they've softened. Pour in the broth and bring to a rolling boil. Add in the cauliflower, turkey drumettes, rosemary, bay leaves, salt, black pepper and hot paprika. Partially cover and let it simmer approximately 30 minutes. Fold in the sour cream and stir to combine well.Bon appétit!

280.   Turkey Meatballs with Tangy Basil Chutney

(Ready in about 30 minutes | Servings 6) Per serving: 390 Calories; 27.2g Fat; 1.8g Carbs; 37.4g Protein; 0.3g Fiber

Ingredients

2 tablespoons sesame oil For the Meatballs: 1/2 cup Romano cheese, grated 1 teaspoon garlic, minced 1/2 teaspoon shallot powder 1/4 teaspoon dried thyme 1/2 teaspoon mustard seeds 2 small-sized eggs, lightly beaten 1 ½ pounds ground turkey 1/2 teaspoon sea salt 1/4 teaspoon ground black pepper, or more to taste 3 tablespoons almond meal For the Basil Chutney: 2 tablespoons fresh lime juice 1/4 cup fresh basil leaves 1/4 cup fresh parsley 1/2 cup cilantro leaves 1 teaspoon fresh ginger root, grated 2 tablespoons olive oil 2 tablespoons water 1 tablespoon habanero chili pepper, deveined and minced

Directions

In a mixing bowl, combine all ingredients for the meatballs. Roll the mixture into meatballs and reserve. Heat the sesame oil in a frying pan over a moderate flame. Sear the meatballs for about 8 minutes until browned on all sides. Make the chutney by mixing all the ingredients in your blender or food processor.Bon appétit!

281.   Parmesan Chicken Salad

(Ready in about 20 minutes | Servings 6) Per serving: 183 Calories; 12.5g Fat; 1.7g Carbs; 16.3g Protein; 0.9g Fiber

Ingredients

2 romaine hearts, leaves separated Flaky sea salt and ground black pepper, to taste 1/4 teaspoon chili pepper flakes 1 teaspoon dried basil 1/4 cup Parmesan, finely grated 2 chicken breasts 2 Lebanese cucumbers, sliced For the dressing: 2 large egg yolks 1 teaspoon Dijon mustard 1 tablespoon fresh lemon juice 1/4 cup olive oil 2 garlic cloves, minced

Directions

In a grilling pan, cook the chicken breast until no longer pink or until a meat thermometer registers 165 degrees F. Slice the chicken into strips. Toss the chicken with the other ingredients. Prepare the dressing by whisking all the ingredients. Dress the salad and enjoy! Keep the salad in your refrigerator for 3 to 5 days.

282.   Authentic Turkey Kebabs

(Ready in about 30 minutes | Servings 6) Per serving: 263 Calories; 13.8g Fat; 6.7g Carbs; 25.8g Protein; 1.2g Fiber

Ingredients

1 ½ pounds turkey breast, cubed 3 Spanish peppers, sliced 2 zucchinis, cut into thick slices 1 onion, cut into wedges 2 tablespoons olive oil, room temperature 1 tablespoon dry ranch seasoning

Directions

Thread the turkey pieces and vegetables onto bamboo skewers. Sprinkle the skewers with dry ranch seasoning and olive oil. Grill your kebabs for about 10 minutes, turning them periodically to ensure even cooking. Bon appétit!

283. Sunday Chicken with Cauliflower Salad

(Ready in about 20 minutes | Servings 2) Per serving: 444 Calories; 36g Fat; 5.7g Carbs; 20.6g Protein; 4.3g Fiber

Ingredients

1 teaspoon hot paprika 2 tablespoons fresh basil, snipped 1/2 cup mayonnaise 1 teaspoon mustard 2 teaspoons butter 2 chicken wings 1/2 cup cheddar cheese, shredded Sea salt and ground black pepper, to taste 2 tablespoons dry sherry 1 shallot, finely minced 1/2 head of cauliflower

Directions

Boil the cauliflower in a pot of salted water until it has softened; cut into small florets and place in a salad bowl. Melt the butter in a saucepan over medium-high heat. Cook the chicken for about 8 minutes or until the skin is crisp and browned. Season with hot paprika salt, and black pepper. Whisk the mayonnaise, mustard, dry sherry, and shallot and dress your salad. Top with cheddar cheese and fresh basil.

284. Duck Breasts in Boozy Sauce

(Ready in about 20 minutes | Servings 4) Per serving: 351 Calories; 24.7g Fat; 6.6g Carbs; 22.1g Protein; 0.6g Fiber

Ingredients

1 ½ pounds duck breasts, butterflied 1 tablespoon tallow, room temperature 1 ½ cups chicken consommé 3 tablespoons soy sauce 2 ounces vodka 1/2 cup sour cream 4 scallion stalks, chopped Salt and pepper, to taste

Directions

Melt the tallow in a frying pan over medium-high flame. Sear the duck breasts for about 5 minutes, flipping them over occasionally to ensure even cooking. Add in the scallions, salt, pepper, chicken consommé, and soy sauce. Partially cover and continue to cook for a further 8 minutes. Add in the vodka and sour cream; remove from the heat and stir to combine well. Bon appétit!

285. Authentic Aioli Baked Chicken Wings

(Ready in about 35 minutes | Servings 4) Per serving: 562 Calories; 43.8g Fat; 2.1g Carbs; 40.8g Protein; 0.4g Fiber

Ingredients

4 chicken wings 1 cup Halloumi cheese, cubed 1 tablespoon garlic, finely minced 1 tablespoon fresh lime juice 1 tablespoon fresh coriander, chopped 6 black olives, pitted and halved 1 ½ tablespoons butter 1 hard-boiled egg yolk 1 tablespoon balsamic vinegar 1/2 cup extra-virgin olive oil 1/4 teaspoon flaky sea salt Sea salt and pepper, to season

Directions

In a saucepan, melt the butter until sizzling. Sear the chicken wings for 5 minutes per side. Season with salt and pepper to taste. Place the chicken wings on a parchment-lined baking pan Mix the egg yolk, garlic, lime juice, balsamic vinegar, olive oil, and salt in your blender until creamy, uniform and smooth. Spread the Aioli over the fried chicken. Now, scatter the coriander and black olives on top of the chicken wings. Bake in the preheated oven at 380 degrees F for 20 to 25 minutes. Top with the cheese and bake an additional 5 minutes until hot and bubbly. Enjoy!

286.   White Cauliflower and Chicken Chowder

(Ready in about 30 minutes | Servings 6) Per serving: 231 Calories; 18.2g Fat; 5.9g Carbs; 11.9g Protein; 1.4g Fiber

Ingredients

1 cup leftover roast chicken breasts 1 head cauliflower, broken into small-sized florets Sea salt and ground white pepper, to taste 2 ½ cups water 3 cups chicken consommé 1 ¼ cups sour cream 1/2 stick butter 1/2 cup white onion, finely chopped 1 teaspoon fresh garlic, finely minced 1 celery, chopped

Directions

In a heavy bottomed pot, melt the butter over a moderate heat. Cook the onion, garlic and celery for about 5 minutes or until they've softened. Add in the salt, white pepper, water, chicken consommé, chicken, and cauliflower florets; bring to a boil. Reduce the temperature to simmer and continue to cook for 30 minutes. Puree the soup with an immersion blender. Fold in sour cream and stir to combine well.Bon appétit!

287.   Zesty Grilled Chicken

Ready in about: 20 minutes + marinating time | Serves: 6 Per serving: Kcal 375, Fat 12g, Net Carbs 3g, Protein 42g

Ingredients

2 lb chicken thighs and drumsticks 1 tbsp coconut aminos 1 tbsp apple cider vinegar A pinch of red pepper flakes Salt and black pepper to taste ½ tsp ground ginger 3 tbsp butter 1 garlic clove, minced 1 tsp lime zest

Directions

In a blender, combine the butter, ½ cup water, salt, ginger, vinegar, garlic, pepper, lime zest, aminos, and pepper flakes and pulse until smooth. Transfer to a bowl and stir in the chicken. Refrigerate for 1 hour. Set the chicken pieces skin side down on a preheated grill pan over medium heat. Cook for 5 minutes, turn, and cook for 5 more minutes. Split among serving plates and enjoy!

288.   Turkey & Bell Pepper One-Pan

Ready in about: 25 minutes | Serves: 4 Per serving: Kcal 448, Fat 32g, Net Carbs 5g, Protein 45g

Ingredients

1 lb turkey breast, skinless, boneless 1 tsp garlic powder 1 tsp chili powder 1 tsp cumin 2 tbsp lime juice Salt and black pepper to taste 1 tsp sweet paprika 2 tbsp coconut oil 1 tsp ground coriander 1 green bell pepper, seeded, sliced 1 red bell pepper, seeded, sliced 1 onion, sliced 1 tbsp fresh cilantro, chopped 1 avocado, sliced 2 limes, cut into wedges

Directions

In a bowl, mix the lime juice, cumin, garlic powder, coriander, paprika, salt, chili powder, and black pepper. Slice the turkey into strips and add them to the bowl. Toss to coat and let sit for 10 minutes. Warm the coconut oil in a pan over medium heat. Add the turkey and cook each side for 3-5 minutes; remove to a plate. In the same pan, stir the bell peppers and onion and cook for 6 minutes. Take the turkey back to the pan and stir well. Sprinkle with cilantro. Serve topped with lime wedges and avocado slices. Enjoy!

289. Chicken & Eggplant Gruyere Gratin

Ready in about: 55 minutes | Serves: 4 Per serving: Kcal 412, Fat 37g, Net Carbs 5g, Protein 34g

Ingredients

3 tbsp butter 1 eggplant, chopped 2 tbsp gruyere cheese, grated Salt and black pepper to taste 2 garlic cloves, minced 1 lb chicken thighs

Directions

Warm butter in a pan over medium heat. Add in the chicken thighs, season with pepper and salt, and cook for 6 minutes on all sides. Lay them in a baking dish. In the same, add garlic and cook for 1 minute. Stir in the eggplant, pepper, and salt and cook for 10 minutes. Pour the mixture over the chicken, top with the gruyere cheese, and set in the preheated to 350°F oven. Bake for 30 minutes. Turn on the oven's broiler, and broil everything for 2 minutes. Split among serving plates and enjoy!

290. Broccoli & Turkey Bacon Crepes

Ready in about: 40 minutes | Serves: 6 Per serving: Kcal 371, Fat 32g, Net Carbs 7g, Protein 25g

Ingredients

6 eggs 1 cup cream cheese 1 tbsp erythritol 1 ½ tbsp coconut flour ⅓ cup Parmesan cheese, grated ½ tsp xanthan gum 1 cup broccoli florets 1 cup mushrooms, sliced 8 oz turkey bacon, cubed 8 oz cheese blend 1 garlic clove, minced 1 onion, chopped 2 tbsp red wine vinegar 2 tbsp butter ½ cup heavy cream 1 tsp Worcestershire sauce ¼ cup chicken stock ½ tsp nutmeg 2 tbsp fresh parsley, chopped Salt and black pepper to taste

Directions

In a bowl, combine 3/4 cup of cream cheese, eggs, erythritol, coconut flour, xanthan gum, Parmesan cheese, and stir until you obtain a crepe batter. Set a pan sprayed with cooking spray over medium heat. Pour some of the batter, spread well into the pan, cook for 2 minutes, flip, and cook for 40 seconds until golden. Do the same with the rest of the batter. Stack all the crepes on a serving plate. In the same pan, melt the butter and sauté onion, garlic, and mushrooms for 3 minutes until tender. Add in the turkey bacon, salt, vinegar, heavy cream, 6 ounces of the cheese blend, remaining cream cheese, nutmeg, black pepper, broccoli, stock, and Worcestershire sauce. Cook for 7 minutes. Fill each crepe with the mixture, roll up each one, and arrange on a baking dish. Scatter over the remaining cheese blend and cook under the broiler for 5 minutes. Arrange the crepes on serving plates, garnish with chopped parsley, and serve.

291. Turkey & Green Bean Stew with Salsa Verde

Ready in about: 30 minutes | Serves: 6 Per serving: Kcal 193, Fat 11g, Net Carbs 2g, Protein 27g

Ingredients

4 cups leftover turkey, chopped 2 cups green beans 2 garlic cloves, minced Salt and black pepper to taste 2 tbsp olive oil ½ cup salsa verde 1 tsp red pepper flakes 1 onion, chopped 1 tbsp fresh cilantro, chopped

Directions

Warm the olive oil in a pan over medium heat. Add in the onion and garlic and sauté for 3 minutes until soft, stirring occasionally. Stir in red pepper flakes, salsa verde, salt, and black pepper for 1 minute. Pour in 2 cups of water and bring to a boil. Simmer for 10 minutes. Add in the turkey and green beans and cook for 10 more minutes. Spoon the stew onto bowls. Top with cilantro and serve.

292.   Chili Turkey Patties with Cucumber Salsa

Ready in about: 30 minutes | Serves: 4 Per serving: Kcal 475, Fat: 38g, Net Carbs: 5g, Protein: 26g

Ingredients

Turkey 2 spring onions, thinly sliced 1 lb ground turkey 1 egg 2 garlic cloves, minced 1 chili pepper, deseeded and diced 2 tbsp ghee Cucumber salsa 1 tbsp apple cider vinegar 1 tbsp chopped dill 2 cucumbers, grated 1 cup sour cream 1 jalapeño pepper, minced 2 tbsp olive oil

Directions

Place all turkey ingredients except the ghee in a bowl. Mix to combine. Make patties out of the mixture. Melt the ghee in a skillet over medium heat. Cook the patties for 3 minutes per side; remove to a plate. Place all salsa ingredients in a bowl and mix to combine. Serve the cakes topped with salsa.

293.   Chipotle Turkey Meatballs

Ready in about: 15 minutes | Serves: 4 Per serving: Kcal 310, Fat: 26g, Net Carbs: 2g, Protein: 22g

Ingredients

1 lb ground turkey 2 tbsp sun-dried tomatoes, chopped 2 tbsp chipotle hot sauce ½ tsp garlic powder 1 egg Salt and black pepper to taste ¼ cup almond flour 2 tbsp olive oil ½ cup mozzarella cheese, shredded

Directions

Mix everything except the olive oil and chipotle sauce with your hands in a bowl. Form the mixture into 16 small balls. Heat the olive oil in a skillet over medium heat. Cook the meatballs for 4-5 minutes per each side. Place on paper towels to remove excess fat. Serve drizzled with chipotle sauce.

294.   Turkey Cakes with Sautéed Green Cabbage

Ready in about: 30 minutes | Serves: 4 Per serving: Kcal: 443, Fat: 25g, Net Carbs: 5.8g, Protein: 31g

Ingredients

1 lb ground turkey 1 egg 1 onion, chopped Salt and black pepper to taste 1 tsp dried thyme 3 tbsp butter ½ head green cabbage, shredded ½ cup almond flour 2 tbsp fresh parsley, chopped

Directions

Combine the ground turkey, egg, almond flour, thyme, salt, and pepper in a mixing bowl. Mix well and create cakes from the mixture. Melt the butter in a large pan over medium heat and fry the cakes on all sides until cooked thoroughly, about 6-8 minutes. Place on a plate and cover with foil to keep warm. In the same pan, add and sauté the green cabbage for 8-10 minutes until tender. Season with salt and pepper. Sprinkle with parsley. Plate the turkey cakes and cabbage and serve.

295.   Mushroom & Cabbage Turkey Au Gratin

Ready in about: 55 minutes | Serves: 6 Per serving: Kcal 351, Fat 15.8g, Net Carbs 8.2g, Protein 36.9g

Ingredients

2 lb turkey breast, skinless, boneless 1 lb mushrooms, sliced 3 cups green cabbage, shredded 3 tbsp olive oil 1 tsp fresh dill, chopped 1 onion, chopped 1 cup Parmesan cheese, grated Salt and black pepper to taste 2 garlic cloves, minced

Directions

Set a saucepan over medium heat. Add in the turkey and cover with salted water. Bring to a boil and simmer for 20 minutes. Remove to a baking dish and let it sit for a few minutes. Cut it and set aside. Warm the olive oil in a pan over medium heat and sauté the onion and garlic for 3 minutes. Stir in mushrooms, green cabbage, dill, salt, and pepper for 5 minutes. Pour the mixture into the baking dish and stir to combine. Top with Parmesan cheese. Place in the oven. Bake for 20 minutes at 390°F. Serve.

296.   Cheesy Turkey & Broccoli Traybake

Ready in about: 30 minutes | Serves: 4 Per serving: Kcal: 365, Fat: 28g, Net Carbs: 2.6g, Protein: 29g

Ingredients

1 lb turkey breast, cooked, shredded 2 tbsp olive oil 1 head broccoli, cut into florets ½ cup sour cream ½ cup heavy cream 1 cup Monterrey Jack cheese, grated 4 tbsp pork rinds, crushed Salt and black pepper to taste ½ tsp paprika Preheat oven to 450°F.

Directions

Boil water in a pan. Add in broccoli and cook for 8 minutes. In a bowl, mix the ground turkey, sour cream, olive oil, and broccoli and stir. Transfer the mixture to a greased baking tray. Sprinkle heavy cream over the dish, top with seasonings, and coat with the Monterrey Jack cheese. Cover with pork rinds. Place in the oven and cook for 20-25 minutes. Place on a plate and serve.

297.   Spicy Turkey Cucumber Bites

Ready in about: 5 minutes | Serves: 6 Per serving: Kcal 170, Fat 14g, Net Carbs 0g, Protein 10g

Ingredients

2 cucumbers, cut into 1-inch slices 2 cups leftover turkey, diced ¼ jalapeño pepper, minced 1 tbsp Dijon mustard ⅓ cup mayonnaise Salt and black pepper to taste

Directions

Cut mid-level holes in cucumber slices with a knife and set aside. Combine turkey, jalapeno pepper, mustard, mayonnaise, salt, and pepper and mix well. Fill cucumber holes with the mixture and serve.

298. Garlick & Cheese Turkey Slices

Ready in about: 20 minutes | Serves: 4 Per serving: Kcal 416; Fat: 26g, Net Carbs: 3.2g, Protein: 40.7g

Ingredients

2 tbsp olive oil 1 lb turkey breasts, sliced 2 garlic cloves, minced ½ cup heavy cream ⅓ cup chicken broth 1 tbsp tomato paste 1 cup cheddar cheese, shredded

DirectionsSet a pan over medium heat and warm the oil. Add in turkey and fry for 6-8 minutes, stirring often; set aside. Stir the garlic in the pan for 30 seconds. Pour in broth, tomato paste, and heavy cream. Cook until thickened, about 2-3 minutes. Return the turkey to the pan and spread shredded cheddar cheese over. Let sit for 5 minutes covered or until the cheese melts. Serve instantly.

299. Turkey Ham and Mozzarella Pate

(Ready in about 10 minutes | Servings 6) Per serving: 212 Calories; 18.8g Fat; 2g Carbs; 10.6g Protein; 1.6g Fiber

Ingredients

4 ounces turkey ham, chopped 2 tablespoons fresh parsley, roughly chopped 2 tablespoons flaxseed meal 4 ounces mozzarella cheese, crumbled 2 tablespoons sunflower seeds

Directions

Thoroughly combine the ingredients, except for the sunflower seeds, in your food processor. Spoon the mixture into a serving bowl and scatter the sunflower seeds over the top.

300. Old-Fashioned Turkey Chowder

(Ready in about 35 minutes | Servings 4) Per serving: 350 Calories; 25.8g Fat; 5.5g Carbs; 20g Protein; 0.1g Fiber

Ingredients

2 tablespoons olive oil 2 tablespoons yellow onions, chopped 2 cloves garlic, roughly chopped 1/2 pound leftover roast turkey, shredded and skin removed 1 teaspoon Mediterranean spice mix 3 cups chicken bone broth 1 ½ cups milk 1/2 cup double cream 1 egg, lightly beaten 2 tablespoons dry sherry

Directions

Heat the olive oil in a heavy-bottomed pot over a moderate flame. Sauté the onion and garlic until they've softened. Stir in the leftover roast turkey, Mediterranean spice mix, and chicken bone broth; bring to a rapid boil. Partially cover and continue to cook for 20 to 25 minutes. Turn the heat to simmer. Pour in the milk and double cream and continue to cook until it has reduced slightly. Fold in the egg and dry sherry; continue to simmer, stirring frequently, for a further 2 minutes.Bon appétit!

301. Boozy Glazed Chicken

(Ready in about 1 hour + marinating time | Servings 4) Per serving: 307 Calories; 12.1g Fat; 2.7g Carbs; 33.6g Protein; 1.5g Fiber

Ingredients

2 pounds chicken drumettes 2 tablespoons ghee, at room temperature Sea salt and ground black pepper, to taste 1 teaspoon Mediterranean seasoning mix 2 vine-ripened tomatoes, pureed 3/4 cup rum 3 tablespoons coconut aminos A few drops of liquid Stevia 1 teaspoon chile peppers, minced 1 tablespoon minced fresh ginger 1 teaspoon ground cardamom 2 tablespoons fresh lemon juice, plus wedges for serving

Directions Toss the chicken with the melted ghee, salt, black pepper, and Mediterranean seasoning mix until well coated on all sides. In another bowl, thoroughly combine the pureed tomato puree, rum, coconut aminos, Stevia, chile peppers, ginger, cardamom, and lemon juice. Pour the tomato mixture over the chicken drumettes; let it marinate for 2 hours. Bake in the preheated oven at 410 degrees F for about 45 minutes. Add in the reserved marinade and place under the preheated broiler for 10 minutes.Bon appétit!

302. Easy Chicken Tacos

(Ready in about 20 minutes | Servings 4) Per serving: 535 Calories; 33.3g Fat; 4.8g Carbs; 47.9g Protein; 1.9g Fiber

Ingredients

1 pound ground chicken 1 ½ cups Mexican cheese blend 1 tablespoon Mexican seasoning blend 2 teaspoons butter, room temperature 2 small-sized shallots, peeled and finely chopped 1 clove garlic, minced 1 cup tomato puree 1/2 cup salsa 2 slices bacon, chopped

Directions Melt the butter in a saucepan over moderately high flame. Now, cook the shallots until tender and fragrant. Then, sauté the garlic, chicken, and bacon for about 5 minutes, stirring continuously and crumbling with a fork. Add the in Mexican seasoning blend. Fold in the tomato puree and salsa; continue to simmer for 5 to 7 minutes over medium-low heat; reserve. Line a baking pan with wax paper. Place 4 piles of the shredded cheese on the baking pan and gently press them down with a wide spatula to make "taco shells". Bake in the preheated oven at 365 degrees F for 6 to 7 minutes or until melted. Allow these taco shells to cool for about 10 minutes.

303. Classic Chicken Salad

(Ready in about 20 minutes | Servings 4) Per serving: 353 Calories; 23.5g Fat; 5.8g Carbs; 27.8g Protein; 2.7g Fiber

Ingredients

1 medium shallot, thinly sliced 1 tablespoon Dijon mustard 1 tablespoon fresh oregano, chopped 1/2 cup mayonnaise 2 cups boneless rotisserie chicken, shredded 2 avocados, pitted, peeled and diced Salt and black pepper, to taste 3 hard-boiled eggs, cut into quarters

Directions

Toss the chicken with the avocado, shallots, and oregano. Add in the mayonnaise, mustard, salt and black pepper; stir to combine enjoy!

304. Chicken Fillet with Brussels Sprouts

(Ready in about 20 minutes | Servings 4) Per serving: 273 Calories; 15.4g Fat; 4.2g Carbs; 23g Protein; 6g Fiber

Ingredients

3/4 pound chicken breasts, chopped into bite-sized pieces 1/2 teaspoon ancho chile powder 1/2 teaspoon whole black peppercorns 1/2 cup onions, chopped 1 cup vegetable broth 2 tablespoons olive oil 1 ½ pounds Brussels sprouts, trimmed and cut into halves 1/4 teaspoon garlic salt 1 clove garlic, minced 2 tablespoons port wine

Directions

Heat 1 tablespoon of the oil in a frying pan over medium-high heat. Sauté the Brussels sprouts for about 3 minutes or until golden on all sides. Salt to taste and reserve. Heat the remaining tablespoon of olive oil. Cook the garlic and chicken for about 3 minutes. Add in the onions, vegetable broth, wine, ancho chile powder, and black peppercorns; bring to a boil. Then, reduce the temperature to simmer and continue to cook for 4 to 5 minutes longer. Add the reserved Brussels sprouts back to the frying pan.Bon appétit!

305. Easy Roasted Turkey Drumsticks

(Ready in about 1 hour 40 minutes | Servings 4) Per serving: 362 Calories; 22.3g Fat; 5.6g Carbs; 34.9g Protein; 3.3g Fiber

Ingredients

2 turkey drumsticks 1 ½ tablespoons sesame oil 1 tablespoon poultry seasoning For the Sauce: 1 ounce Cottage cheese 1 ounce full-fat sour cream 1 small-sized avocado, pitted and mashed 2 tablespoons fresh parsley, finely chopped 1 teaspoon fresh lemon juice 1/3 teaspoon sea salt

Directions

Pat the turkey drumsticks dry and sprinkle them with the poultry seasoning. Brush a baking pan with the sesame oil. Place the turkey drumsticks on the baking pan. Roast in the preheated oven at 350 degrees F for about 1 hour 30 minutes, rotating the pan halfway through the cooking time. In the meantime, make the sauce by whisking all the sauce ingredients.Bon appétit!

306. Creamy Tomato and Chicken Chowder

(Ready in about 35 minutes | Servings 6) Per serving: 238 Calories; 15.5g Fat; 6.1g Carbs; 36g Protein; 1.3g Fiber

Ingredients

3 chicken legs, boneless and chopped 1 teaspoon ginger-garlic paste 2 cups tomato bisque 2 cups water 2 tablespoons olive oil Sea salt and ground black pepper, to taste 1 onion, chopped 1/2 cup celery, thinly sliced 1 chili pepper, deveined and minced 1 tablespoon flax seed meal 1/2 cup Greek-style yogurt

Directions

Heat the olive oil in a stockpot over a moderately high flame. Sear the chicken legs for about 8 minutes. Season with salt and black pepper and reserve. In the same stockpot, cook the onion, celery, and chili pepper until they've softened. Add in the ginger-garlic paste, tomato bisque, and water. Turn the heat to simmer and continue to cook for 30 minutes more until thoroughly cooked. Fold in the flax seed meal and yogurt and continue to cook, stirring frequently, for 4 to 5 minutes more.

307. Turkey Wings with Gravy

(Ready in about 6 hours | Servings 6) Per serving: 280 Calories; 22.2g Fat; 4.3g Carbs; 15.8g Protein; 0.8g Fiber

Ingredients

2 pounds turkey wings 1/2 teaspoon cayenne pepper 4 garlic cloves, sliced 1 large onion, chopped Salt and pepper, to taste 1 teaspoon dried marjoram 1 tablespoon butter, room temperature 1 tablespoon Dijon mustard For the Gravy: 1 cup double cream Salt and black pepper, to taste 1/2 stick butter 3/4 teaspoon guar gum

Directions

Rub the turkey wings with the Dijon mustard and 1 tablespoon of butter. Preheat a grill pan over medium-high heat. Sear the turkey wings for 10 minutes on all sides. Transfer the turkey to your Crock pot; add in the garlic, onion, salt, pepper, marjoram, and cayenne pepper. Cover and cook on low setting for 6 hours. Melt 1/2 stick of the butter in a frying pan. Add in the cream and whisk until cooked through. Next, stir in the guar gum, salt, and black pepper along with cooking juices. Let it cook until the sauce has reduced by half.

308. Flatbread with Chicken Liver Pâté

(Ready in about 2 hours 15 minutes | Servings 4) Per serving: 395 Calories; 30.2g Fat; 3.6g Carbs; 17.9g Protein; 0.5g Fiber

Ingredients

1 yellow onion, finely chopped 10 ounces chicken livers 1/2 teaspoon Mediterranean seasoning blend 4 tablespoons olive oil 1 garlic clove, minced For Flatbread: 1 cup lukewarm water 1/2 stick butter 1/2 cup flax meal 1 ½ tablespoons psyllium husks 1 ¼ cups almond flour

Directions

Pulse the chicken livers along with the seasoning blend, olive oil, onion and garlic in your food processor; reserve. Mix the dry ingredients for the flatbread. Mix in all the wet ingredients. Whisk to combine well. Let it stand at room temperature for 2 hours. Divide the dough into 8 balls and roll them out on a flat surface. In a lightly greased pan, cook your flatbread for 1 minute on each side or until golden.Bon appétit!

309. Grilled Chicken Salad with Avocado

(Ready in about 20 minutes | Servings 4) Per serving: 408 Calories; 34.2g Fat; 4.8g Carbs; 22.7g Protein; 3.1g Fiber

Ingredients

1/3 cup olive oil 2 chicken breasts Sea salt and crushed red pepper flakes 2 egg yolks 1 tablespoon fresh lemon juice 1/2 teaspoon celery seeds 1 tablespoon coconut aminos 1 large-sized avocado, pitted and sliced

Directions

Grill the chicken breasts for about 4 minutes per side. Season with salt and pepper, to taste. Slice the grilled chicken into bite-sized strips. To make the dressing, whisk the egg yolks, lemon juice, celery seeds, olive oil and coconut aminos in a measuring cup.Bon appétit!

310. Creamed Greek-Style Soup

(Ready in about 30 minutes | Servings 4) Per serving: 256 Calories; 18.8g Fat; 5.4g Carbs; 15.8g Protein; 0.2g Fiber

Ingredients

1/2 stick butter 1/2 cup zucchini, diced 2 garlic cloves, minced 4 ½ cups roasted vegetable broth Sea salt and ground black pepper, to season 1 ½ cups leftover turkey, shredded 1/3 cup double cream 1/2 cup Greek-style yogurt

Directions

In a heavy-bottomed pot, melt the butter over medium-high heat. Once hot, cook the zucchini and garlic for 2 minutes until they are fragrant. Add in the broth, salt, black pepper, and leftover turkey. Cover and cook for 25 minutes, stirring periodically. Then, fold in the cream and yogurt. Continue to cook for 5 minutes more or until thoroughly warmed.Enjoy!

311.Spinach Chicken Cheesy Bake

Ready in about: 45 minutes | Serves: 4 Per serving: Kcal 340, Fat 30.2g, Net Carbs 3.1g, Protein 15g

Ingredients

1 lb chicken breasts 1 tsp mixed spice seasoning Pink salt and black pepper to taste 2 loose cups baby spinach 3 tsp olive oil 4 oz cream cheese 1 ¼ cups mozzarella cheese, grated 4 tbsp water Preheat oven to 370°F.

Directions

Season chicken with spice mix, salt, and black pepper. Pat with your hands to have the seasoning stick on the chicken. Put in the casserole dish and layer spinach over the chicken. Mix the oil with cream cheese, mozzarella, salt, and pepper and stir in water a tablespoon at a time. Pour the mixture over the chicken and cover the casserole dish with aluminium foil. Bake for 20 minutes. Remove the foil and continue cooking for 15 minutes until a nice golden brown color is formed on top. Take out and allow sitting for 5 minutes. Serve warm with braised asparagus.

312. Roasted Chicken Breasts with Capers

Ready in about: 65 minutes | Serves: 6 Per serving: Kcal 430, Fat 23g, Net Carbs 3g, Protein 33g

Ingredients

2 medium lemons, sliced 3 chicken breasts, halved Salt and black pepper to taste ¼ cup almond flour 3 tbsp olive oil 2 tbsp capers, rinsed 1 ¼ cups chicken broth 2 tbsp fresh parsley, chopped 1 tbsp butter Preheat oven to 350°F.

Directions

Line a baking sheet with parchment paper. Lay the lemon slices on the baking sheet and drizzle with some olive oil. Roast for 25 minutes until the lemon rinds brown. Cover the chicken with plastic wrap, place them on a flat surface, and gently pound with the rolling pin to flatten to about ½-inch thickness. Remove the plastic wraps and season with salt and pepper. Dredge the chicken in the almond flour on each side, and shake off any excess flour. Set aside. Heat the remaining olive oil in a skillet over medium heat. Fry the chicken on both sides until golden brown, about 8 minutes. Pour in the broth and let it boil until it becomes thick in consistency, 12 minutes. Stir in the capers, butter, and roasted lemons and simmer on low heat for 10 minutes. Turn the heat off. Pour the sauce over the chicken and garnish with parsley to serve.

313.   Chicken in White Wine Sauce

Ready in about: 40 minutes | Serves: 4 Per serving: Kcal 345, Fat 12g, Net Carbs 4g, Protein 24g

Ingredients

1 ½ chicken thighs Salt and black pepper to taste 2 shallots, chopped 2 tbsp canola oil 4 pancetta strips, chopped 2 garlic cloves, minced 10 oz white mushrooms, halved 1 cup white wine 1 cup whipping cream

Directions

Warm the canola oil a pan over medium heat. Cook the pancetta for 3 minutes. Add in the chicken, sprinkle with pepper and salt, and cook until brown, about 5 minutes. Remove to a plate. In the same pan, sauté shallots, mushrooms, and garlic for 6 minutes. Return the pancetta and chicken to the pan. Stir in the white wine and 1 cup of water and bring to a boil. Reduce the heat and simmer for 20 minutes. Pour in the whipping cream and warm without boiling. Serve with steamed asparagus.

314.   Creamy Stuffed Chicken with Parma Ham

Ready in about: 40 minutes | Serves: 4 Per serving: Kcal 485, Fat 35g, Net Carbs 2g, Protein 26g

Ingredients

4 chicken breasts 2 tbsp olive oil 2 cloves garlic, minced 2 shallots, finely chopped 1 tsp dried mixed herbs 8 slices Parma ham 4 oz cream cheese, softened 1 lemon, zested Salt to taste Preheat oven to 350°F.

Directions

Heat the oil in a skillet over medium heat. Sauté garlic and shallots for 3 minutes. Stir the cream cheese, mixed herbs, salt, and lemon zest for 2 minutes. Remove and let cool. Score a pocket in each chicken breast, fill the holes with the cheese mixture, and cover with the cut-out chicken. Wrap each breast with 2 ham slices and secure the ends with a toothpick. Lay the chicken parcels on a greased baking sheet. Bake for 20 minutes. Remove and let it rest for 4 minutes. Serve.

315.   Chicken Wings with Herb Chutney

Ready in about: 35 minutes + marinating time | Serves: 4 Per serving: Kcal 243, Fat 15g, Net Carbs 3.5g, Protein 22g

Ingredients

12 chicken wings, cut in half 1 tbsp turmeric 1 tbsp cumin 3 tbsp fresh ginger, grated 2 tbsp cilantro, chopped ½ tsp paprika Salt and black pepper to taste 4 tbsp olive oil Juice of ½ lime 2 tbsp fresh thyme, chopped ¾ cup cilantro, chopped 1 jalapeño pepper, chopped

Directions

In a bowl, stir 1 tbsp ginger, cumin, paprika, salt, 2 tbsp olive oil, black pepper, and turmeric. Place in the chicken wings pieces and toss to coat. Marinate in the fridge for 20 minutes. Remove before grilling. Heat the grill, place in the marinated wings, and cook for 25 minutes, turning from time to time. Remove and set to a serving plate. Blitz thyme, remaining ginger, salt, jalapeno, black pepper, lime juice, cilantro, remaining olive oil, and 1 tbsp water in a blender. Drizzle the chicken wings with the sauce and serve.

316. Eggplant & Tomato Braised Chicken Thighs

Ready in about: 45 minutes | Serves: 4 Per serving: Kcal 468, Fat 39.5g, Net Carbs 2g, Protein 26g

Ingredients

2 tbsp ghee 1 lb chicken thighs Salt and black pepper to taste 2 garlic cloves, minced 1 (14 oz) can whole tomatoes 1 eggplant, diced

Directions

Melt ghee in a saucepan over medium heat. Season the chicken with salt and black pepper and fry for 4 minutes on each side until golden brown. Remove to a plate. Sauté the garlic in the ghee for 2 minutes. Pour in the tomatoes and cook covered for 8 minutes. Add in the eggplant and sauté for 4 minutes. Adjust the seasoning with salt and black pepper. Stir and add the chicken. Coat with sauce and simmer for 3 minutes. Serve chicken with sauce on a bed of squash pasta.

317. Sweet Chili Grilled Chicken

Ready in about: 30 minutes | Serves: 6 Per serving: Kcal 265, Fat 9g, Net Carbs 3g, Protein 26g

Ingredients

2 lb chicken breasts 4 cloves garlic, minced 2 tbsp fresh oregano, chopped ½ cup lemon juice 2/3 cup olive oil 1 tbsp erythritol Salt and black pepper to taste 3 small chilies, minced

Directions

Preheat grill to high heat. In a bowl, mix the garlic, oregano, lemon juice, olive oil, chilies, and erythritol. Cover the chicken with plastic wraps and use the rolling pin to pound to ½-inch thickness. Remove the wrap and brush the spice mixture on the chicken on all sides. Place on the grill and cook for 15 minutes, flip, and continue cooking for 10 more minutes. Remove to a plate and serve with salad.

318. Bacon & Chicken Cottage Pie Cups

Ready in about: 55 minutes | Serves: 4 Per serving: Kcal 571, Fat 45g, Net Carbs 8.2g, Protein 41g

Ingredients

1 onion, chopped 4 bacon slices, chopped 3 tbsp butter 1 carrot, chopped 3 garlic cloves, minced Salt and black pepper to taste ¾ cup crème fraîche ½ cup chicken stock 12 oz chicken breasts, cubed 2 tbsp Dijon mustard ¾ cup cheddar cheese, shredded For the dough ¾ cup almond flour 3 tbsp cream cheese, softened 1 ½ cups mozzarella cheese, grated 1 egg 1 tsp onion powder 1 tsp garlic powder

Directions

Melt the butter in a pan over medium heat. Sauté the onion, garlic, salt, pepper, bacon, and carrot for 5 minutes. Add in the chicken and cook for 3 minutes. Stir in the crème fraîche, mustard, and stock and cook for 7 minutes. Mix in the cheddar cheese. Microwave mozzarella and cream cheeses for 1 minute. Stir in the garlic powder, salt, pepper, almond flour, onion powder, and egg. Knead the dough well, split into 4 pieces, and flatten each one into a circle. Set the chicken mixture into 4 greased ramekins, top with dough circles, and place in the oven. Cook for 25 minutes at 370º F. Serve chilled.

319.   Chicken & Broccoli Stir-Fry

Ready in about: 30 minutes | Serves: 4 Per serving: Kcal 286, Fat 10.1g, Net Carbs 3.4g, Protein 17.3g

Ingredients

2 chicken breasts, cut into strips 2 tbsp olive oil 1 cup unsalted cashew nuts 2 cups broccoli florets 1 white onion, thinly sliced Salt and black pepper to taste

Directions

Toast the cashew nuts in a dry skillet over medium heat for 2-3 minutes, shaking occasionally. Remove to a plate. Heat the olive oil in the pan and sauté the onion for 4 minutes until soft; set aside. Add the chicken to the pan. Cook for 4 minutes. Include the broccoli, salt, and black pepper. Stir and cook for 5-6 minutes until tender and add in the onion. Stir once more, cook for 1 minute, and turn the heat off. Serve the chicken stir-fry topped with the cashew nuts.

320.   Cheesy Chicken Bake with Zucchini

Ready in about: 40 minutes | Serves: 6 Per serving: Kcal: 489, Fat: 37g, Net Carbs: 4.5g, Protein: 21g

Ingredients

2 lb chicken breasts, cubed 3 tbsp butter 1 cup green bell peppers, sliced 1 cup yellow onions, sliced 1 zucchini, cubed 2 garlic cloves, minced 1 tsp dried dill Salt and black pepper to taste 8 oz cream cheese, softened ½ cup mayonnaise 2 tbsp Worcestershire sauce 2 cups cheddar cheese, shredded Preheat oven to 370°F.

Directions

Melt the butter in a pan over medium heat. Add in the chicken and cook until lightly browned, about 5 minutes. Put in onions, zucchini, garlic, and bell peppers and sauté for 5-6 minutes until tender, stirring occasionally. Season with salt, black pepper, and dill, stir, and set aside. In a bowl, mix cream cheese, mayonnaise, and Worcestershire sauce. Stir in the chicken-vegetable mix. Transfer to a greased baking dish. Sprinkle with the cheddar cheese and bake for 30 minutes. Serve.

321.   Roasted Stuffed Chicken with Tomato Basil Sauce

Ready in about: 35 minutes | Serves: 6 Per serving: Kcal 338, Fat: 28g, Net Carbs: 2.5g, Protein: 37g

Ingredients

4 oz cream cheese 3 oz mozzarella slices, sliced 10 oz spinach ⅓ cup shredded mozzarella cheese 2 tbsp olive oil 1 cup tomato-basil sauce 3 whole chicken breasts Salt and black pepper to taste Preheat oven to 400°F.

Directions

Combine the cream cheese, shredded mozzarella, and spinach in a bowl. Microwave for 90 seconds. Cut the chicken a couple of times horizontally and stuff with the mixture. Brush with olive oil. Place on a lined baking dish and bake in the oven for 25 minutes. Pour the tomato-basil sauce over and top with mozzarella slices. Return to the oven and cook for an additional 5 minutes.

322.   Chicken with Creamed Turnip Greens

Ready in about: 35 minutes | Serves: 4 Per serving: Kcal 446, Fat: 38g, Net Carbs: 2.6g, Protein: 18g

Ingredients

1 lb chicken thighs 2 tbsp coconut oil 2 tbsp coconut flour 12 oz turnip greens, chopped 1 tsp oregano 1 cup heavy cream 1 cup chicken broth 2 tbsp butter

Directions

Warm the coconut oil in a skillet over medium heat. Brown the chicken on all sides, about 6-8 minutes. Set aside. Add and melt the butter and whisk in the flour. Whisk in heavy cream and chicken broth. Bring to a boil. Stir in oregano. Add the turnip greens to the skillet and cook until wilted, about 3-4 minutes. Add the thighs in the skillet and cook for an additional 15 minutes. Serve warm.

323.   Lemon Chicken Bake

Ready in about: 55 minutes | Serves: 6 Per serving: Kcal 274, Fat 9g, Net Carbs 4.5g, Protein 25g

Ingredients

6 chicken breasts 1 parsnip, cut into wedges Salt and black pepper to taste 2 lemons, juiced and zested Lemon rinds from 2 lemons 1 cup chicken stock In a baking dish, add the chicken alongside pepper and salt.

Directions

Sprinkle with lemon juice and broth. Toss to coat. Add in parsnip, lemon rinds, and lemon zest and put in the oven. Bake for 45 minutes at 370°F. Get rid of the lemon rinds, split the chicken onto plates, sprinkle sauce from the baking dish over. Serve.

324.   Sticky Cranberry Chicken Wings

Ready in about: 50 minutes | Serves: 6 Per serving: Kcal 152, Fat 8.5g, Net Carbs 1.6g, Protein 17.6g

Ingredients

4 tbsp unsweetened cranberry puree 2 lb chicken wings 3 tbsp olive oil Salt to taste 4 tbsp chili sauce Lemon juice from 1 lemon Preheat oven to 400°F.

Directions

In a bowl, mix cranberry puree, olive oil, salt, chili sauce, and lemon juice. Add in the wings and toss to coat. Place the chicken under the broiler, and cook for 45 minutes, turning once halfway. Remove the chicken after and serve warm with a cranberry dipping sauce.

325.   Grilled Chicken Wings

Ready in about: 15 minutes + chilling time | Serves: 4 Per serving: Kcal 216, Fat 11.5g, Net Carbs 4.3g, Protein 18.5g

Ingredients

2 lb chicken wings Juice from 1 lemon ½ cup fresh parsley, chopped 2 garlic cloves, minced 1 serrano pepper, chopped 3 tbsp olive oil Salt and black pepper to taste ½ cup ranch dip 1 tsp fresh cilantro, chopped

Directions

In a bowl, stir together lemon juice, garlic, salt, serrano pepper, cilantro, olive oil, and black pepper. Place in the chicken wings and toss to coat. Refrigerate for 2 hours. Preheat grill to high heat. Add in the chicken wings. Cook each side for 6 minutes. Remove to a plate and serve with ranch dip. Enjoy!

326.   Chicken in Creamy Mushroom Sauce

Ready in about: 40 minutes | Serves: 4 Per serving: Kcal 448, Fat 38.2g, Net Carbs 2g, Protein 22g

Ingredients

2 tbsp ghee 4 chicken breasts, cut into chunks Salt and black pepper to taste 1 packet white onion soup mix 2 cups chicken broth 15 baby Bella mushrooms, sliced 1 cup heavy cream 2 tbsp fresh parsley, chopped

Directions

Melt ghee in a saucepan over medium heat, season the chicken with salt and black pepper, and brown on all sides for 6 minutes in total. Put on a plate. In a bowl, stir the onion soup mix and chicken broth. Add the mixture to the saucepan and simmer for 3 minutes. Add in the mushrooms and chicken. Cover. Simmer for another 20 minutes. Stir in heavy cream and cook for 3 minutes. Adjust the seasoning. Ladle the chicken with creamy sauce and mushrooms over bed of cauli mash. Garnish with parsley and serve.

327.   Chicken with Baked Cheese Slices

Ready in about: 30 minutes | Serves: 4 Per serving: Kcal 445, Fat 34g, Net Carbs 4g, Protein 39g

Ingredients

2 tbsp butter 1 tsp garlic, minced 1 lb chicken breasts 1 tsp creole seasoning ¼ cup scallions, chopped ½ cup tomatoes, chopped ½ cup chicken stock ¼ cup whipping cream ½ cup Monterey Jack cheese, grated ¼ cup fresh cilantro, chopped Salt and black pepper to taste 4 oz cream cheese, softened 8 eggs 1 tsp garlic powder Set a pan over medium heat and warm 1 tbsp butter.

Directions

Add chicken, sprinkle with creole seasoning, and cook each side for 2 minutes; remove to a plate. Melt the rest of the butter, stir in garlic and tomatoes, and cook for 4 minutes. Return the chicken to the pan and pour in the stock. Simmer for 15 minutes. Place in the whipping cream, scallions, salt, Monterey Jack cheese, and pepper and cook for 2 minutes. In a blender, combine the cream cheese with garlic powder, salt, eggs, and pepper and pulse until smooth. Spread the mixture on a lined baking sheet and bake in the oven for 10 minutes at 325ºF. Allow the cheese sheet to cool down, place on a cutting board, roll, and cut into medium slices. Split them among bowls and top with chicken mixture. Sprinkle with chopped cilantro and serve.

328. Chicken Paella with Chorizo

Ready in about: 65 minutes | Serves: 6 Per serving: Kcal 440, Fat 28g, Net Carbs 3g, Protein 22g

Ingredients

2 lb chicken drumsticks 12 oz chorizo, chopped 1 onion, chopped 4 oz jarred piquillo peppers, diced 2 tbsp olive oil ½ cup chopped parsley 1 tsp smoked paprika 2 tbsp tomato puree ½ cup white wine 1 cup chicken broth 4 cups cauli rice 1 cup green beans, chopped 1 lemon, cut in wedges Salt and black pepper to taste Preheat oven to 350°F.

Directions

Heat the olive oil in a pan over medium heat. Season the chicken with salt and pepper and fry on both sides for 8-10 minutes until lightly brown. Remove to a plate. Add the chorizo and onion to the hot oil and sauté for 4 minutes. Include in tomato puree, piquillo peppers, and paprika. Let simmer for 2 minutes. Add in the broth and cook for 6 minutes until it is slightly reduced. Stir in cauli rice, white wine, green beans, and parsley, and lay the chicken on top. Transfer the pan to the oven and bake for 20-25 minutes. Let the paella to sit for 10 minutes. Arrange the lemon wedges on top and serve.

329. Lemon & Rosemary Chicken in a Skillet

Ready in about: 20 minutes + marinating time | Serves: 4 Per serving: Kcal 477, Fat: 31g, Net Carbs: 2.5g, Protein: 31g

Ingredients

8 chicken thighs Salt and black pepper to taste 1 lemon, juiced and zested 4 tbsp olive oil 1 tbsp fresh rosemary, chopped 1 garlic clove, minced

Directions

Combine 2 tbsp of the olive oil, lemon juice, lemon zest, garlic, rosemary, salt, and pepper in a bowl. Add in the chicken thighs and toss to coat. Place in the fridge to marinate for at least 1 hour. Heat the remaining olive oil in a skillet over medium heat. Add the chicken along with the juices and cook until crispy, about 4-5 minutes per side. Remove to a plate and serve with green salad

330. Pancetta & Chicken Casserole

Ready in about: 40 minutes | Serves: 4 Per serving: Kcal 313, Fat 18g, Net Carbs 3g, Protein 26g

Ingredients

8 pancetta strips, chopped ⅓ cup Dijon mustard Salt and black pepper to taste 1 onion, chopped 2 tbsp olive oil 1 ½ cups chicken stock 1 lb chicken breasts ¼ tsp sweet paprika In a bowl, combine paprika, salt, pepper, and mustard.

Directions

Massage the chicken with the mixture. Set a pan over medium heat, stir in the pancetta, and cook until it browns, about 5 minutes. Remove to a plate. Place oil in the same pan and add the chicken breasts. Cook each side for 2 minutes and set aside. Pour the stock in the pan and bring to a simmer. Stir in black pepper, pancetta, salt, and onion. Return the chicken to the pan, stir gently, and simmer for 20 minutes over medium heat, turning the meat halfway through. Split the chicken on serving plates, sprinkle the sauce over it, and serve.

331. Fried Chicken Breasts

Ready in about: 20 minutes + marinating time| Serves: 4 Per serving: Kcal 387, Fat 16g, Net Carbs 2.5g, Protein 23g

Ingredients

2 chicken breasts, cut into strips 1 cup pork rinds, crushed 4 tbsp coconut oil 16 oz jarred pickle juice 2 eggs, whisked

Directions

In a bowl, combine chicken with pickle juice. Refrigerate for 2 hours. Set the eggs in one bowl and pork rinds in a separate one. Dip the chicken in the eggs and then in pork rinds. Put a pan over medium heat and warm oil. Fry the chicken for 3 minutes per side and remove to a plate. Serve.

332. Chicken Gumbo

Ready in about: 40 minutes | Serves: 4 Per serving: Kcal 361, Fat 22g, Net Carbs 6g, Protein 26g

Ingredients

2 sausages, sliced 2 chicken breasts, cubed 1 celery stalk, chopped ½ tsp dried oregano 2 bell peppers, seeded and chopped 1 onion, chopped 2 cups tomatoes, chopped 4 cups chicken broth ½ tsp dried thyme 2 garlic cloves, minced 1 tsp dry mustard 1 tsp cayenne pepper Salt and black pepper to taste ½ tsp cajun seasoning 2 tbsp olive oil

Directions

In a pot over medium heat, warm the olive oil. Add the sausages and chicken and cook for 5-6 minutes; set aside. Add the onion, garlic, celery, and bell peppers and sauté for 5 minutes. Stir in dry mustard, oregano, thyme, cayenne pepper, and cajun seasoning for 1 minute. Pour in the broth and tomatoes. Cook for 10 minutes. Return the sausages and chicken, adjust the seasoning with salt and pepper and bring to a boil. Reduce the heat and simmer for 20 minutes covered. Serve hot divided between bowls.

333. Ranch Chicken Meatballs

Ready in about: 25 minutes | Serves: 4 Per serving: Kcal 456, Fat 31g, Net Carbs 2.1g, Protein 32g

Ingredients

1 lb ground chicken Salt and black pepper to taste 2 tbsp ranch dressing ½ cup almond flour ¼ cup mozzarella cheese, grated 1 tbsp Italian seasoning ¼ cup hot sauce 1 egg

Directions

In a bowl, combine chicken, pepper, ranch dressing, Italian seasoning, almond flour, mozzarella cheese, salt, and egg and mix well. Form into golf ball-sized meatballs. Arrange them on a lined baking tray and bake in the oven for 16 minutes at 480°F. Remove to a bowl and serve with hot sauce.

334.   Habanero Chicken Wings

Ready in about: 40 minutes | Serves: 4 Per serving: Kcal 416, Fat 25g, Net Carbs 2g, Protein 26g

Ingredients

2 lb chicken wings Salt and black pepper to taste 3 tbsp coconut aminos 3 tbsp rice vinegar 1 tbsp stevia ¼ cup chives, chopped ½ tsp xanthan gum 2 dried habanero peppers, chopped Spread the chicken wings on a lined baking sheet and sprinkle with 2 tbsp water, pepper and salt. Bake in the oven for 30 minutes at 370°F.

Directions

Put a pan over medium heat and add in the remaining ingredients. Bring to a boil and cook for 2 minutes. Pour the sauce over the chicken and bake for 10 minutes. Serve.

335.   Chicken Breasts with Cheddar & Pepperoni

Ready in about: 40 minutes | Serves: 4 Per serving: Kcal 387, Fat 21g, Net Carbs 4.5g, Protein 32g

Ingredients

12 oz canned tomato sauce 2 tbsp olive oil 4 chicken breast halves Salt and black pepper to taste ½ tsp dried oregano 4 oz cheddar cheese, sliced 1 tsp garlic powder 2 oz pepperoni, sliced Preheat oven to 390°F.

Directions

In a bowl, mix chicken with oregano, salt, garlic, and pepper. Heat the olive oil in a pan over medium heat. Add in the chicken and cook each side for 2 minutes. Remove to a baking dish. Top with the cheddar cheese, spread the sauce, and cover with pepperoni slices. Bake for 30 minutes. Roasted

336.   Quattro Formaggi Stuffed Chicken Breasts

Ready in about: 40 minutes | Serves: 6 Per serving: Kcal 565, Fat 37g, Net Carbs 2g, Protein 51g

Ingredients

2 lb chicken breasts 2 oz mozzarella cheese, cubed 2 oz mascarpone cheese, softened 4 oz cheddar cheese, cubed 2 oz provolone cheese, cubed 1 zucchini, shredded Salt and black pepper to taste 1 garlic clove, minced 2 oz smoked bacon slices, chopped

Directions

Sprinkle black pepper and salt to the zucchini, squeeze well, and place in a bowl. Stir in the smoked bacon, mascarpone, cheddar cheese, provolone cheese, mozzarella cheese, black pepper, and garlic. Cut slits into chicken breasts, apply black pepper and salt, and stuff with the zucchini and cheese mixture. Set on a lined baking sheet, place in the oven at 400°F, and bake for 45 minutes. Serve

337. Chicken Stew with Sun-Dried Tomatoes

Ready in about: 60 minutes | Serves: 4 Per serving: Kcal 224, Fat 11g, Net Carbs 6g, Protein 23g

Ingredients

1 carrot, chopped 2 tbsp olive oil 1 celery stalk, chopped 2 cups chicken stock 1 shallot, chopped 1 lb chicken thighs 2 garlic cloves, minced ½ tsp dried rosemary 2 oz sun-dried tomatoes, chopped 1 cup spinach ¼ tsp dried thyme ½ cup heavy cream Salt and black pepper to taste A pinch of xanthan gum

Directions

In a pot, heat the olive oil over medium heat and add garlic, carrot, celery, and shallot. Season with salt and pepper and sauté for 5-6 minutes until tender. Stir in the chicken and cook for 5 minutes. Pour in the stock, tomatoes, rosemary, and thyme and simmer for 30 minutes covered. Stir in xanthan gum, cream, and spinach and cook for 5 minutes. Adjust the seasonings. Serve the stew into bowls.

338. Chicken & Zucchini Bake

Ready in about: 45 minutes | Serves: 4 Per serving: Kcal 235, Fat 11g, Net Carbs 2g, Protein 35g

Ingredients

1 zucchini, chopped Salt and black pepper to taste 1 tsp garlic powder 2 tbsp avocado oil 1 lb chicken breasts, sliced 1 tomato, cored and chopped ½ tsp dried oregano ½ tsp dried basil ½ cup mozzarella cheese, shredded

Directions

Apply pepper, garlic powder, and salt to the chicken. Set a pan over medium heat and warm avocado oil. Add in the chicken slices and cook until golden, 5 minutes. Remove to a baking dish. To the same pan, add zucchini, tomato, pepper, basil, oregano, and salt and cook for 2 minutes. Spread over the chicken. Bake in the oven for 20 minutes at 330°F. Sprinkle the mozzarella over the chicken, return to the oven, and bake for 5 minutes until the cheese is melted and bubbling. Serve with green salad.

339. Chicken & Bacon Rolls

Ready in about: 45 minutes | Serves: 4 Per serving: Kcal 623, Fat 48g, Net Carbs 5g, Protein 38g

Ingredients

1 tbsp fresh chives, chopped 8 oz blue cheese, crumbled 1 lb chicken breasts, halved 12 bacon slices 2 tomatoes, chopped Salt and black pepper to taste

Directions

Set a pan over medium heat. Add in the bacon and cook until halfway done; remove to a plate. In a bowl, stir blue cheese, chives, tomatoes, pepper, and salt. Use a meat tenderizer to flatten the chicken breasts, season, and lay blue cheese mixture on top. Roll them up and wrap in bacon slices. Place the wrapped chicken breasts in a greased baking dish and roast in the oven for 30 minutes at 370°F. Serve warm.

340.   Baked Chicken with Acorn Squash & Goat's Cheese

Ready in about: 60 minutes | Serves: 6 Per serving: Kcal 235, Fat 16g, Net Carbs 5g, Protein 12g

Ingredients

6 chicken breasts, butterflied 1 lb acorn squash, cubed Salt and black pepper to taste 1 cup goat's cheese, crumbled ½ tsp dried parsley 3 tbsp olive oil

Directions

Arrange the chicken breasts and squash in a baking dish. Season with salt, black pepper, and parsley. Drizzle with olive oil and pour a cup of water. Cover with aluminium foil and bake in the oven for 30 minutes at 420ºF. Discard the foil, scatter goat's cheese, and bake for 15-20 minutes. Serve and enjoy!

341.   Almond-Crusted Chicken Breasts

Ready in about: 60 minutes | Serves: 4 Per serving: Kcal 485, Fat 32g, Net Carbs 1g, Protein 41g

Ingredients

4 bacon slices, cooked, crumbled 4 chicken breasts 1 tbsp water ½ cup olive oil 1 egg, whisked Salt and black pepper to taste 1 cup asiago cheese, shredded ¼ tsp garlic powder 1 cup ground almonds

Directions

In a bowl, combine almonds with pepper, salt, and garlic. Place egg in a separate bowl and mix with the water. Season with pepper and salt. Dip each piece into the egg and then into the almond mixture. Warm oil a pan and cook the chicken breasts until golden brown. Remove to a baking pan. Bake in the oven for 20 minutes at 360ºF. Scatter with cheese and bacon and roast for 5-10 minutes. Serve warm

342.   Chicken Thighs with Broccoli & Green Onions

Ready in about: 25 minutes | Serves: 2 Per serving: Kcal 387, Fat 23g, Net Carbs 5g, Protein 27g

Ingredients

2 boneless chicken thighs, cut into strips 1 tbsp olive oil 1 tsp red pepper flakes ½ tsp onion powder ½ tbsp fresh ginger, grated ¼ cup tamari sauce ½ tsp garlic powder ½ tsp xanthan gum ½ cup green onions, chopped 1 head broccoli, cut into florets

Directions

Warm the oil in a pan over medium heat. Add in chicken, green onions, and ginger and sauté for 4 minutes. Stir in the onion powder, pepper flakes, garlic powder, xanthan gum, and erythritol for 1 minute. Pour in 1 cup water and tamari sauce. Simmer for 15 minutes. Add in broccoli. Cook for 6 minutes. Serve.

343. Chicken with Green Sauce

Ready in about: 35 minutes | Serves: 4 Per serving: Kcal 236, Fat 9g, Net Carbs 2.3g, Protein 18g

Ingredients

2 tbsp butter 4 scallions, chopped 4 chicken breasts Salt and black pepper to taste 6 oz sour cream 2 tbsp fresh dill, chopped

Directions

Melt butter in a pan with the butter over medium heat. Add in the chicken, season with pepper and salt, and fry for 2-3 per side until golden. Transfer to a baking dish. Cook in the oven for 15 minutes at 390°F. To the pan, add scallions and cook for 2 minutes. Pour in the sour cream, warm through without boil. Slice the chicken and place it on a platter with green sauce spooned over. Top with fresh dill and serve.

344. Roasted Chicken with Herbs

Ready in about: 50 minutes | Serves: 6 Per serving: Kcal 367, Fat 15g, Net Carbs 1.1g, Protein 33g

Ingredients

1 (4-pound) whole chicken ½ tsp onion powder Salt and black pepper to taste 2 tbsp olive oil 1 tsp dry thyme 1 tsp dry rosemary 1 ½ cups chicken broth 2 tsp guar gum 2 tbsp fresh parsley, chopped

Directions

Rub chicken with oil, salt, rosemary, thyme, pepper, and onion powder. Place it in a baking dish and pour in the stock. Bake for 40 minutes at 380°F. Remove the chicken to a platter. Add the guar gum and 1 cup water in a pan over medium heat. Cook for 2-3 minutes until thickened. Season with salt and black pepper and stir in the parsley. Carve the chicken and top with the sauce to serve.

345. Turkey Enchilada Bowl

Ready in about: 30 minutes | Serves: 4 Per serving: Kcal: 568, Fat: 40.2g, Net Carbs: 5.9g, Protein: 38g

Ingredients

1 lb boneless, skinless turkey thighs, cut into pieces 2 tbsp coconut oil ¾ cup red enchilada sauce 1 onion, chopped 3 oz canned diced green chiles 1 avocado, diced 1 cup mozzarella cheese, shredded ¼ cup pickled jalapeños, chopped ½ cup sour cream 1 tomato, diced

Directions

Warm the coconut oil in a large pan over medium heat. Add in the turkey and cook until browned on the outside, about 5-6 minutes. Stir in onion, chiles, ¼ cup water, and enchilada sauce. Cover with a lid. Allow simmering for 20 minutes until the turkey is cooked through. Spoon the turkey onto a serving bowl and top with the sauce, mozzarella cheese, sour cream, tomato, and avocado. Serve.

346.   Red Wine Chicken

Ready in about: 40 minutes | Serves: 4 Per serving: Kcal 314, Fat 12g, Net Carbs 4g, Protein 27g

Ingredients

2 tbsp butter 1 lb chicken breasts, halved 2 garlic cloves, minced Salt and black pepper to taste 1 cup chicken stock 1 tbsp stevia ½ cup red wine 2 tomatoes, sliced 6 mozzarella cheese slices

Directions

Set a pan over medium heat and warm butter. Add the chicken, season with pepper and salt, and cook until brown, 5-6 minutes. Stir in the stevia, garlic, chicken stock, and red wine and cook for 10 minutes. Remove to a lined baking sheet and arrange mozzarella cheese slices on top. Bake in the preheated to 370°F oven for 20 minutes until the cheese melts. Lay tomato slices over chicken pieces and serve.

347.   Pressure Cooker Mexican Turkey Soup

Ready in about: 35 minutes | Serves: 4 Per serving: Kcal 387, Fat 24g, Net Carbs 6g, Protein 38g

Ingredients

½ lb turkey breast, cubed 4 cups chicken stock 1 onion, chopped 1 cup canned chunky salsa 8 oz cheddar cheese, shredded ¼ tsp cayenne red pepper 4 oz canned diced green chilies 1 tsp fresh cilantro, chopped 2 tbsp olive oil

Directions

Set the pressure cooker to Sauté and warm the olive oil. Cook the turkey and onion for 5-6 minutes, stirring occasionally. Stir in the salsa, green chilies, cayenne pepper, and chicken stock and seal the lid. Press Pressure Cook and set the cooking time to 15 minutes. When ready, do a quick pressure release. Stir in the cheddar cheese until it is melted, about 2 minutes. Sprinkle with cilantro and serve.

348.   Spicy Eggs with Turkey Ham

Ready in about: 15 minutes | Serves: 2 Per serving: Kcal 462; Fat: 40.6g, Net Carbs: 7.1g, Protein: 16.9g

Ingredients

2 tbsp olive oil ½ cup onions, chopped 1 tsp garlic, minced 1 tsp serrano pepper, minced Salt and black pepper to taste 5 oz turkey ham, chopped 4 eggs, whisked 1 thyme sprig, chopped ½ cup olives, pitted and sliced

Directions

Over medium heat, set a skillet and warm oil. Add in onion and sauté for 4 minutes until tender. Stir in garlic, salt, ham, black pepper, and serrano pepper and cook for 5-6 more minutes. Add in eggs and sprinkle with thyme. Cook for 5 minutes. Garnish with sliced olives before serving.

349. Buttered Duck Breast

Ready in about: 30 minutes | Serves: 2 Per serving: Kcal 547, Fat 46g, Net Carbs 2g, Protein 35g

Ingredients

1 medium duck breast, skin scored 1 tbsp heavy cream 2 tbsp butter Salt and black pepper to taste 1 cup kale ¼ tsp fresh sage

DIRECTIONS

Warm half of the butter in a pan over medium heat. Add in sage and heavy cream and cook for 2 minutes. Stir in the kale and cook for 1 minute. Melt the remaining butter in another pan over medium heat. Add in the duck as the skin side faces down. Cook for 4 minutes, flip, and cook for 3 minutes. Set the duck breast on a flat surface and slice. Arrange the slices on a platter and drizzle over the sauce to serve.

350. Turkey & Cheese Stuffed Peppers

Ready in about: 40 minutes | Serves: 4 Per serving: Kcal 486, Fat 17g, Net Carbs 8.6g, Protein 51g

Ingredients

4 bell peppers, tops removed 3 oz cream cheese, softened 1 carrot, chopped 2 tbsp olive oil 1 tbsp hot sauce ¾ cup blue cheese, crumbled 1 onion, chopped 1 lb ground turkey Salt and black pepper to taste

Directions

Warm the olive oil in a saucepan over medium heat and sauté the onion and carrot for 3-4 minutes. Stir in the ground turkey and cook for 5-6 minutes. Season with salt and pepper and remove to a bowl. Let it cool slightly. Add in the hot sauce and cream cheese and stir well. Stuff the peppers with the mixture. Arrange them on a lined baking sheet. Place in the preheated to 425ºF oven and bake for 20 minutes. Top with the blue cheese and add back to the oven. Bake for 5 minutes until the cheese melts. Serve.

351. Turkey Salad with Spinach & Raspberries

Ready in about: 25 minutes | Serves: 4 Per serving: Kcal 451, Fat 33g, Net Carbs 6g, Protein 28g

Ingredients

1 tbsp swerve sugar 1 red onion, chopped ¼ cup vinegar ¼ cup olive oil ¼ cup water 1 ¾ cups raspberries 1 tbsp Dijon mustard Salt and black pepper to taste 10 oz baby spinach 1 lb turkey breast, boneless, halved 4 oz goat cheese, crumbled ½ cup pecans, halved

Directions

In a blender, combine swerve sugar, vinegar, 1 cup of the raspberries, black pepper, mustard, water, onion, half of the olive oil, and salt and pulse until smooth. Strain the dressing into a bowl and set aside. Warm the remaining oil in a pan over medium heat. Season the turkey with salt and pepper. Place it skin-side down into the pan. Cook for 12-14 minutes, flipping once. Place the spinach in a platter and top with the remaining raspberries, pecans, goat cheese, and dressing. Slice the turkey and put over the salad.

352.   Duck & Vegetable Casserole

Ready in about: 20 minutes | Serves: 2 Per serving: Kcal 433, Fat 21g, Net Carbs 8g, Protein 53g

Ingredients

½ lb duck breast, skin on and sliced 2 zucchinis, sliced 1 tbsp coconut oil 2 green onions, chopped 1 carrot, chopped 1 green bell pepper, chopped Salt and black pepper to taste 1 garlic clove, minced

Directions

Warm the coconut oil in a pan over medium heat. Add in the duck and cook each side for 3 minutes. Remove to a plate. To the pan, add the green onions and garlic and cook for 2 minutes. Place in the zucchini, bell pepper, salt, pepper, and carrot and cook for 10 minutes. Pour over the duck and serve.

353.   Coconut Turkey Chili with Kale

Ready in about: 30 minutes | Serves: 4 Per serving: Kcal 295, Fat 15.2g, Net Carbs 4.2g, Protein 25g

Ingredients

1 lb turkey breast, cubed 1 cup kale, chopped 20 oz canned diced tomatoes 2 tbsp coconut oil 2 tbsp coconut cream 2 garlic cloves, minced 1 onion, sliced 1 tsp ground coriander 1 tbsp fresh ginger, grated 1 tbsp turmeric Salt and black pepper to taste ½ tsp chili powder

Directions

Warm the olive oil in a pan over medium heat and. Add in the turkey, onion, garlic, and ginger and cook for 5 minutes. Stir in tomatoes, turmeric, coriander, salt, pepper, and chili powder and for 10 minutes. Pour in the coconut cream and kale and simmer for 5 more minutes. Serve warm.

354.   Turkey & Leek Soup

Ready in about: 45 minutes | Serves: 4 Per serving: Kcal 305, Fat 11g, Net Carbs 3g, Protein 15g

Ingredients

1 celery stalk, chopped 2 leeks, chopped 2 tbsp butter 4 cups chicken stock Salt and black pepper to taste ¼ cup fresh parsley, chopped 3 cups zoodles ½ lb turkey breast, skinless, boneless

Directions

Melt the butter in a pot over medium heat. Chop the turkey into cubes and add it to the pot along with leeks and celery. Cook for 5 minutes. Pour in the stock, season with salt and pepper, and cook for 30 minutes. Mix in the zoodles and cook for 5 more minutes. Serve topped with parsley in bowls and enjoy!

355. Duck and Eggplant Casserole

(Ready in about 45 minutes | Servings 4) Per serving: 562 Calories; 49.5g Fat; 6.7g Carbs; 22.5g Protein; 2.1g Fiber

Ingredients

1 pound ground duck meat 1 ½ tablespoons ghee, melted 1/3 cup double cream 1/2 pound eggplant, peeled and sliced 1 ½ cups almond flour Salt and black pepper, to taste 1/2 teaspoon fennel seeds 1/2 teaspoon oregano, dried 8 eggs

Directions

Mix the almond flour with salt, black, fennel seeds, and oregano. Fold in one egg and the melted ghee and whisk to combine well. Press the crust into the bottom of a lightly-oiled pie pan. Cook the ground duck until no longer pink for about 3 minutes, stirring continuously. Whisk the remaining eggs and double cream. Fold in the browned meat and stir until everything is well incorporated. Pour the mixture into the prepared crust. Top with the eggplant slices. Bake for about 40 minutes. Cut into four pieces Bon appétit!

356. Cilantro Chicken Breasts with Mayo-Avocado Sauce

Ready in about: 25 minutes | Serves: 4 Per serving: Kcal 398, Fat 32g, Net Carbs 4g, Protein 24g

Ingredients

Mayo-avocado sauce 1 avocado, pitted ½ cup mayonnaise Salt to taste Chicken 2 tbsp ghee 4 chicken breasts Pink salt and black pepper to taste 2 tbsp fresh cilantro, chopped ½ cup chicken broth

Directions Spoon the avocado into a bowl and mash with a fork. Add in mayonnaise and salt and stir until a smooth sauce is derived. Pour sauce into a jar and refrigerate. Melt the ghee in a large skillet over medium heat. Season chicken with salt and pepper and fry for 4 minutes on each side until golden brown. Remove. Pour the broth in the same skillet and add the cilantro. Bring to simmer covered for 3 minutes and return the chicken. Cover and cook on low heat for 5 minutes until the liquid has reduced and chicken is fragrant. Place the chicken only into serving plates and spoon the mayo-avocado sauce over. Serve.

357. Stuffed Chicken Breasts with Cucumber Noodle Salad

Ready in about: 60 minutes | Serves: 4 Per serving: Kcal: 453, Fat: 31g, Net Carbs: 6g, Protein: 43g

Ingredients

Chicken 4 chicken breasts 1 cup baby spinach ¼ cup goat cheese ¼ cup cheddar cheese, shredded 4 tbsp butter, melted Salt and black pepper to taste Tomato sauce 1 tbsp butter 1 shallot, chopped 2 garlic cloves, chopped ½ tbsp liquid stevia 2 tbsp tomato paste 14 oz canned crushed tomatoes Salt and black pepper to taste 1 tsp dried basil 1 tsp dried oregano Salad 2 cucumbers, spiralized 2 tbsp olive oil 1 tbsp white wine vinegar Preheat oven to 400°F.

Directions Place a pan over medium heat. Warm 2 tbsp of butter and sauté spinach until it shrinks. Season with salt and pepper. Transfer to a bowl containing goat cheese, stir, and set aside. Cut the chicken breasts lengthwise and stuff with the cheese mixture. Set into a baking dish. On top, spread the cheddar cheese and add 2 tbsp of butter. Bake until cooked through for 25-30 minutes. Warm 1 tbsp of the butter in a pan over medium heat. Add in garlic and shallot and cook for 3 minutes until soft. Stir in herbs, tomato paste, stevia, tomatoes, salt, and pepper and cook for 15 minutes. Arrange the cucumbers on a serving platter, season with salt, pepper, olive oil, and vinegar. Top with the chicken and pour over the sauce. Serve.

358.   Garlic & Ginger Chicken with Peanut Sauce

Ready in about: 20 minutes + marinating time | Serves: 6 Per serving: Kcal 492, Fat: 36g, Net Carbs: 3g, Protein: 35g

Ingredients

Chicken ingredients 1 tbsp wheat-free soy sauce 1 tbsp sugar-free fish sauce 1 tbsp lime juice 1 tsp cilantro, chopped 1 minced garlic 1 tsp minced ginger 1 tbsp olive oil 1 tbsp rice wine vinegar 1 tsp cayenne pepper 1 tbsp erythritol 6 chicken thighs Peanut sauce ½ cup peanut butter 1 tsp minced garlic 1 tbsp lime juice 2 tbsp water 1 tsp minced ginger 1 tbsp jalapeño pepper, chopped 2 tbsp rice wine vinegar 2 tbsp erythritol 1 tbsp fish sauce

Directions

Combine all chicken ingredients in a large Ziploc bag. Seal the bag and shake to combine. Refrigerate for 1 hour. Remove from the fridge about 15 minutes before cooking. Preheat the grill to medium heat. Cook the chicken for 7 minutes per side until golden brown. Remove to a serving plate. Whisk together all the sauce ingredients in a mixing bowl. Serve the chicken drizzled with peanut sauce.

359.   Chicken & Squash Traybake

Ready in about: 50 minutes | Serves: 4 Per serving: Kcal: 411, Fat: 15g, Net Carbs: 5.5g, Protein: 31g

Ingredients

1 ½ lb chicken thighs 1 lb butternut squash, cubed ½ cup black olives, pitted ¼ cup olive oil 5 garlic cloves, sliced ¼ tbsp dried oregano Preheat oven to 400°F.

Directions

Place the chicken in a greased baking dish with the skin down. Place the garlic, olives, and butternut squash around the chicken. Drizzle with olive oil. Sprinkle with black pepper, salt, and oregano. Bake in the oven for 45 minutes until golden brown. Serve warm.

360.   Poulet en Papillote

Ready in about: 60 minutes | Serves: 4 Per serving: Kcal 364, Fat 16.5g, Net Carbs 4.8g, Protein 25g

Ingredients

4 chicken breasts, scored 4 tbsp white wine 1 tbsp olive oil 4 tbsp butter, sliced 3 cups mixed mushrooms, teared up 1 medium celeriac, peeled, sliced 3 cloves garlic, minced 4 sprigs thyme, chopped 3 lemons, juiced Salt and black pepper to taste 2 tbsp Dijon mustard Preheat oven to 450°F.

Directions

Arrange the celeriac on a baking sheet, drizzle it with olive oil, and bake for 20 minutes; set aside. In a bowl, mix the chicken, roasted celeriac, mushrooms, garlic, thyme, lemon juice, salt, pepper, and mustard. Make 4 large cuts of foil, fold them in half, and fold them in half again. Tightly fold the two open edges together to create bags. Distribute the chicken mixture among the bags, top with white wine and butter. Seal the last open end securely, making sure not to pierce the bags. Put them on a baking tray and bake for 25 minutes. Remove the chicken from the bags and serve.

361.   Fried Chicken with Coconut Sauce

Ready in about: 30 minutes | Serves: 6 Per serving: Kcal 491, Fat 35g, Net Carbs 3.2g, Protein 58g

Ingredients

3 tbsp coconut oil 2 lb chicken breasts 1 cup chicken stock 1 ¼ cups leeks, chopped 1 tbsp lime juice ¼ cup coconut cream 1 tsp red pepper flakes 2 tbsp green onions, chopped Salt and black pepper to taste

Directions

Put a pan over medium heat and warm oil. Add in the chicken and cook each side for 2 minutes. Set aside. Place the leeks in the pan and cook for 4 minutes. Stir in stock, pepper flakes, salt, pepper, coconut cream, and lime juice. Take the chicken back to the pan and cook covered for 15 minutes. Serve warm.

362.Spanish Chicken

Ready in about: 50 minutes | Serves: 4 Per serving: Kcal 415, Fat 33g, Net Carbs 4g, Protein 25g

Ingredients

½ cup mushrooms, chopped 1 lb chorizo, chopped 2 tbsp avocado oil 4 cherry peppers, chopped 1 red bell pepper, seeded, chopped 1 onion, peeled and sliced 2 garlic cloves, minced 2 cups tomatoes, chopped 4 chicken thighs Salt and black pepper to taste 1 cup chicken stock 1 tsp turmeric 1 tbsp white wine vinegar 1 tsp dried oregano 2 tbsp fresh parsley, chopped

Directions

Warm the avocado oil in a pan over medium heat. Stir in the chorizo and cook for 5-6 minutes until browned; remove to a bowl. Place the chicken thighs in the chorizo fat and cook each side for 3 minutes. Season with salt and black pepper and set aside on a bowl. In the same pan, add the onion, garlic, bell pepper, cherry peppers, and mushrooms and cook for 4 minutes. Pour in the stock, turmeric, tomatoes, vinegar, and oregano. Return the chorizo and chicken and place the pan in the oven. Bake for 30 minutes at 400°F. Garnish with chopped parsley and serve.

363.   Lime Chicken Wings

Ready in about: 30 minutes | Serves: 4 Per serving: Kcal 365, Fat: 25g, Net Carbs: 4g, Protein: 21g

Ingredients

1 tsp garlic powder 1 lime, zested and juiced ½ tsp ground cilantro 1 tbsp fish sauce 2 tbsp butter ¼ tsp xanthan gum 3 tbsp swerve sweetener 20 chicken wings Salt and black pepper to taste

Directions

Combine lime juice and zest, fish sauce, cilantro, swerve sweetener, garlic powder, and 1 cup of water in a saucepan over medium heat. Bring to a boil. Cover, lower the heat, and let simmer for 10 minutes. Stir in the butter and xanthan gum. Set aside. Season the wings with salt and pepper. Preheat the grill and cook for 5 minutes per side. Serve topped with the sauce.

364.   One-Pot Chicken with Mushrooms

Ready in about: 35 minutes | Serves: 6 Per serving: Kcal 447, Fat: 37g, Net Carbs: 1g, Protein: 31g

Ingredients

2 cups mushrooms, sliced ½ tsp onion powder ½ tsp garlic powder ¼ cup butter 1 tsp Dijon mustard 1 tbsp tarragon, chopped 2 lb chicken thighs Salt and black pepper to taste Season the thighs with salt, pepper, garlic and onion powders.

Directions

Melt the butter in a skillet over medium heat. Cook the chicken until browned; set aside. Add mushrooms to the same fat and cook for 5 minutes. Stir in Dijon mustard and ½ cup of water. Return the chicken to the skillet. Season with salt and pepper, reduce the heat, and cover with a lid. Let simmer for 15 minutes. Stir in tarragon. Serve warm.

365.   Chicken Breasts with Walnut Crust

Ready in about: 30 minutes | Serves: 4 Per serving: Kcal 322, Fat 18g, Net Carbs 1.5g, Protein 35g

Ingredients

1 egg, whisked Salt and black pepper to taste 2 tbsp coconut oil 1 ½ cups walnuts, ground 1 lb chicken breast halves 1 lemon, sliced Season the chicken with salt and pepper.

Directions

Dip in the egg first and then in walnuts. Warm the coconut oil in a pan over medium heat and brown the chicken for 5-6 minutes in total. Remove to a baking sheet, set in the oven, and bake for 10 minutes at 350° F. Serve topped with lemon slices.

366.   Chicken & Green Cabbage Casserole

Ready in about: 50 minutes | Serves: 4 Per serving: Kcal 231, Fat 15g, Net Carbs 6g, Protein 25g

Ingredients

3 cups cheddar cheese, grated 10 oz green cabbage, shredded 1 lb chicken breasts, cubed 1 cup mayonnaise 1 tbsp coconut oil, melted 1 cup chicken stock Salt and black pepper to taste

Directions

Juice of 1 lemon Apply oil to a baking dish and set the chicken pieces to the bottom. Spread green cabbage, followed by half of the cheddar cheese. In a bowl, combine the mayonnaise with pepper, stock, lemon juice, and salt. Pour the mixture over the chicken, spread the rest of the cheese, and cover with aluminum foil. Bake for 30 minutes in the oven at 350°F. Open the aluminum foil and cook for 10 more minutes. Serve.

367.   Kale & Ricotta Stuffed Chicken Breasts

Ready in about: 25 minutes | Serves: 4 Per serving: Kcal 305, Fat 12g, Net Carbs 4g, Protein 23g

Ingredients

10 oz kale, trimmed and chopped 4 chicken breasts Salt and black pepper to taste 4 oz cream cheese, softened ½ cup ricotta cheese, crumbled 1 garlic clove, minced 2 tbsp avocado oil ½ cup white wine 2 tbsp butter

Directions

Warm avocado oil in a pan over medium heat. Add in kale, garlic, salt, and pepper and sauté for 5 minutes until wilted. Remove to a bowl and let it cool. Add in the ricotta cheese and cream cheese and stir well. Put the chicken breasts on a working surface, cut a pocket in each one, and stuff them with the mixture. Melt the butter in the pan over medium heat and add the stuffed chicken. Cook each side for 5 minutes. Transfer to a baking tray, drizzle with white wine and 2 tablespoons of water, and place in the preheated to 420°F oven. Bake for 10 minutes. Remove and arrange on a serving plate. Serve sliced.

368.   Chicken with Asparagus & Root Vegetables

Ready in about: 35 minutes | Serves: 4 Per serving: Kcal 497, Fat 31g, Net Carbs 7.4g, Protein 37g

Ingredients

2 cups whipping cream 1 lb chicken breasts, chopped 3 tbsp butter 1 onion, chopped 1 carrot, chopped 4 cups chicken stock Salt and black pepper to taste 1 bay leaf 1 turnip, chopped 1 parsnip, chopped 17 oz asparagus, trimmed 2 tsp fresh thyme, chopped

Directions

Put a pan over medium heat and warm butter. Sauté the onion, carrot, turnip, parsnip, and chicken for 5-6 minutes. Pour in the chicken stock and bay leaf. Bring to a boil and simmer for 20 minutes. Add in the asparagus and cook for 7 minutes. Discard the bay leaf. Stir in the whipping cream and adjust the seasoning with salt and pepper. Scatter with fresh thyme and serve.

369.   Roast Chicken with Herb Stuffing

Ready in about: 120 minutes | Serves: 6 Per serving: Kcal 432, Fat: 32g, Net Carbs: 5.1g, Protein: 30g

Ingredients

5-pound whole chicken 1 tbsp fresh oregano, chopped 1 tbsp fresh thyme, chopped Salt and black pepper to taste 1 tbsp fresh parsley, chopped 2 tbsp olive oil 2 lb Brussels sprouts 1 lemon, cut into wedges 4 tbsp butter, softened

Directions

Preheat oven to 420°F. Season the chicken with salt and pepper and brush with some butter. Stuff it with oregano, thyme, and lemon. Place ina greased baking dish, pour in 1 cup water, and roast for 15 minutes. Reduce the heat to 325°F, spread the remaining butter all over, and bake for 40 more minutes. Warm the olive oil in a pan over medium heat and add the Brussels sprouts. Season with salt and pepper and sauté for 8-10 minutes until tender. Sprinkle with parsley. Remove the chicken from the oven and let sit for 10 minutes. Carve and place on a serving platter. Serve with Brussels sprouts.

370. Baked Pecorino Toscano Chicken

Ready in about: 50 minutes | Serves: 4 Per serving: Kcal 346, Fat 24g, Net Carbs 6g, Protein 20g

Ingredients

4 chicken breasts, halved ½ cup mayonnaise ½ cup buttermilk Salt and black pepper to taste ¾ cup Pecorino cheese, grated 8 mozzarella cheese slices Place the chicken in a greased baking dish.

Directions

In a bowl, mix mayonnaise, buttermilk, cheese, salt, and pepper. Spread half of the mixture over the chicken. Arrange the mozzarella slices over, and finish with a layer of the remaining mixture. Pour in ½ cup of water. Bake in the oven for 35-40 minutes at 370°F.

371. Rosemary Turkey Pie

Ready in about: 40 minutes +chilling time | Serves: 4 Per serving: Kcal 325, Fat 23g, Net Carbs 5.6g, Protein 21g

Ingredients

2 cups chicken stock 1 cup turkey meat, cooked, chopped Salt and black pepper to taste 1 tbsp fresh rosemary, chopped ½ cup kale, chopped ½ cup butternut squash, chopped ½ cup Monterey jack cheese, grated ¼ tsp smoked paprika ¼ tsp xanthan gum For the crust ¼ cup butter ¼ tsp xanthan gum 2 cups almond flour A pinch of salt 1 egg ¼ cup cheddar cheese

Directions

Set a greased pot over medium heat. Place in the turkey and squash and cook for 10 minutes. Stir in stock, Monterey Jack cheese, rosemary, black pepper, smoked paprika, kale, and salt. In a bowl, combine ½ cup stock from the pot with ¼ teaspoon xanthan gum, and transfer everything to the pot; set aside. In a separate bowl, stir flour, ¼ teaspoon xanthan gum, and salt. Whisk in the butter, cheddar cheese, and egg until a pie crust dough forms. Shape into a ball, wrap in plastic foil, and refrigerate for 30 minutes. Spray a baking dish with cooking spray and sprinkle pie filling on the bottom. Set the dough on a working surface and roll it into a circle. Top the filling with the circle. Ensure well pressed and seal edges, set in an oven at 350°F, and bake for 35 minutes. Allow the pie to cool, and enjoy.

372. Turkey Pastrami & Mascarpone Pinwheels

Ready in about: 40 minutes | Serves: 4 Per serving: Kcal 266, Fat 24g, Net Carbs 0g, Protein 13g

Ingredients

10 canned pepperoncini peppers, sliced and drained Cooking spray 8 oz mascarpone cheese 10 oz turkey pastrami, sliced

Directions

Lay a 12 x 12 plastic wrap on a flat surface and arrange the pastrami all over slightly overlapping each other. Spread the cheese on top of the salami layers and arrange the pepperoncini on top. Hold two opposite ends of the plastic wrap and roll the pastrami. Twist both ends to tighten and refrigerate for 2 hours. Unwrap the salami roll and slice into 2-inch pinwheels. Serve.

373.   Zucchini Spaghetti with Turkey Bolognese Sauce

Ready in about: 30 minutes | Serves: 6 Per serving: Kcal 273, Fat: 16g, Net Carbs: 3.8g, Protein: 19g

Ingredients

2 cups sliced mushrooms 2 tsp olive oil 1 lb ground turkey 3 tbsp pesto sauce 1 cup diced onion 2 cups broccoli florets 6 cups zucchini, spiralized Salt and black pepper to taste

Directions

Heat the olive oil in a skillet. Add zucchini and cook for 2-3 minutes, stirring continuously; set aside. Add turkey to the skillet and cook until browned, about 7-8 minutes. Transfer to a plate. Add onion, broccoli, and mushrooms in the turkey fat and sauté for 5-6 minutes until tender. Return the turkey to the skillet, and stir in the pesto, salt, and pepper. Simmer for 15 minutes. Stir in zucchini pasta and serve.

Fish and Seafood

374.   Easy Cod Fritters

(Ready in about 20 minutes | Servings 5) Per serving: 326 Calories; 21.7g Fat; 5.8g Carbs; 25.6g Protein; 1g Fiber

Ingredients

2 ½ cups cod fish, cooked 1/2 cup almond flour 1/2 cup Romano cheese, preferably freshly grated 3 tablespoons olive oil Sea salt and pepper, to taste 1 teaspoon butter, room temperature 1/2 teaspoon dried oregano 1/2 teaspoon dried thyme 1/4 cup onion, chopped 3 cups broccoli, cut into rice-sized chunks 2 eggs, whisked

Directions

Melt the butter in a pan over medium-high flame. Once hot, cook the broccoli for 5 to 6 minutes, until crisp-tender. Let it cool completely. Add in the cooked fish, salt, pepper, oregano, thyme, onion, eggs, almond flour, and cheese; mix until everything is well incorporated. Form the mixture into 10 patties. In a frying pan, heat the oil over a moderately high heat. Cook your fritters for 4 to 5 minutes per side.Bon appétit!

375.   Cod Fish Fillets with French Salad

(Ready in about 15 minutes + marinating time | Servings 4) Per serving: 425 Calories; 27.2g Fat; 6.1g Carbs; 38.3g Protein; 3g Fiber

Ingredients

4 white cod fish fillets 1 tablespoon olive oil 2 tablespoons fresh lemon juice 1 teaspoon garlic, minced 2 tablespoons scallions, chopped Salt and pepper, to taste For French Salad: 1 cup arugula 1 head Iceberg lettuce 2 tablespoons dandelion 1/4 cup red wine vinegar 1/4 cup extra-virgin olive oil 1 cup chicory 1 cup frissee Salt and ground black pepper, to your liking

Directions

Toss the cod fish fillets with the olive oil, lemon juice, garlic, scallions salt, and pepper; allow it to marinate for 2 hours in your refrigerator. Sear the fish fillets in the preheated skillet over moderately high heat; basting with the marinade. Toss all ingredients for the salad in a salad bowl.

376.   Cheesy Salmon Dip

(Ready in about 10 minutes | Servings 10) Per serving: 109 Calories; 6.3g Fat; 1.3g Carbs; 11.4g Protein; 0.1g Fiber

Ingredients

10 ounces salmon 4 hard-boiled egg yolks, finely chopped 1/4 cup fresh scallions, chopped 5 ounces Ricotta cheese 5 ounces full-fat cream cheese Salt and freshly ground black pepper, to your liking 1/2 teaspoon hot paprika

Directions

Grill the salmon for about 10 minutes until browned and flakes easily with a fork. Cut into small chunks. Mix all ingredients until everything is well incorporated. Storing Place the cheesy salmon dip in airtight containers or Ziploc bags; keep in your refrigerator for up to 4 days.

377.   Mediterranean-Style Tuna Salad with Bocconcini

(Ready in about 10 minutes | Servings 4) Per serving: 273 Calories; 11.7g Fat; 6.7g Carbs; 34.2g Protein; 4.1g Fiber

Ingredients

1 pound tuna steak 8 ounces bocconcini 1 teaspoon sesame oil 1 teaspoon balsamic vinegar 1 tablespoon fish sauce 1/2 cup radicchio, sliced 1 tomato, diced 1/2 cup black olives, pitted and sliced 2 teaspoons tahini paste 1/2 teaspoon chili pepper, finely chopped 1 head Romaine lettuce 2 garlic cloves, minced 1/2 cup onion, thinly sliced 2 bell peppers, sliced 1 Lebanese cucumber, sliced

Directions

Grill the tuna over medium-high heat for about 4 minutes per side. Flake the fish with a fork. Mix the vegetables in a salad bowl. In a small mixing dish, thoroughly combine the tahini, sesame oil, vinegar, and fish sauce. Dress the salad.Enjoy!

378.   Zingy Tuna Steaks with Spinach

(Ready in about 20 minutes | Servings 6) Per serving: 444 Calories; 38.2g Fat; 4.7g Carbs; 21.9g Protein; 1g Fiber

Ingredients

2 pounds tuna steaks 3 cups spinach 1 tablespoon Dijon mustard 3 tablespoons peanut oil Salt and pepper, to season 1/2 cup radishes, thinly sliced 1 fresh lemon, sliced 1 cup green onions, thinly sliced

Directions

Brush each tuna steaks with peanut oil and season them with salt and pepper. Arrange the tuna steaks on a foil-lined baking pan. Top with lemon slices, cover with foil and roast at 400 degrees F for about 10 minutes. Bon appétit!

379.   Mackerel and Vegetable Casserole

(Ready in about 30 minutes | Servings 4) Per serving: 301 Calories; 14g Fat; 6g Carbs; 33.3g Protein; 3.2g Fiber

Ingredients

1 pound mackerel steaks, chopped 1/2 stick butter Salt and black pepper, to your liking 1/4 cup fish consommé 1 cup goat cheese, shredded 1/2 cup fresh scallions, chopped 1/2 cup celery, thinly sliced 1 cup parsnip, thinly sliced 2 cloves garlic, thinly sliced 2 shallots, thinly sliced 2 tomatoes, thinly sliced

Directions

In a frying pan, melt the butter in over a moderately high heat. Cook the vegetables until they are just tender and fragrant. Add in the clam juice and tomatoes and cook for a further 5 minutes. Place the sautéed vegetables in a lightly-greased casserole dish. Lower the mackerel steaks on top of the vegetable layer. Sprinkle with salt and pepper. Bake in the preheated oven at 420 degrees F for about 15 minutes. Top with shredded cheese and bake for a further 5 to 6 minutes or until it is hot and bubbly. Bon appétit!

380.   Clams with Garlic-Tomato Sauce

(Ready in about 25 minutes | Servings 4) Per serving: 134 Calories; 7.8g Fat; 5.9g Carbs; 8.3g Protein; 1g Fiber

Ingredients

40 littleneck clams For the Sauce: 2 tomatoes, pureed 2 tablespoons olive oil 1 shallot, chopped Sea salt and freshly ground black pepper, to taste 1/2 teaspoon paprika 1/3 cup port wine 2 garlic cloves, pressed 1/2 lemon, cut into wedges

Directions

Grill the clams until they are open, for 5 to 6 minutes. In a frying pan, heat the olive oil over moderate heat. Cook the shallot and garlic until tender and fragrant. Stir in the pureed tomatoes, salt, black pepper and paprika and continue to cook an additional 10 to 12 minutes or until thoroughly cooked. Heat off and add in the port wine; stir to combine. Garnish with fresh lemon wedges. Bon appétit!

381. Salad with Crispy-Skinned Snapper

(Ready in about 15 minutes | Servings 4) Per serving: 507 Calories; 42.8g Fat; 6g Carbs; 24.4g Protein; 2.7g Fiber

Ingredients

4 snapper fillets with skin 6 ounces Feta cheese, crumbled Sea salt and ground black pepper, to taste 1 teaspoon ground mustard seeds 1/2 teaspoon celery seeds 2 cups arugula 2 tablespoons butter, melted 2 cups lettuce leaves, torn into pieces 1 carrot, thinly sliced 1 cup spring onions, thinly sliced 1/2 cup black olives, pitted and sliced 10 grape tomatoes, halved For the Vinaigrette: 1/3 cup extra-virgin olive oil 1 teaspoon Dijon mustard 1 lime, juiced and zested 1 teaspoon ginger- garlic paste 1 teaspoon dried basil 2 tablespoons fresh mint, finely chopped Sea salt and ground black pepper, to taste

Directions

In a grill pan, melt the butter over a moderately high flame. Cook the fish for 5 to 6 minutes; flip the fish fillets over and cook them for 5 minutes more. Toss all ingredients for the salad. Whisk all ingredients for the vinaigrette and dress the salad.Top with the fish fillets, serve, and enjoy!

382. Red Snapper Soup

(Ready in about 20 minutes | Servings 4) Per serving: 316 Calories; 14.3g Fat; 6.6g Carbs; 32.7g Protein; 1.7g Fiber

Ingredients

1 pound red snapper, chopped 1 cup tomato puree 3 cups chicken stock 1/4 cup Marsala wine 2 thyme sprigs, chopped 1/2 teaspoon dried rosemary 1/2 stick butter, melted 1 medium leek, finely chopped 2 garlic cloves, minced 1/4 cup fresh parsley, chopped Sea salt and ground black pepper, to taste

Directions

In a heavy-bottomed pot, melt the butter over a moderately high heat. Cook the leek and garlic for 3 to 4 minutes or until tender and fragrant. Add in the parsley, tomato puree, chicken stock, wine, red snapper, and rosemary; bring to a rolling boil. Turn the heat to simmer; continue to simmer until the thoroughly cooked for a further 15 to 20 minutes. Season with salt and pepper to taste. Enjoy!

383. Rich and Spicy Seafood Stew

(Ready in about 25 minutes | Servings 4) Per serving: 296 Calories; 8.6g Fat; 5.5g Carbs; 41.4g Protein; 4.3g Fiber

Ingredients

1/2 pound sole, cut into 2-inch pieces 1/3 pound halibut, cut into 2-inch pieces 1/2 cup Marsala wine 1/8 teaspoon hot sauce, or more to taste 1 tablespoon lard, room temperature 1 cup shallots, chopped 1 teaspoon garlic, smashed Sea salt and black pepper, to taste 4 cups chicken bone broth 1 cup tomato sauce 2 thyme sprigs, chopped

Directions

In a large-sized pot, melt the lard over medium-high heat. Cook the shallots and garlic until they've softened. Add in the salt, black pepper, chicken bone broth, tomato sauce, and thyme and; continue to cook an additional 15 minutes. Add in the fish, wine and hot sauce; bring to a boil. Reduce the heat to simmer. Let it simmer for 4 to 5 minutes longer, stirring periodically. Enjoy!

384.   Greek Salad with Grilled Halloumi

(Ready in about 15 minutes | Servings 4) Per serving: 199 Calories; 10.6g Fat; 6.1g Carbs; 14.2g Protein; 1.1g Fiber

Ingredients

1 pound halibut steak 1 cup cherry tomatoes, halved 1 onion, thinly sliced 1 tablespoon lemon juice 1 Lebanese cucumbers, thinly sliced 1/2 cup radishes, thinly sliced 2 tablespoons sunflower seeds 1 ½ tablespoons extra-virgin olive oil 1/2 head butterhead lettuce 1 cup Halloumi cheese Sea salt and pepper, to taste

Directions

Cook the halibut steak on preheated grill for 5 to 6 minutes per side. until the fish flakes easily with a fork. Grill the halloumi cheese and slice into small pieces. Toss the grilled halloumi cheese with the remaining ingredients and set aside.Serve with chilled salad and enjoy!

385.   Sour Cream Salmon with Parmesan

Ready in about: 25 minutes | Serves: 4 Per serving: Kcal 288, Fat 23.4g, Net Carbs 1.2g, Protein 16.2g

Ingredients

1 cup sour cream 1 tbsp fresh dill, chopped ½ lemon, zested and juiced Pink Salt and black pepper to taste 4 salmon steaks ½ cup Parmesan cheese, grated Preheat oven to 400°F.

Directions

In a bowl, mix the sour cream, dill, lemon zest, juice, salt, and pepper. Season the fish with salt and black pepper, drizzle lemon juice on both sides of the fish, and arrange them on a lined baking sheet. Spread the sour cream mixture on each fish and sprinkle with Parmesan cheese. Bake the fish for 15 minutes and after broil the top for 2 minutes with a close watch for a nice brown color. Plate the fish and serve with buttery green beans.

386.   Steamed Salmon with Creamy Cucumber Sauce

Ready in about: 30 minutes | Serves: 4 Per serving: Kcal 458, Fat 30.4g, Net Carbs 2.6g, Protein 39.1g

Ingredients

4 salmon fillets, skin on 10 oz broccoli florets 2 tbsp olive oil 1 cucumber, diced 1 cup crème fraiche ¼ tsp lemon juice Salt and black pepper to taste 2 tbsp fresh dill

Directions

Combine the cucumber, crème fraiche, fresh dill, and lemon juice in a bowl. Season with salt and stir thoroughly. Cover and place in the refrigerator to chill until ready to use. Fill a large pot halfway up with water and place in a steamer basket; bring to a boil. Add in the broccoli florets and season with salt. Steam the broccoli for 6 minutes, until they are tender-crisp but still vibrant green. Transfer to a bowl and drizzle with olive oil; tent with foil to keep warm. Put the salmon in the basket, skin side down and sprinkle with salt and pepper. Cook for 8-10 minutes until the fish flakes easily. Serve the salmon topped with cucumber sauce and broccoli on the side.

387.   Creamy Hoki with Almond Bread Crust

Ready in about: 50 minutes | Serves: 4 Per serving: Kcal 386, Fat 27g, Net Carbs 3.5g, Protein 28.5g

Ingredients

1 cup flaked smoked hoki, boneless 1 cup cubed hoki fillets, cubed 4 eggs 3 tbsp almond flour 1 onion, sliced 2 cups sour cream 1 tbsp chopped parsley 1 cup pork rinds, crushed 1 cup grated cheddar cheese Salt and black pepper to taste 2 tbsp butter

Directions

Boil the eggs in salted water in a pot over medium heat for 10 minutes. Run the eggs under cold water and peel the shells. After, place on a cutting board and chop them. Melt the butter in a saucepan over medium heat and sauté the onion for 4 minutes. Turn the heat off and stir in the almond flour to form a roux. Turn the heat back on and cook the roux until golden brown and stir in the sour cream until the mixture is smooth. Season with salt and pepper and stir in the parsley. Preheat oven to 360°F. Spread the smoked and cubed fish on a greased baking dish, sprinkle the eggs on top, and spoon the sauce over. In a bowl, mix pork rinds and cheddar cheese and spread over the sauce. Bake the casserole in the oven for 20 minutes until the top is golden and the sauce and cheese are bubbly. Remove the bake after and serve with a steamed green vegetable mix.

388.   Blackened Fish Tacos with Slaw

Ready in about: 20 minutes | Serves: 4 Per serving: Kcal 268, Fat: 20g, Net Carbs: 3.5g, Protein: 13.8g

Ingredients

1 tbsp olive oil 1 tsp chili powder 2 tilapia fillets 1 tsp paprika 4 low carb tortillas Slaw ½ cup red cabbage, shredded 1 tbsp lemon juice 1 tsp apple cider vinegar 1 tbsp olive oil Salt and black pepper to taste

Directions

Season the tilapia with chili powder and paprika. Heat the olive oil in a skillet over medium heat. Add tilapia and cook until blackened, about 3 minutes per side. Cut into strips. Divide the tilapia between the tortillas. Combine all slaw ingredients in a bowl and top the fish to serve.

389.   Sicilian-Style Sardines with Zoodles

Ready in about: 10 minutes | Serves: 2 Per serving: Kcal 355, Fat: 31g, Net Carbs: 6g, Protein: 20g

Ingredients

4 cups zoodles (zucchini spirals) 2 oz cubed bacon 4 oz canned sardines, chopped ½ cup canned tomatoes, chopped 1 tbsp capers 1 garlic clove, minced

Directions

Pour some of the sardine oil into a pan over medium heat. Add the garlic and sauté for 1 minute. Stir in bacon and cook for 2 more minutes. Pour in the tomatoes and simmer for 5 minutes. Add zoodles and sardines and cook for 3 minutes. Transfer to a serving plate and top with capers. Serve.

390. Cod in Garlic Butter Sauce

Ready in about: 20 minutes | Serves: 6 Per serving: Kcal 264, Fat 17.3g, Net Carbs 2.3g, Protein 20g

Ingredients

2 tsp olive oil 6 Alaska cod fillets Salt and black pepper to taste 4 tbsp butter 3 cloves garlic, minced ⅓ cup lemon juice 3 tbsp white wine 2 tbsp chopped chives Heat the oil in a skillet over medium heat.

Directions

Season the cod with salt and black pepper. Fry the fillets in the oil for 4 minutes on one side, flip, and cook for 1 minute. Take out, plate, and set aside. In the same skillet over, Melt the butter and sauté the garlic for 3 minutes. Add the lemon juice, white wine, and chives. Season with salt and black pepper and cook for 3 minutes until the wine slightly reduces. Put the fish in a platter, spoon the sauce over, and serve with buttered green beans.

391. Coconut Crab Patties

Ready in about: 15 minutes | Serves: 4 Per serving: Kcal 215, Fat: 11.5g, Net Carbs: 3.6g, Protein: 15.3g

Ingredients

2 tbsp coconut oil 1 tbsp lemon juice 1 lb lump crab meat 2 tsp Dijon mustard 1 egg, beaten 1 ½ tbsp coconut flour

DirectionsIn a bowl, add all the ingredients except the oil and mix well. Make patties out of the mixture. Melt the coconut oil in a skillet over medium heat. Add the crab patties and cook for about 2-3 minutes per side.

392. Lemon Garlic Shrimp

Ready in about: 22 minutes | Serves: 6 Per serving: Kcal 258, Fat 22g, Net Carbs 2g, Protein 13g

Ingredients

½ cup butter, divided 2 lb shrimp, peeled and deveined Salt and black pepper to taste ¼ tsp sweet paprika 3 garlic cloves, minced 1 lemon, zested and juiced

DirectionsMelt the butter in a skillet over medium heat. Season the shrimp with salt, pepper, and paprika and add to the butter. Cook for 4 minutes on both sides until pink. Set aside. Include the lemon zest, juice, garlic, and 3 tbsp water to the skillet. Return the shrimp and cook for 2 minutes. Serve warm.

393. Italian-Style Seafood Stew

(Ready in about 20 minutes | Servings 4) Per serving: 209 Calories; 12.6g Fat; 6.6g Carbs; 15.2g Protein; 2g Fiber

Ingredients

2 tablespoons lard, room temperature 1/2 teaspoon lime zest 1/2 pound shrimp 1/2 pound scallops 1 teaspoon Italian seasonings blend Salt and ground black pepper, to taste 1 leek, chopped 2 garlic cloves, pressed 1 cup tomato puree 1 celery stalk, chopped 3 cups fish stock 2 tablespoons port wine

Directions

Melt the lard in a large pot over a moderately high heat. Sauté the leek and garlic until they've softened. Stir in the pureed tomatoes and continue to cook for about 10 minutes. Add in the remaining ingredients and bring to a boil. Turn the heat to a simmer and continue to cook for 4 to 5 minutes. Enjoy!

394. Creole Tuna with Lemon

(Ready in about 40 minutes | Servings 4) Per serving: 266 Calories; 11.5g Fat; 5.6g Carbs; 34.9g Protein; 0.7g Fiber

Ingredients

4 tuna fillets 1/4 cup scallions, chopped 2 garlic cloves, minced 1/3 cup fresh lemon juice 1/3 cup coconut aminos 3 teaspoons olive oil 1 teaspoon lemon thyme Salt and ground black pepper 1 teaspoon dried rosemary

Directions

Place all ingredients in a ceramic dish; cover and let it marinate for about 30 minutes in the refrigerator. Grill the tuna fillets for about 15 minutes, basting with the reserved marinade.

395. Pepper Boats with Herring

(Ready in about 10 minutes | Servings 4) Per serving: 120 Calories; 5.4g Fat; 5.8g Carbs; 12.3g Protein; 1.6g Fiber

Ingredients

4 pickled peppers, slice into halves 8 ounces canned herring, drained 1 teaspoon Dijon mustard 1 celery, chopped 1 cup onions, chopped Salt and freshly ground black pepper, to taste 1 tablespoon fresh coriander, chopped

Directions

Broil the bell pepper for 5 to 6 minutes until they've softened. Cut into halves and discard the seeds. In a mixing bowl, thoroughly combine the herring, Dijon mustard, celery, onions, salt, black pepper, and fresh coriander. Mix to combine well. Spoon the mixture into the bell pepper halves.Reheat the thawed peppers at 200 degrees F until they are completely warm. Enjoy!

396. Old-Fashioned Seafood Chowder

(Ready in about 15 minutes | Servings 5) Per serving: 404 Calories; 30g Fat; 5.3g Carbs; 23.9g Protein; 0.3g Fiber

Ingredients

1/2 stick butter 3/4 pound prawns, peeled and deveined 1/2 pound crab meat 2 tablespoons scallions, chopped 1 tablespoon tomato sauce 1 teaspoon Mediterranean spice mix 1 egg, lightly beaten 2 garlic cloves, minced 1/3 cup port wine 1 quart chicken bone broth 2 cups double cream

Directions

In a heavy bottomed pot, melt the butter over a moderately high flame. Sauté the scallions and garlic until they've softened. Add in the prawns, crab meat, wine, and chicken bone broth. Continue to cook until thoroughly heated for 5 to 6 minutes. Decrease the heat to low; add in the remaining ingredients and continue to simmer for 5 minutes more.Enjoy!

397.   Chinese-Style Mackerel Chowder

(Ready in about 30 minutes | Servings 6) Per serving: 165 Calories; 5.5g Fat; 4g Carbs; 25.4g Protein; 0.5g Fiber

Ingredients

1 ¼ pounds mackerel, cut into small pieces 1 tablespoon peanut oil 1 chili pepper, deveined and sliced 1 tablespoon coconut aminos 1/4 cup fresh mint, chopped 2 ½ cups hot water 1 teaspoon Five-spice powder 1/2 cup white onions, sliced 1 garlic clove, smashed 1 celery rib, diced 1 bell pepper, deveined and sliced 3/4 cup heavy cream

Directions

Heat the oil in a large pot over a moderately high heat. Cook the onion and garlic until they are just tender or about 3 minutes. Stir in the celery, peppers, coconut aminos, water, and Five-spice powder. Reduce to a simmer, and cook, partially covered, for 15 minutes. Fold in the fish chunks and continue to simmer an additional 15 minutes or until cooked through. Add in the heavy cream and remove from heat.Serve with fresh mint leaves and enjoy!

398.   Colorful Prawn Salad

(Ready in about 10 minutes + chilling time | Servings 6) Per serving: 209 Calories; 9.5g Fat; 6.8g Carbs; 20.2g Protein; 0.4g Fiber

Ingredients

1 medium-sized lemon, cut into wedges 2 pounds prawns 1/2 cup mayonnaise 1/2 cup cream cheese 1/2 teaspoon stone-ground mustard 1 tablespoon dry sherry 1 tablespoon balsamic vinegar Salt and black pepper 4 scallion stalks, chopped 1 Italian pepper, sliced 1 cucumber, sliced 1 ½ cups radishes, sliced 1 tablespoon Sriracha sauce

Directions

Bring a pot of a lightly salted water to a boil over high heat. Add in the lemon and prawns and cook approximately 3 minutes, until they are opaque. Drain and rinse your prawns. In a salad bowl, toss the remaining ingredients until well combined.Top with the prepared prawns and serve!

399.   Salmon and Ricotta Stuffed Tomatoes

(Ready in about 30 minutes | Servings 6) Per serving: 303 Calories; 22.9g Fat; 6.8g Carbs; 17g Protein; 1.6g Fiber

Ingredients

6 tomatoes, pulp and seeds removed 1 ½ cups Ricotta cheese 10 ounces salmon 1 cup scallions, finely chopped 2 garlic cloves, minced 2 tablespoons coriander, chopped 1/2 cup aioli 1 teaspoon Dijon mustard Sea salt and ground black pepper, to taste

Directions

Grill your salmon for about 10 minutes until browned and flakes easily with a fork. Cut into small chunks. Thoroughly combine the salmon, scallions, garlic, coriander, aioli, mustard, salt, and pepper in a bowl. Spoon the filling into tomatoes. Bake in the preheated oven at 390 degrees F for 17 to 20 minutes until they are thoroughly cooked.Enjoy!

400.   Haddock and Vegetable Skewers

(Ready in about 15 minutes | Servings 4) Per serving: 257 Calories; 12.5g Fat; 7g Carbs; 27.5g Protein; 0.9g Fiber

Ingredients

1 pound haddock, cut into small cubes Salt and pepper, to taste 1/2 teaspoon basil 2 tablespoons olive oil 1 red onion, cut into wedges 1 zucchini, diced 1 cup cherry tomatoes 2 tablespoons coconut aminos

Directions

Start by preheating your grill on high. Toss the haddock and vegetables with salt, pepper, basil, olive oil, and coconut aminos. Alternate the seasoned haddock, onion, zucchini and tomatoes on bamboo skewers. Grill your skewers for 5 minutes for medium-rare, flipping them occasionally to ensure even cooking.Bon appétit!

401.   Avocado and Shrimp Salad

(Ready in about 10 minutes + chilling time | Servings 6) Per serving: 236 Calories; 14.3g Fat; 5.3g Carbs; 16.3g Protein; 3g Fiber

Ingredients

1 cup butterhead lettuce 1 avocado, pitted and sliced 1/2 cup aioli 1 pound shrimp, peeled and deveined 1/2 cup cucumber, chopped 1 shallot, thinly sliced 1 tablespoon soy sauce 2 teaspoons fresh lemon juice

Directions

Cook your shrimp in a pot of salted water for about 3 minutes. Drain and reserve. In a salad bowl, mix all ingredients, except for the lettuce leaves. Gently stir to combine. Enjoy!

402.   Classic Fish Tart

(Ready in about 45 minutes | Servings 6) Per serving: 416 Calories; 34.2g Fat; 5.5g Carbs; 19.5g Protein; 1.5g Fiber

Ingredients

For the Crust:

1 teaspoon baking powder Flaky salt, to taste 1/2 stick butter 1 cup almond meal 3 tablespoons flaxseed meal 2 teaspoons ground psyllium husk powder 2 eggs 2 tablespoons almond milk For the Filling: 10 ounces cod fish, chopped 2 eggs 1 teaspoon Mediterranean spice mix 1 ½ cups Colby cheese, shredded 1 teaspoon stone-ground mustard 1/2 cup cream cheese 1/2 cup mayonnaise

Directions

Thoroughly combine all the crust ingredients. Press the crust into a parchment-lined baking pan. Bake the crust in the preheated oven at 365 degrees F for about 15 minutes. In a mixing dish, combine the ingredients for the filling. Spread the mixture over the pie crust and bake for a further 25 minutes.Enjoy!

403. Trout with Authentic Chimichurri Sauce

(Ready in about 15 minutes | Servings 6) Per serving: 265 Calories; 20.9g Fat; 4g Carbs; 17.1g Protein; 0.7g Fiber

Ingredients

2 tablespoons butter 6 trout fillets Sea salt and ground black pepper, to taste 1/2 teaspoon curry powder 1/2 teaspoon mustard seeds For Chimichurri Sauce: 1/3 cup apple cider vinegar Kosher salt and pepper, to taste 2 garlic cloves, minced 1/2 cup yellow onion, finely chopped 1 chili pepper, finely chopped 1/2 cup fresh cilantro, minced 1 tablespoon fresh basil leaves, snipped 1/3 cup olive oil

Directions

In a cast-iron skillet, melt the butter over a moderately high heat. Season the trout fillets with salt, pepper, curry powder, and mustard seeds. Cook the trout fillets for about 5 minutes per side. To make the Chimichurri sauce, pulse the remaining ingredients in your food processor until well mixed.

404. Herby Salmon in Creamy Sauce

Ready in about: 15 minutes | Serves: 2 Per serving: Kcal 468, Fat: 40g, Net Carbs: 1.5g, Protein: 22g

Ingredients

2 salmon fillets 1 tsp dried tarragon 1 tsp dried dill 3 tbsp butter ¼ cup heavy cream Salt and black pepper to taste

Directions

Season the salmon with some dill and tarragon. Warm butter in a pan over medium heat. Add salmon and cook for 4 minutes on both sides. Set aside. In the same pan, add the remaining dill and tarragon. Cook for 30 seconds to infuse the flavors. Whisk in the heavy cream, season with salt and black pepper, and cook for 2-3 minutes. Serve the salmon topped with the sauce.

405. Trout & Fennel Parcels

Ready in about: 20 minutes | Serves: 4 Per serving: Kcal 234, Fat 9.3g, Net Carbs 2.8g, Protein 17g

Ingredients

1 lb deboned trout, butterflied Salt and black pepper to taste 3 tbsp olive oil + extra for tossing 4 sprigs thyme 4 butter cubes 1 fennel bulb, thinly sliced 1 medium red onion, sliced 8 lemon slices 3 tsp capers Preheat oven to 400°F.

Directions

Cut out parchment paper wide enough for each trout. In a bowl, toss the fennel and onion with a little bit of olive oil and share into the middle parts of the papers. Place the fish on each veggie mound, top with a drizzle of olive oil each, salt, pepper, 1 sprig of thyme, and 1 cube of butter. Lay the lemon slices on the fish. Wrap and close the packets securely and place them on a baking sheet. Bake in the oven for 15 minutes. Garnish the fish with capers and serve.

406.   Tuna Steaks with Shirataki Noodles

Ready in about: 30 minutes | Serves: 4 Per serving: Kcal 310, Fat 18.2g, Net Carbs 2g, Protein 22g

Ingredients

1 pack (7 oz) miracle noodle angel hair 1 red bell pepper, seeded and halved 4 tuna steaks Salt and black pepper to taste 2 tbsp olive oil 2 tbsp pickled ginger 2 tbsp chopped cilantro 1 tbsp olive oil

Directions

In a colander, rinse the shirataki noodles with running cold water. Bring a pot of salted water to a boil. Blanch the noodles for 2 minutes. Drain and transfer to a dry skillet over medium heat. Dry roast for a minute until opaque. Grease a grill grate with olive oil and preheat to medium heat. Season the red bell pepper and tuna with salt and pepper, brush with olive oil, and grill covered for 3 minutes on each side. Transfer to a plate to cool. Assemble the noodles, tuna, and bell pepper into a serving platter. Top with pickled ginger and garnish with cilantro. Serve with roasted sesame sauce.

407.   Salmon Panzanella

Ready in about: 22 minutes | Serves: 4 Per serving: Kcal 338, Fat 21.7g, Net Carbs 3.1g, Protein 28.5g

Ingredients

1 lb skinned salmon, cut into 4 steaks each 1 cucumber, peeled, seeded, cubed Salt and black pepper to taste 8 black olives, pitted and chopped 1 tbsp capers, rinsed 2 large tomatoes, diced 3 tbsp red wine vinegar ¼ cup red onion, thinly sliced 3 tbsp olive oil 2 slices zero carb bread, cubed Preheat a grill to 350°F.

Directions

In a bowl, mix the cucumber, olives, pepper, capers, tomatoes, wine vinegar, onion, olive oil, and bread. Let sit for a few minutes to incorporate the flavors. Season the salmon with salt and pepper. Grill them on both sides for 8 minutes in total. Serve the salmon with the veggies' salad.

408.   Tilapia with Olives & Tomato Sauce

Ready in about: 30 minutes | Serves: 4 Per serving: Kcal 282, Fat: 15g, Net Carbs: 6g, Protein: 23g

Ingredients

4 tilapia fillets 2 garlic cloves, minced ½ tsp dried oregano 14 oz canned tomatoes, diced 2 tbsp olive oil ½ red onion, chopped 2 tbsp fresh parsley, chopped ¼ cup Kalamata olives

Directions

Heat olive oil in a skillet over medium heat and cook the onion for 3 minutes. Add garlic and oregano and cook for 30 seconds. Stir in tomatoes and bring the mixture to a boil. Reduce the heat and simmer for 5 minutes. Add olives and tilapia and cook for about 8 minutes. Serve the tilapia with tomato sauce.

409. Grilled Shrimp with Chimichurri Sauce

Ready in about: 10 minutes + marinating time | Serves: 4 Per serving: Kcal 283, Fat: 20.3g, Net Carbs: 3.5g, Protein: 16g

Ingredients

1 lb shrimp, peeled and deveined 2 tbsp olive oil Juice of 1 lime Chimichurri ½ tsp salt ¼ cup olive oil 2 garlic cloves ¼ cup red onions, chopped ¼ cup red wine vinegar ½ tsp pepper 2 cups parsley ¼ tsp red pepper flakes

Directions

Process the chimichurri ingredients in a blender until smooth; set aside. Combine the shrimp, olive oil, and lime juice in a bowl. Let marinate in the fridge for 30 minutes. Preheat the grill to medium heat. Add shrimp and cook for about 2 minutes per side. Serve shrimp drizzled with the chimichurri sauce.

410. Shrimp in Curry Sauce

Ready in about: 15 minutes | Serves: 2 Per serving: Kcal 560, Fat: 41g, Net Carbs: 4.3g, Protein: 24.4g

Ingredients

½ oz Parmesan cheese, grated 1 egg, beaten ¼ tsp curry powder 2 tsp almond flour ½ lb shrimp, shelled 3 tbsp coconut oil Sauce 2 tbsp curry leaves 2 tbsp butter ½ onion, diced ½ cup heavy cream ½ oz cheddar cheese, shredded

Directions

Combine all dry ingredients for the batter. Melt the coconut oil in a skillet over medium heat. Dip the shrimp in the egg first, and then coat with the dry mixture. Fry until golden and crispy, about 5-6 minutes. Melt the butter in the skillet. Add onion and cook for 3 minutes. Stir in curry leaves for 30 seconds. Mix in heavy cream and cheddar cheese and cook until thickened, 2 minutes. Add shrimp. Stir to coat. Serve.

411. Coconut Curry Mussels

Ready in about: 25 minutes | Serves: 6 Per serving: Kcal 356, Fat 20.6g, Net Carbs 0.3g, Protein 21.1g

Ingredients

3 lb mussels, cleaned, de-bearded 1 cup minced shallots 3 tbsp minced garlic 1 ½ cups coconut milk 2 cups dry white wine 2 tsp red curry powder ⅓ cup coconut oil ⅓ cup chopped green onions ⅓ cup chopped parsley

Directions

Pour the wine into a saucepan and cook the shallots and garlic over medium heat, 5 minutes. Stir in the coconut milk and red curry powder and cook for 3 minutes. Add the mussels and steam for 7 minutes or until their shells are opened. Then, use a slotted spoon to remove to a bowl leaving the sauce in the pan. Discard any closed mussels at this point. Stir the coconut oil into the sauce, turn the heat off, and stir in the parsley and green onions. Serve the mussels immediately with a butternut squash mash.

412. Cheesy Tuna Pâté

(Ready in about 10 minutes | Servings 6) Per serving: 181 Calories; 10.4g Fat; 2.1g Carbs; 19g Protein; 1g Fiber

Ingredients

2 (6-ounce) cans tuna in oil, drained 1 tablespoon fresh Italian parsley, chopped 1/2 cup Cottage cheese 1 ounce sunflower seeds, ground 1 ounce sesame seeds, ground 1/2 teaspoon mustard seeds

Directions

Add all of the above ingredients to a bowl of your blender or food processor. Blend until everything is well combined.

413. Old Bay Sea Bass Chowder

(Ready in about 30 minutes | Servings 4) Per serving: 170 Calories; 5.8g Fat; 5.7g Carbs; 20g Protein; 1.9g Fiber

Ingredients

1 ¼ pounds sea bass, skin removed, cut into small chunks 2 carrots, chopped 1/4 cup port wine 1/2 cup sour cream Sea salt and ground black pepper, to taste 1 teaspoon Old Bay seasonings 3 teaspoons olive oil 1 onion, chopped 1 celery rib, chopped 3 cups boiling water 1/2 cup fish stock

Directions In a heavy-bottomed pot, heat the olive oil over a moderately high flame. Once hot, cook the fish for about 10. Stir in the onion, celery, carrot, spices, water, and fish stock and bring to a boil. Turn the heat to medium-low. Let it simmer for 15 to 20 minutes more or until thoroughly cooked. Afterwards, add in the port wine and sour cream. Remove form the heat and stir to combine well.Bon appétit!

414. Swordfish with Mashed Cauliflower

(Ready in about 35 minutes | Servings 4) Per serving: 404 Calories; 22.2g Fat; 5.7g Carbs; 43.5g Protein; 3g Fiber

Ingredients

1 ½ tablespoons extra-virgin olive oil 1 tablespoon freshly squeezed lemon juice 1 pound swordfish cutlets, about 3/4 inch thick 1/2 cup fresh basil, roughly chopped Flaky sea salt and ground black pepper, to taste 1 ½ teaspoons Greek herb mix 1/4 cup Romano cheese, freshly grated 1 pound cauliflower, broken into florets 1/4 cup double cream 2 tablespoons butter

Directions Whisk the extra-virgin olive oil with the lemon juice. Grill the fish cutlets for about 15 minutes, basting them with the lemon mixture. Season with salt, black pepper, and Greek herb mix. Reserve, keeping them warm. Boil the cauliflower in a lightly salted water until crisp-tender. Mash the cauliflower with a potato masher. Fold in the other ingredients and stir to combine well.

415. Easy Halibut Steaks

(Ready in about 35 minutes | Servings 2) Per serving: 308 Calories; 10.9g Fat; 2g Carbs; 46.5g Protein; 0.8g Fiber

Ingredients

2 halibut steaks 1 teaspoon garlic, finely minced 1/3 cup freshly squeezed lime juice 1 teaspoon dry rosemary 1 teaspoon dry thyme 4 tablespoons fresh chives, chopped 2 teaspoons sesame oil, room temperature Flaky sea salt and white pepper, to taste

Directions

Place the fresh lime juice, sesame oil, salt, white pepper, rosemary, thyme, chives, garlic, and halibut steak in a ceramic dish; let it marinate for about 30 minutes. Grill the halibut steaks approximately 15 minutes, turning occasionally and basting with the reserved marinade.Bon appétit!

416.   Sherry and Butter Prawns

(Ready in about 10 minutes + marinating time | Servings 4) Per serving: 294 Calories; 14.3g Fat; 3.6g Carbs; 34.6g Protein; 1.4g Fiber

Ingredients

1 ½ pounds king prawns, peeled and deveined 2 tablespoons dry sherry 1 teaspoon dried basil 1/2 teaspoon mustard seeds 1 ½ tablespoons fresh lemon juice 1 teaspoon cayenne pepper, crushed 1 tablespoon garlic paste 1/2 stick butter, at room temperature

Directions

Whisk the dry sherry with cayenne pepper, garlic paste, basil, mustard seeds, lemon juice and prawns. Let it marinate for 1 hour in your refrigerator. In a frying pan, melt the butter over medium-high flame, basting with the reserved marinade. Sprinkle with salt and pepper to taste. Enjoy!

417.   Super Easy Fish Cakes

(Ready in about 30 minutes | Servings 6) Per serving: 234 Calories; 10.6g Fat; 2.5g Carbs; 31.2g Protein; 0.2g Fiber

Ingredients

1 ½ pounds tilapia fish, deboned and flaked 2 tablespoons sesame oil 1/2 cup Cottage cheese, at room temperature 2 eggs, lightly beaten 1/4 cup almond meal 1/4 tablespoons flax meal 2 teaspoons brown mustard Sea salt and pepper, to taste 2 tablespoons fresh basil, chopped

Directions

Mix the flakes fish with the eggs, almond and flax meal, cheese, mustard, salt, pepper, and basil. Form the mixture into 12 patties. Now, place the patties on a parchment-lined baking sheet. Spritz them with sesame oil. Bake in the preheated oven at 395 degrees F approximately 25 minutes, rotating the pan occasionally once. Bon appétit!

418.   Crabmeat and Vegetable Bowl

(Ready in about 10 minutes | Servings 4) Per serving: 232 Calories; 15.6g Fat; 6g Carbs; 18.9g Protein; 2g Fiber

Ingredients

12 ounces lump legs 10 Kalamata olives, pitted and halved 1/4 cup fresh scallions, chopped 2 ounces thinly sliced bacon, chopped 4 cups spinach 1 large-sized tomato, diced 3 tablespoons olive oil 1 tablespoon peanut butter 1/2 lime, zested and juiced Flaky sea salt and ground black pepper, to your liking 1/4 cup fresh parsley, chopped

Directions

Start by preheating your grill to 225 degrees F for indirect cooking. Place the crab legs on the grill grates. Close the lid and grill for about 30 minutes or until done. To prepare the dressing, whisk the oil, peanut butter, lime juice, salt, and pepper. Toss the remaining ingredients and dress your salad. Bon appétit!

419.   Creamed Halibut Fillets with Brown Mushrooms

(Ready in about 20 minutes | Servings 4) Per serving: 585 Calories; 30.5g Fat; 5.5g Carbs; 66.8g Protein; 1.1g Fiber

Ingredients

4 halibut fillets 1 ½ cups chicken stock 1/2 cup fresh scallions, chopped 1 cup sour cream 2 tablespoons olive oil 1 medium-sized leek, chopped 1/2 pound brown mushrooms, thinly sliced 2 garlic cloves, chopped Sea salt and freshly ground black pepper, to taste 1 tablespoon butter

Directions

Heat the olive oil in a saucepan over a moderately high heat. Cook the leek until tender and translucent. Add in the mushrooms, garlic, salt, and black pepper and continue to cook for 5 minutes more or until the mushrooms release liquid. Add in the halibut fillets and continue to cook over medium-high heat approximately 5 minutes on each side. Add in the butter, chicken stock, and scallions; bring to a boil. Immediately reduce the heat and let it cook for 10 minutes more or until heated through. Add in the sour cream, remove from the heat and stir to combine well.Bon appétit!

420.   Amberjack Fillets with Cheese Sauce

(Ready in about 20 minutes | Servings 6) Per serving: 285 Calories; 20.4g Fat; 1.2g Carbs; 23.8g Protein; 0.1g Fiber

Ingredients

6 amberjack fillets 1/4 cup fresh tarragon chopped 2 tablespoons olive oil, at room temperature Sea salt and ground black pepper, to taste For the Sauce: 1/3 cup vegetable broth 3/4 cup double cream 1/3 cup Romano cheese, grated 3 teaspoons butter, at room temperature 2 garlic cloves, finely minced

Directions

In a non-stick frying pan, heat the olive oil until sizzling. Once hot, fry the amberjack for about 6 minutes per side or until the edges are turning opaque. Sprinkle them with salt, black pepper, and tarragon. Reserve. To make the sauce, melt the butter in a saucepan over moderately high heat. Sauté the garlic until tender and fragrant or about 2 minutes. Add in the vegetable broth and cream and continue to cook for 5 to 6 minutes more; heat off. Stir in the Romano cheese and continue stirring in the residual heat for a couple of minutes more.Bon appétit!

421.   Refreshing Prawn Salad

(Ready in about 10 minutes | Servings 6) Per serving: 196 Calories; 8.3g Fat; 6.5g Carbs; 21.4g Protein; 1.6g Fiber

Ingredients

2 pounds tiger prawns, peeled leaving tails intact Sea salt and freshly ground black pepper, to taste 1 celery rib, sliced 1 cup white onions, chopped 1 Lebanese cucumber, chopped 1/2 head Iceberg lettuce, torn into pieces ¼ cup fresh basil, chopped Juice from 1 fresh lime ¼ cup capers, drained 1/2 cup mayonnaise

Directions

Boil the tiger prawns in a large pot of salted water for about 3 minutes. Drain well and let it cool completely. Toss the remaining ingredients in a large bowl; toss to combine well. Top with the tiger prawns and serve immediately!

422.   Family Seafood Bowl

(Ready in about 10 minutes | Servings 4) Per serving: 260 Calories; 13.6g Fat; 5.9g Carbs; 28.1g Protein; 1.5g Fiber

Ingredients

1 pound sea scallops, halved horizontally 1/2 cup Kalamata olives, pitted and sliced 2 cups arugula 1/2 tablespoon Dijon mustard 1 teaspoon garlic, chopped 1 cup cherry tomatoes, halved 1 Lebanese cucumber, sliced 1/4 cup extra-virgin olive oil 2 tablespoons fresh lime juice Sea salt and pepper, to season

Directions Boil the scallops in a pot of a lightly salted water for about 3 minutes or until opaque; place them in a serving bowl. To make the salad, toss the remaining ingredients until everything is well combined.. Enjoy!

423.   Avocado and Herring Fat Bombs

(Ready in about 5 minutes | Servings 4) Per serving: 316 Calories; 24.4g Fat; 5.9g Carbs; 17.4g Protein; 4.2g Fiber

Ingredients

1 avocado, pitted and peeled 1/2 cup scallions, chopped 1 teaspoon capers 1 can herring Salt and black pepper, to taste 3 ounces sunflower seeds 1/2 teaspoon hot paprika

Directions In a mixing bowl, combine all ingredients until well incorporated. Roll the mixture into 8 balls.Bon appétit!

424.   Smoky Sardine Salad

(Ready in about 10 minutes | Servings 4) Per serving: 195 Calories; 14.7g Fat; 6g Carbs; 7.8g Protein; 3.1g Fiber

Ingredients

1 head of Iceberg lettuce 1 pound fresh sardines, chopped 1 red onion, chopped 1 celery, thinly sliced 1/2 cup cucumber, thinly sliced Sea salt and ground black pepper, to taste 3/4 cup mayonnaise 1/2 teaspoon smoked paprika 1/4 cup fresh scallions, roughly chopped

Directions Pat your sardines dry with a kitchen paper towel. Place your sardines in a baking dish; roast them in the preehated oven at 390 degrees F for 20 minutes. Toss the remaining ingredients in a salad bowl.Top your salad with the sardines and enjoy!

425.   Pan-Seared Halibut with Herb Sauce

(Ready in about 20 minutes | Servings 4) Per serving: 273 Calories; 19.2g Fat; 4.3g Carbs; 22.6g Protein; 0.7g Fiber

Ingredients

2 tablespoons butter, at room temperature 4 halibut steaks 1 teaspoon garlic 1 ½ tablespoons extra-virgin olive oil 1/2 cup white onions, chopped 1 tablespoon fish sauce Salt and ground black pepper, to taste 1 tablespoon soy sauce 2 cloves garlic, finely minced 3 tablespoons fish consommé 2 tablespoons fresh coriander, chopped 1/4 cup Italian parsley, finely chopped 1 tablespoon fresh lemon juice

Directions

Melt the butter in a saucepan over medium-high heat. Once hot, sear the halibut for 6 to 7 minutes until cooked all the way through. Reserve. In the same pan, sauté the onions and garlic until tender and fragrant. Add in the fish consommé along with the coriander, fish sauce, and reserved halibut steaks; continue to cook, partially covered, for 5 to 6 minutes. Whisk the remaining ingredients for the herb sauce.

426. Oven-Baked Sole Fillets

(Ready in about 30 minutes | Servings 4) Per serving: 195 Calories; 8.2g Fat; 0.5g Carbs; 28.7g Protein; 0.6g Fiber

Ingredients

2 tablespoons olive oil 1/2 tablespoon Dijon mustard 1 teaspoon garlic paste 1/2 tablespoon fresh ginger, minced 1/2 teaspoon porcini powder Salt and ground black pepper, to taste 1/2 teaspoon paprika 4 sole fillets 1/4 cup fresh parsley, chopped

Directions

Combine the oil, Dijon mustard, garlic paste, ginger, porcini powder, salt, black pepper and paprika. Rub this mixture all over sole fillets. Place the sole fillets in a lightly oiled baking pan. Bake in the preheated oven at 400 degrees F for about 20 minutes.Serve with fresh parsley.

427. Green Salad with Crab Mayo

(Ready in about 15 minutes | Servings 4) Per serving: 293 Calories; 27.1g Fat; 6.3g Carbs; 9.3g Protein; 3.3g Fiber

Ingredients

For the Crab Mayo:

1 pound crabmeat 2 egg yolks Coarse sea salt and ground black pepper, to season 1 teaspoon garlic, pressed 1/2 teaspoon basil 1/2 tablespoon Dijon mustard 3/4 cup extra-virgin olive oil 1/2 teaspoon Sriracha sauce 2 tablespoons fresh lime juice For the Salad: A bunch of scallions, chopped 1 cup radishes, sliced 1 head Romaine lettuce 1 cup Arugula 1 Spanish pepper, julienned

Directions

Mix the egg yolks and mustard in your blender; pour in the oil in a tiny stream, and continue to blend. Now, add in the Sriracha sauce, lime juice, salt, black pepper, garlic, basil, and crabmeat. Toss the remaining ingredients in a salad bowl. Add in prepared crab mayo sauce and gently stir to combine.Serve well-chilled.

428. Shrimp with Mignonette Sauce

(Ready in about 15 minutes | Servings 4) Per serving: 252 Calories; 7.3g Fat; 5.3g Carbs; 36.6g Protein; 2.5g Fiber

Ingredients

1 ½ tablespoons butter, melted 1 large onion, chopped 1 teaspoon garlic, minced 1 cup tomato puree Salt and pepper, to taste 1 ½ pounds shrimp, shelled and deveined 2 tablespoons dry sherry For Mignonette Sauce: 1/2 cup onion, chopped 1 teaspoon black pepper, coarsely ground 1/2 cup white wine vinegar

Directions

Melt the butter in a sauté pan over a moderately high heat. Then, cook the onion and garlic until they are tender and fragrant. Add in the tomato puree and season with salt and pepper to taste; add in shrimp and continue to cook until thoroughly cooked. Remove from heat and add in dry sherry. Wisk all ingredients for Mignonette sauce. Bon appétit!

429. Classic Tuna and Avocado Salad

(Ready in about 20 minutes | Servings 4) Per serving: 244 Calories; 12.7g Fat; 5.3g Carbs; 23.4g Protein; 4.4g Fiber

Ingredients

1 ½ pounds tuna steaks 1 avocado, pitted, peeled and diced Salt and ground black pepper, to taste 2 tablespoons fresh lemon juice 1 head lettuce 1/2 cup black olives, pitted and sliced 2 Italian peppers, deveined and sliced 1 cup grape tomatoes, halved 1 shallot, chopped 1/4 cup mayonnaise

Directions

Grill the tuna steaks for about 15 minutes; cut into chunks. In a salad bowl, mix lettuce, peppers, tomatoes, shallot, and avocado. Then, make the dressing by mixing the mayonnaise, salt, pepper and lime juice. Dress the salad and toss to combine. Top with black olives.Top your salad with the tuna chunks and serve!

430. Seafood Gumbo with a Twist

(Ready in about 25 minutes | Servings 4) Per serving: 481 Calories; 26.9g Fat; 5g Carbs; 46.6g Protein; 1.3g Fiber

Ingredients

2 tablespoons lard, melted 2 breakfast sausages, cut crosswise into 1/2-inch-thick slices 2 garlic cloves, finely minced 1 yellow onion, chopped 1 cup tomatoes, pureed 1 tablespoon fish sauce 3/4 cup fish consommé 1/3 cup port wine 1/2 pound tilapia, cut into chunks 20 sea scallops 2 tablespoons fresh coriander, chopped

Directions

In a stock pot, melt the lard over medium-high heat. Cook the sausages for about 5 minutes until no longer pink; reserve. Now, sauté the onion and garlic until they've softened; reserve. Add in the pureed tomatoes, fish sauce, fish consommé and wine; let it simmer for another 15 minutes. Add in the tilapia, scallops, coriander, and reserved sausages. Continue to simmer, partially covered, for 5 to 6 minutes.Garnish with coriander and enjoy!

431. Chinese-Style Mackerel

(Ready in about 35 minutes | Servings 4) Per serving: 415 Calories; 28g Fat; 4.4g Carbs; 34.5g Protein; 1.8g Fiber

Ingredients

For the Fish: 1 pound mackerel fillets 1/3 cup Shaoxing wine Sea salt and ground black pepper, to taste ½ teaspoon cayenne pepper 2 tablespoons avocado oil 2 tablespoons coconut aminos

For the Mushroom Coulis: 1 ½ ounces sesame oil 1 Spanish pepper, deveined and chopped Salt and ground black pepper, to taste 1/2 shallot, peeled and chopped 1/4 teaspoon cardamom 2 ounces button mushrooms, chopped 3 tablespoons Shaoxing wine

Directions In a wok, heat the avocado oil over a moderately high heat. Season the fish with salt, black pepper, and cayenne pepper. Cook the fish for about 10 minutes until golden brown; reserve. Add in 1/3 cup of Shaoxing wine and coconut aminos; bring to a boil. Turn the heat to simmer and continue to cook for 4 to 5 minutes. Add the mackerel fillets back to the pan, and continue to cook for 4 minutes longer. To make the mushroom coulis, heat sesame oil in a wok that is preheated over a moderate flame. Now, cook the shallots until tender and translucent or about 3 minutes. Turn the heat to simmer and stir in the peppers and mushrooms along with 3 tablespoons of Shaoxing wine; cook for 10 minutes longer or until the vegetables have softened. Add in salt, black pepper, and cardamom. Puree the sautéed mixture in your blender until creamy and uniform.Enjoy!

432.   Cod Fish with Broccoli and Chutney

(Ready in about 30 minutes | Servings 4) Per serving: 291 Calories; 9.5g Fat; 3.5g Carbs; 42.5g Protein; 3g Fiber

Ingredients

1 pound broccoli, cut into florets 1 teaspoon paprika 1 ½ pounds cod fish 2 Spanish peppers, thinly sliced 1 onion, thinly sliced 2 tablespoons sesame oil Sea salt and freshly ground black pepper, to taste For Tomato Chutney: 1 cup tomatoes, chopped 1 teaspoon sesame oil 2 garlic cloves, sliced Sea salt and ground black pepper, to taste

Directions

In a frying pan, heat 2 tablespoons of sesame oil over a moderately high flame. Stir in the broccoli florets, Spanish peppers, and onion until they've softened; season with salt, black pepper, and paprika; reserve. In the same pan, sear the fish for 4 to 5 minutes per side. To make the chutney, heat 1 teaspoon of sesame oil in a frying pan over a moderately high heat. Sauté the garlic until just browned or about 1 minute. Add in the chopped tomatoes and continue to cook, stirring periodically, until cooked through. Season with salt and pepper to taste.Enjoy

433.   Spicy Fish Curry

(Ready in about 25 minutes | Servings 6) Per serving: 270 Calories; 16.9g Fat; 5.6g Carbs; 22.3g Protein; 1.5g Fiber

Ingredients

2 pounds pollock, cut into large pieces 1 teaspoon fresh garlic, minced Salt and black pepper, to taste 1 cup coconut milk 4 Roma tomatoes, pureed 2 tablespoons sesame oil 1 cup white onions, chopped 8 fresh curry leaves 2 tablespoons fresh lime juice 2 green chilies, minced 1/2 tablespoon fresh ginger, grated 1 teaspoon mustard seeds 1 tablespoon ground coriander

Directions

Drizzle the fish with lime juice. Heat the sesame oil in a frying pan over a moderately high flame. Cook the onion, curry leaves and garlic for 3 to 4 minutes until tender and aromatic. Add in the ginger, salt, pepper, tomatoes, mustard seeds, and ground coriander. Let it simmer for 12 minutes or until thoroughly cooked. Add in the fish and coconut milk and continue to cook, partially covered, for 6 to 7 minutes longer.Bon appétit!

434.   Pistachio-Crusted Salmon with Asparagus

Ready in about: 35 minutes | Serves: 4 Per serving: Kcal 474, Fat: 31, Net Carbs: 3.8g, Protein: 44.4g

Ingredients

4 salmon fillets Salt and black pepper to taste 1 tbsp Dijon mustard 2 tbsp crushed pork rinds ½ cup crushed pistachios 2 tbsp fresh dill, chopped 2 tbsp olive oil 1 lemon, cut into wedges 1 lb asparagus spears Preheat oven to 370ºF.

Directions

In a small bowl, combine the pork rinds, pistachios, and 1 tbsp of olive oil; stir with a fork to combine. Brush the salmon with Dijon mustard and season with salt and pepper. Press down the pistachio mixture on the salmon to form a crust. Coat the asparagus with the remaining olive oil and season with salt and pepper in a bowl. Lay the salmon on a greased baking dish. Arrange the asparagus around the salmon, and bake in the oven for 15-20 minutes until the salmon is flaky to the touch. Top with chopped dill and serve with lemon wedges on the side.

435.   Spicy Sea Bass with Hazelnuts

Ready in about: 20 minutes | Serves: 2 Per serving: Kcal 467, Fat: 31g, Net Carbs: 2.8g, Protein: 40g

Ingredients

2 sea bass fillets 2 tbsp butter, melted ⅓ cup roasted hazelnuts A pinch of cayenne pepper Preheat oven to 425°F.

Directions

Line a baking dish with waxed paper. Brush the butter over the fish. Process the cayenne pepper and hazelnuts in a food processor to achieve a smooth consistency. Coat the sea bass with the hazelnut mixture. Place in the oven and bake for about 15 minutes. Serve with mashed parsnips.

436.   Red Cabbage Tilapia Bowl

Ready in about: 20 minutes | Serves: 4 Per serving: Kcal 269, Fat 23.4g, Net Carbs 4g, Protein 16.5g

Ingredients

2 cups cauli rice 2 tsp ghee 4 tilapia fillets, cut into cubes Salt and chili pepper to taste ¼ head red cabbage, shredded 1 ripe avocado, pitted and chopped

Directions

Sprinkle cauli rice in a bowl with a little water and microwave for 3 minutes. Fluff after with a fork and set aside. Melt ghee in a skillet over medium heat, rub the tilapia with the taco seasoning, salt, and chili pepper and fry until brown on all sides, about 8 minutes. Transfer to a plate and set aside. Share the cauli rice, cabbage, fish, and avocado in 4 serving bowls. Serve with chipotle lime sour cream dressing.

437.   Seared Scallops with Chorizo and Asiago Cheese

Ready in about: 15 minutes | Serves: 4 Per serving: Kcal 491, Fat 32g, Net Carbs 5g, Protein 36g

Ingredients

2 tbsp ghee 16 fresh scallops 8 oz chorizo, chopped 1 red bell pepper, sliced 1 cup red onions, finely chopped 1 cup asiago cheese, grated Salt and black pepper to taste

Directions

Melt half of the ghee in a skillet over medium heat, and cook the onion and bell pepper for 5 minutes until tender. Add the chorizo and stir-fry for another 3 minutes. Remove and set aside. Pat dry the scallops with paper towels and season with salt and pepper. Add the remaining ghee to the skillet and sear the scallops for 2 minutes on each side to have a golden brown color. Add the chorizo mixture back and warm through. Transfer to serving platter and top with asiago cheese.

438.   Sushi Shrimp Rolls

Ready in about: 10 minutes | Serves: 4 Per serving: Kcal 216, Fat: 10g, Net Carbs: 1g, Protein: 18.7g

Ingredients

2 cups cooked and chopped shrimp 1 tbsp sriracha sauce 1 cucumber, julienned 4 hand roll nori sheets ¼ cup mayonnaise ¼ cup sugar-free soy sauce

Directions

Combine shrimp, mayonnaise, cucumber, and sriracha sauce in a bowl. Lay out a single nori sheet on a flat surface and spread about 1/4 of the shrimp mixture. Roll the nori sheet as desired. Repeat with the other ingredients. Serve with sugar-free soy sauce.

439.   Shrimp Stuffed Zucchini

Ready in about: 50 minutes | Serves: 4 Per serving: Kcal 135, Fat 14.4g, Net Carbs 3.2g, Protein 24.6g

Ingredients

4 medium zucchinis 1 lb small shrimp, peeled, deveined 1 tbsp onion paste 2 tsp cold butter ¼ cup tomatoes, chopped Salt and black pepper to taste 1 cup pork rinds, crushed 1 tbsp basil leaves, chopped 2 tbsp butter, melted Preheat oven to 350°F.

Directions

Trim off the top and bottom ends of the zucchinis. Lay them flat on a chopping board and cut a ¼-inch off the top to create a boat for the stuffing. Scoop out the seeds and set aside. Melt the cold butter in a skillet and sauté the onion, zucchini flesh, and tomato for 6 minutes. Transfer the mixture to a bowl and add the shrimp, half of the pork rinds, basil, salt, and pepper and mix well. Stuff the zucchini boats with the mixture. Sprinkle the top of the boats with the remaining pork rinds and drizzle the melted butter over them. Place on a baking sheet and bake for 15-20 minutes. The shrimp should no longer be pink by this time. Remove the zucchinis after and serve with a tomato salad.

440.   Cholula Shrimp Spread

(Ready in about 10 minutes + chilling time | Servings 8) Per serving: 108 Calories; 5.4g Fat; 5g Carbs; 8.2g Protein; 0.5g Fiber

Ingredients

12 ounces shrimp, canned and drained 1 tablespoon Cholula 1/2 cup mayonnaise 2 teaspoons green garlic, finely minced Sea salt and ground black pepper, to taste 1 teaspoon cayenne pepper 1/2 teaspoon dried rosemary

Directions

In a mixing bowl, stir all ingredients until well incorporated. Cover and transfer to your refrigerator until thoroughly chilled.Bon appétit!

441. Middle-Eastern Salmon with Nabulsi Cheese

(Ready in about 20 minutes | Servings 6) Per serving: 354 Calories; 20.2g Fat; 4.5g Carbs; 39.6g Protein; 0.5g Fiber

Ingredients

6 salmon fillets 1 garlic clove, finely minced 1 cup Nabulsi cheese, crumbled 3 tablespoons mayonnaise Coarse salt and black pepper, to taste 1 teaspoon Za'atar 1 cup cauliflower 1/2 cup shallots, thinly sliced 1 tablespoon fresh lemon juice 2 tablespoons sesame oil

Directions

Toss the salmon fillets with salt, pepper, and Za'atar. Place the salmon fillets on a parchment-lined baking pan; scatter the cauliflower, shallot, and garlic around the fish fillets. Wrap with the foil and bake in the preheated oven at 390 degrees F for 10 to 12 minutes or until the salmon fillets flake easily with a fork. Remove the foil. Mix the Nabulsi cheese, mayonnaise, lemon juice, and sesame oil. Pour the cheese mixture over the fish and vegetables. Bake for a further 5 minutes or until the top is hot and bubbly. Bon appétit!

442. Halibut with Creamed Cauliflower

(Ready in about 25 minutes | Servings 4) Per serving: 508 Calories; 22.9g Fat; 4.7g Carbs; 68.6g Protein; 1.4g Fiber

Ingredients

4 halibut fillets 1 head of cauliflower, broken into florets 2 tablespoons butter 1 lemon, cut into wedges 1 cup Cheddar cheese, shredded 1/2 teaspoon dried oregano 1/2 teaspoon dried rosemary Sea salt and ground black pepper, to taste

Directions

Parboil the cauliflower in a pot of lightly salted water until crisp-tender. Place in a lightly buttered baking pan; brush with melted butter, too. Season with salt and pepper to taste. Scatter the shredded Cheddar cheese on top of the cauliflower layer and bake at 385 degrees F approximately 15 minutes. Grill the halibut steaks until golden and crisp on top. Sprinkle with oregano and rosemary; salt to taste. Enjoy! Serve with lemon wedges. Bon appétit!

443. Tilapia with Spicy Dijon Sauce

(Ready in about 15 minutes + marinating time | Servings 4) Per serving: 228 Calories; 13g Fat; 6.5g Carbs; 13.7g Protein; 1.1g Fiber

Ingredients

1 tablespoon butter, room temperature 2 chili peppers, deveined and minced 1 cup heavy cream 1 teaspoon Dijon mustard 1 pound tilapia fish, cubed Sea salt and ground black pepper, to taste 1 cup white onions, chopped 1 teaspoon garlic, pressed 1/2 cup dark rum

Directions

Toss the tilapia with salt, pepper, onions, garlic, chili peppers and rum. Let it marinate for 2 hours in your refrigerator. In a grill pan, melt the butter over a moderately high heat. Sear the fish in hot butter, basting with the reserved marinade. Add in the mustard and cream and continue to cook until everything is thoroughly cooked, for 2 to 3 minutes.Bon appétit!

444.   Saucy Tuna with Brussels Sprouts

(Ready in about 25 minutes | Servings 4) Per serving: 372 Calories; 27.8g Fat; 5.6g Carbs; 26.5g Protein; 2.2g Fiber

Ingredients

1 pound tuna 1 tablespoon fresh lemon juice 1/4 cup extra-virgin olive oil 1 tomato, chopped Sea salt and freshly ground black pepper, to taste 1 teaspoon dried rosemary   1/2 cup fish stock 1/2 pounds Brussels sprouts 1/4 cup parsley 2 garlic cloves, crushed 1/3 cup pine nuts, chopped

Directions

Brush a non-stick skillet with cooking spray. Once hot, cook the tuna steaks for about 4 minutes per side; sprinkle with salt, pepper, and rosemary; set aside. In the same skillet, cook Brussels sprouts; adding the fish stock to prevent over cooking. Then, sauté for about 5 minutes or until the Brussels sprouts are crisp-tender. Add in the chopped tomatoes and continue to cook for 3 minutes more. Fold in the reserved tuna steaks. Process the parsley, garlic, pine nuts, lemon juice, and olive oil in your food processor or blender until it reaches a paste consistency. Reserve.Bon appétit!

445.   Salmon and Cheese Stuffed Peppers

(Ready in about 25 minutes | Servings 4) Per serving: 273 Calories; 13.9g Fat; 5.1g Carbs; 28.9g Protein; 2.1g Fiber

Ingredients

4 bell peppers 1 pound salmon fillets, boneless 1 onion, finely chopped 1/2 teaspoon garlic, pressed 1/3 cup mayonnaise 1/3 cup black olives, pitted and chopped Sea salt and pepper, to taste 1/2 teaspoon dried oregano 1/2 teaspoon dried oregano 1 cup cream cheese

Directions

Broil the bell pepper for 5 to 6 minutes until they've softened. Now, remove the seeds and membranes and cut the peppers in half. Cook the salmon in a lightly oiled grill pan for 5 to 6 minutes per side until the fish flakes easily with a fork. Add in the other ingredients; stir to combine well. Divide the salmon mixture between the peppers and bake in the preheated oven at 380 degrees F for about 15 minutes or until heated through.Reheat the thawed stuffed peppers at 200 degrees F until they are completely warm.

446.   Parmesan Crusted Cod

(Ready in about 15 minutes | Servings 4) Per serving: 222 Calories; 12.6g Fat; 0.9g Carbs; 27.9g Protein; 0.3g Fiber

Ingredients

1 pound cod fillets, cut into 4 servings 2 tablespoons olive oil 1/2 teaspoon paprika 3/4 cup grated Parmesan cheese Flaky sea salt and ground black pepper, to taste

Directions

In a shallow mixing dish, combine the salt pepper, paprika, and Parmesan cheese, Press the cod fillets into this Parmesan mixture. Heat the olive oil in a nonstick skillet over medium-high flame. Cook the cod fillets for 12 to 15 minutes or until opaque.Bon appétit!

Vegetarian,Soup Stew and Salad

447.   Summer Cheese Ball

(Ready in about 25 minutes | Servings 2) Per serving: 133 Calories; 9.9g Fat; 6.8g Carbs; 6g Protein; 0.7g Fiber

Ingredients

1 Lebanese cucumber, chopped 2 tablespoons pine nuts, chopped 1 teaspoon salt 1 ounce Feta cheese 1 ounce Neufchatel 1 tablespoon fresh basil, chopped

Directions

Salt the chopped cucumber and place it in a colander. Let it stand for 30 minutes; press the cucumber to drain away the excess liquid and transfer to a mixing bowl. Mix in the cheese and basil. Shape the mixture into a ball and top with chopped nuts.Enjoy!

448.   Greek-Style Roasted Asparagus

(Ready in about 15 minutes | Servings 6) Per serving: 128 Calories; 9.4g Fat; 2.9g Carbs; 6.4g Protein; 2.9g Fiber

Ingredients

1 cup Halloumi cheese, crumbled 1 red onion, chopped 2 garlic cloves, minced 1 ½ pounds asparagus spears 2 tablespoons extra-virgin olive oil Salt and black pepper, to the taste

Directions

Brush your asparagus with extra-virgin olive oil. Toss with the onion, garlic, salt, and black pepper. Roast in the preheated oven at 395 degrees F for about 15 minutes.Enjoy!

449.   Cheddar and Mushroom-Stuffed Peppers

(Ready in about 30 minutes | Servings 6) Per serving: 319 Calories; 18.8g Fat; 5.6g Carbs; 10.3g Protein; 1.9g Fiber

Ingredients

6 bell peppers, seeds and tops removed 1/2 cup Cheddar cheese, grated ½ cup tomato puree 3/4 pound Cremini mushrooms, chopped 2 tablespoons olive oil 1 onion, chopped 1 teaspoon garlic, minced 2 tablespoons fresh cilantro, chopped 1 teaspoon mustard seeds Salt to taste

Directions

In a frying pan, heat the olive oil over a moderately-high flame. Sauté the onion and garlic until they are tender and aromatic. Add in the Cremini mushrooms and continue to cook for a further 5 minutes or until the mushrooms release the liquid. Add in the cilantro, mustard seeds, and salt; stir to combine. Divide this filling between bell peppers. Place the peppers in a lightly greased casserole dish. Pour the tomato sauce around stuffed peppers. Bake at 385 degrees F for about 22 minutes or until heated through.

450. Creole Cheesy Spinach

(Ready in about 10 minutes | Servings 4) Per serving: 208 Calories; 13.5g Fat; 6g Carbs; 14.5g Protein; 5.1g Fiber

Ingredients

2 pounds spinach, torn into pieces 1/2 stick butter Sea salt and pepper, to taste 1/4 teaspoon caraway seeds 1 cup Creole cream cheese 1 teaspoon garlic, pressed

Directions

Melt the butter in a saucepan over medium-high heat; now, sauté the garlic until tender and fragrant. Add the spinach, salt, pepper, and caraway seeds; continue to cook for about 6 minutes until warmed through.Enjoy!

451. Spicy and Aromatic Chinese Cabbage

(Ready in about 15 minutes | Servings 4) Per serving: 53 Calories; 3.7g Fat; 3.2g Carbs; 1.7g Protein; 2.1g Fiber

Ingredients

3/4 pound Chinese cabbage, cored and cut into chunks 1 teaspoon Chinese Five-spice powder Salt and Sichuan pepper, to taste 1 tablespoon sesame oil 1 shallot, sliced 1/2 teaspoon chili sauce, sugar-free 2 tablespoons rice wine 1 tablespoon soy sauce

Directions

Heat the sesame oil in a wok a moderately-high heat. Sauté the shallot until tender and translucent. Add in the Chinese cabbage and continue to cook for about 3 minutes. Partially cover and add in the remaining ingredients; continue to cook for 5 minutes more.Bon appétit!

452. Old-Fashioned Cabbage with Bacon and Eggs

(Ready in about 15 minutes | Servings 4) Per serving: 173 Calories; 10.6g Fat; 5.6g Carbs; 14.2g Protein; 1.6g Fiber

Ingredients

2 cups cabbage, shredded 2 teaspoons red wine 4 eggs 4 rashers of bacon, chopped 1 cup red onions, minced 1 teaspoon garlic, smashed 1 bay laurel 1 thyme sprig 1 rosemary sprig Kosher salt and black pepper, to taste

Directions Cook the bacon in a nonstick skillet over medium-high heat; reserve. Sauté the red onions and garlic in 1 tablespoon of bacon grease. Add in the cabbage and continue to cook, stirring frequently, until it has softened or about 4 minutes. Add a splash of wine to deglaze the pan. Add in the spices and continue to cook for a further 2 minutes. Fry the eggs in 1 tablespoon of bacon grease. Add in the reserved bacon and top with fried eggs.Bon appétit!

453. Greek-Style Zucchini Patties

(Ready in about 15 minutes | Servings 6) Per serving: 153 Calories; 11.8g Fat; 6.6g Carbs; 6.4g Protein; 1.1g Fiber

Ingredients

1 pound zucchinis, shredded 1 cup Halloumi cheese, shredded 1/2 cup onion, finely chopped 1 teaspoon garlic, finely minced 2 tablespoons butter 1 egg, whisked 2 celery stalks, shredded 2 tablespoons cilantro, chopped Sea salt and pepper, to taste

Directions

Thoroughly combine all ingredients in a mixing bowl. Form the mixture into 12 patties and arrange them on a parchment-lined baking sheet. Bake in the preheated oven at 365 degrees F for 12 minutes, rotating the pan once or twice.Enjoy!

454.   Spicy Salad with Macadamia Nuts

(Ready in about 5 minutes | Servings 4) Per serving: 184 Calories; 16.8g Fat; 4g Carbs; 2.1g Protein; 1.4g Fiber

Ingredients

1 cup radishes, thinly sliced 2 cups butterhead lettuce, torn into bite-sized pieces 1 Lebanese cucumber, sliced 1 bell pepper, sliced 1 white onion, sliced 1 ounce macadamia nuts, chopped Sea salt, to season 1 tablespoon sunflower seeds 1/2 lemon, freshly squeezed 3 tablespoons olive oil 1/2 teaspoon Sriracha sauce

Directions

In a mixing bowl, toss all ingredients until well combined. Taste and adjust seasonings.

455.   Cream of Cauliflower Soup

(Ready in about 20 minutes | Servings 4) Per serving: 260 Calories; 22.5g Fat; 4.1g Carbs; 7.2g Protein; 4.2g Fiber

Ingredients

3 cups cauliflower, cut into florets 1 cup avocado, pitted and chopped Salt and pepper, to taste 1 thyme sprig 1 cup coconut milk, unsweetened 3 cups roasted vegetable broth

Directions In a heavy-bottomed pot, simmer the vegetable broth over medium-high heat. Add in the cauliflower and continue to simmer for 10 to 15 minutes more. Add in the coconut milk, avocado, salt, pepper, and thyme. Partially cover and continue to cook for a further 5 minutes. Puree the mixture in your blender.Enjoy!

456.   Greek-Style Vegetables

(Ready in about 15 minutes | Servings 4) Per serving: 318 Calories; 24.3g Fat; 5.1g Carbs; 15.4g Protein; 1.7g Fiber

Ingredients

1/2 pound brown mushrooms, chopped 1 cup broccoli, cut into small florets 1 medium-sized zucchini, chopped 8 ounces feta cheese, cubed 1 teaspoon Greek seasoning mix 2 tablespoons olive oil 1 onion, chopped 1 teaspoon garlic, minced 1 vine-ripened tomato, pureed 1/4 cup white wine

DirectionsIn a medium pot, heat the oil over a moderately-high heat. Sauté the onion and garlic for about 5 minutes, adding a splash of water if needed, until tender and aromatic. Add in the mushrooms, broccoli, zucchini, Greek seasoning mix, tomato puree, and white wine. Continue to cook for 4 to 5 minutes or until they've softened.Enjoy!

457.   Provençal-Style Green Beans

(Ready in about 15 minutes | Servings 4) Per serving: 183 Calories; 16.1g Fat; 4.4g Carbs; 3.2g Protein; 4g Fiber

Ingredients

1 pound green beans 1/2 teaspoon fresh garlic, minced 1/2 teaspoon red pepper flakes Salt and pepper, to taste 1 tablespoon butter, melted 1 celery stalk, shredded For Tapenade: 1 ½ tablespoons capers 2 anchovy fillets 1 tablespoon fresh lime juice 1/2 cup black olives 3 tablespoons extra-virgin olive oil

Directions

Steam the green beans approximately 4 minutes or until crisp-tender. In a saucepan, melt the butter over a moderately-high heat. Sauté the celery and garlic for 4 to 5 minutes or until they are tender and fragrant. Add in green beans and stir to combine. Season with red pepper, salt, and black pepper. To make the tapenade, pulse all ingredients until well combined.

458.   Broccoli with Gruyère Cheese Sauce

(Ready in about 30 minutes | Servings 6) Per serving: 159 Calories; 12.3g Fat; 7.2g Carbs; 5.7g Protein; 5.5g Fiber

Ingredients

2 pounds broccoli, cut into small florets 1/4 teaspoon turmeric powder Sea salt and black pepper, to taste 1 ½ tablespoons olive oil 1/4 cup scallions, chopped 2 tablespoons green garlic, minced   For the Sauce: 1/3 cup sour cream 1/2 cup Gruyère cheese, shredded 1 ½ tablespoons butter

Directions

Parboil the broccoli florets in a large pot of boiling water for about 3 minutes until crisp-tender. Drain. Heat the oil in a frying pan over a moderately-high heat. Once hot, cook the scallions and green garlic for about 2 minutes or until tender and aromatic. Add in the curry turmeric powder, salt, pepper and continue to sauté for 3 minutes more or until aromatic. Add a splash of vegetable broth, partially cover, and continue to cook for 6 to 7 minutes. Add the reserved broccoli back to the pan. In another pan, melt the butter over a moderately-high heat. Add in the sour cream and cheese and stir over low heat for 2 to 3 minutes.Bon appétit!

459.   Mushroom and Cauliflower Quiche

(Ready in about 35 minutes | Servings 4) Per serving: 275 Calories; 21.3g Fat; 5.3g Carbs; 14g Protein; 3g Fiber

Ingredients

1 pound cauliflower florets 1/2 pound brown mushrooms, thinly sliced 1 1/2 cup cream cheese 1 cup Gruyère cheese 1 cup cream of mushroom soup 1 teaspoon Italian herb mix 2 tablespoons butter 4 eggs, lightly beaten 1 teaspoon Dijon mustard

Directions

Melt the butter in a saucepan over medium-high heat. Now, cook the mushrooms until they release the liquid. Add in the cream of mushrooms soup, Italian herb mix, and cauliflower. Continue to sauté until the cauliflower has softened. Spoon the cauliflower mixture into a buttered casserole dish. In a mixing bowl, whisk the eggs, cheese, and Dijon mustard. Spoon the sauce over the top of your casserole. Bake in the preheated oven at 365 degrees F for about 30 minutes or until the top is hot and bubbly. Bon appétit!

460.   Japanese-Style Eringi Mushrooms

(Ready in about 15 minutes | Servings 3) Per serving: 103 Calories; 6.7g Fat; 5.9g Carbs; 2.7g Protein; 3.3g Fiber

Ingredients

8 ounces Eringi mushrooms, trim away about 1-inch of the root section Salt and Sansho pepper, to season 1 ½ tablespoons butter, melted 1 cup onions, finely chopped 2 cloves garlic, minced 2 tablespoons mirin 1/2 cup dashi stock 1 tablespoon lightly toasted sesame seeds

Directions

Melt the butter in a large pan over a moderately-high flame. Cook the onions and garlic for about 4 minutes, stirring continuously to ensure even cooking. Add in the Eringi mushrooms and continue to cook an additional 3 minutes until they are slightly shriveled. Season to taste and add in the mirin and dashi stock; continue to cook an additional 3 minutes.Enjoy!

461.   Artichoke Salad with Mozzarella Cheese

(Ready in about 25 minutes | Servings 6) Per serving: 146 Calories; 9.4g Fat; 6.1g Carbs; 5.8g Protein; 6g Fiber

Ingredients

2 tablespoons olive oil 3 artichoke hearts, defrosted Sea salt and black pepper, to taste 3/4 cup scallions, peeled and finely chopped 12/3 cup arugula 1/3 cup mustard greens 1/3 cup green cabbage 3 tablespoons capers, drained 1 chili pepper, sliced thin 3 teaspoon fresh lemon juice 1 ½ teaspoons deli mustard 2 tablespoons balsamic vinegar 2 tomatoes, sliced 2 ounces Kalamata olives, pitted and sliced 4 ounces Mozzarella cheese, crumbled

Directions

Start by preheating your oven to 350 degrees F. Line a baking sheet with parchment paper or a silicone mat. Brush the artickohe hearts with olive oil. Roast the artichoke hearts in the preheated oven at 360 degrees F for about 20 minutes. Season with salt and pepper to taste. Meanwhile, toss the vegetables with capers, lemon juice, mustard and balsamic vinegar until well combined.

462.   Homemade Cold Gazpacho Soup

Ready in about: 15 minutes + chilling time | Serves: 6 Per serving: Kcal 528, Fat: 45.8g, Net Carbs: 6.5g, Protein: 7.5g

Ingredients

2 small green peppers, roasted 2 large red peppers, roasted 2 avocados, flesh scoped out 2 garlic cloves 2 spring onions, chopped 1 cucumber, chopped 1 cup olive oil 2 tbsp lemon juice 4 tomatoes, chopped 7 oz goat cheese, crumbled 1 small red onion, chopped 2 tbsp apple cider vinegar 1 tsp xylitol Salt to taste

Directions

Place the peppers, tomatoes, avocados, red onion, garlic, lemon juice, olive oil, vinegar, xylitol, and salt in a food processor. Pulse until your desired consistency is reached. Taste and adjust the seasoning. Transfer the mixture to a pot. Stir in cucumber and spring onions. Chill in the fridge for at least 2 hours. Divide the soup between 6 bowls. Serve topped with goat cheese and an extra drizzle of olive oil. Tip: For more protein, add cooked and chopped shrimp to this refreshing delight.

463.   Power Green Soup

Ready in about: 30 minutes | Serves: 6 Per serving: Kcal 392, Fat: 37.6g, Net Carbs: 5.8g, Protein: 4.9g

Ingredients

1 broccoli head, chopped 1 cup spinach 1 onion, chopped 2 garlic cloves, minced ½ cup watercress 5 cups vegetable stock 1 cup coconut milk 1 tbsp ghee Salt and black pepper to taste

Directions

Melt the ghee in a large pot over medium heat. Add onion and garlic and cook for 3 minutes. Add broccoli and cook for an additional 5 minutes. Pour the vegetable stock over and close the lid. Bring to a boil. Reduce the heat. Simmer for 3 minutes. Add spinach and watercress and cook for 3 more minutes. Stir in the coconut cream, salt, and black pepper. Blend the soup with a hand blender. Serve warm.

464.   Creamy Cauliflower Soup with Bacon Chips

Ready in about: 25 minutes | Serves: 4 Per serving: Kcal 402, Fat 37g, Net Carbs 6g, Protein 8g

Ingredients

2 tbsp ghee 1 onion, chopped 2 head cauliflower, cut into florets 2 cups water Salt and black pepper to taste 3 cups almond milk 1 cup white cheddar cheese, grated 3 bacon strips

Directions

Melt the ghee in a saucepan over medium heat and sauté the onion for 3 minutes until fragrant. Include the cauli florets and sauté for 3 minutes until slightly softened. Add the water and season with salt and black pepper. Bring to a boil and then reduce the heat. Cover and simme for 10 minutes. Puree the soup with an immersion blender until the ingredients are evenly Combined. Stir in the almond milk and cheese until the cheese Melts. In a non-stick skillet over high heat, fry the bacon for 5 minutes until crispy. Divide soup between serving bowls, top with crispy bacon, and serve hot.

465.   Slow Cooker Beer Soup with Cheddar & Sausage

Ready in about: 8 hr | Serves: 6 Per serving: Kcal 244, Fat: 17g, Net Carbs: 4g, Protein: 5g

Ingredients

1 cup heavy cream 10 oz sausages, sliced 1 celery stalk, chopped 1 carrot, chopped 2 garlic cloves, minced 4 oz cream cheese, softened 1 tsp red pepper flakes 6 oz low carb beer 2 cups beef stock 1 onion, chopped 1 cup cheddar cheese, grated Salt and black pepper to taste

Directions

Turn on the slow cooker. Add in beef stock, beer, sausages, carrot, onion, garlic, celery, salt, red pepper flakes, and pepper and stir well. Pour in enough water to cover all the ingredients by roughly 2 inches. Close the lid and cook for 6 hours on Low. Open the lid and stir in the heavy cream, cheddar, and cream cheese and cook for 2 more hours. Ladle the soup into bowls and serve. Yummy!

466.   Salsa Verde Chicken Soup

Ready in about: 15 minutes | Serves: 4 Per serving: Kcal 346, Fat: 23g, Net Carbs: 3g, Protein: 25g

Ingredients

½ cup salsa verde 2 cups cooked and shredded chicken 2 cups chicken broth 1 cup cheddar cheese, shredded 4 oz cream cheese, softened ½ tsp chili powder ½ tsp cumin 2 tsp fresh cilantro, chopped Salt and black pepper to taste

Directions

Combine the cream cheese, salsa verde, and broth in a food processor; pulse until smooth. Transfer the mixture to a pot and place over medium heat. Cook until hot, but do not bring to a boil. Add chicken, chili powder, and cumin and cook for about 3-5 minutes or until it is heated through. Stir in cheddar cheese and season with salt and pepper. If it is very thick, add a few tablespoons of water and boil for 1-3 more minutes. Serve hot in bowls sprinkled with fresh cilantro.

467.   Thyme & Wild Mushroom Soup

Ready in about: 25 minutes | Serves: 4 Per serving: Kcal 281, Fat: 25g, Net Carbs: 5.8g, Protein: 6.1g

Ingredients

¼ cup butter ½ cup crème fraiche 12 oz wild mushrooms, chopped 2 tsp thyme leaves 2 garlic cloves, minced 4 cups chicken broth

Directions

Melt the butter in a large pot over medium heat. Add garlic and cook for 1 minute until tender. Add mushrooms and cook for 10 minutes. Pour in the broth over and bring to a boil. Simmer for 10 minutes. Puree the soup with a hand blender until smooth. Stir in crème fraiche. Garnish with thyme to serve.

468.   Brazilian Moqueca (Shrimp Stew)

Ready in about: 25 minutes | Serves: 6 Per serving: Kcal 324, Fat: 21g, Net Carbs: 5g, Protein: 23.1g

Ingredients

1 cup coconut milk 2 tbsp lime juice ¼ cup diced roasted peppers 1 ½ lb shrimp, peeled and deveined ¼ cup olive oil 1 garlic clove, minced 14 oz diced tomatoes 2 tbsp sriracha sauce 1 onion, chopped ¼ cup chopped cilantro 2 tbsp fresh dill, chopped to garnish Salt and black pepper to taste

Directions

Heat the olive oil in a pot over medium heat. Add onion and garlic and cook for 3 minutes until translucent. Stir in tomatoes, shrimp, and cilantro. Cook until the shrimp becomes opaque, about 3-4 minutes. Pour in sriracha sauce and coconut milk, and cook for 2 minutes. Do not bring to a boil. Stir in the lime juice and season with salt and pepper. Spoon the stew in bowls, garnish with fresh dill, and serve.

469.   Cobb Egg Salad in Lettuce Cups

Ready in about: 25 minutes | Serves: 4 Per serving: Kcal 325, Fat 24.5g, Net Carbs 4g, Protein 21g

Ingredients

1 head green lettuce, firm leaves removed for cups 2 chicken breasts, cut into pieces 1 tbsp olive oil Salt and black pepper to taste 6 large eggs 2 tomatoes, seeded, chopped 6 tbsp Greek yogurt Preheat oven to 400°F.

Directions

Put the chicken in a bowl, drizzle with olive oil, and sprinkle with salt and black pepper. Toss to coat. Put the chicken on a baking sheet and spread out evenly. Slide the baking sheet in the oven and bake the chicken until cooked through and golden brown for 8 minutes, stirring once. Boil the eggs in salted water for 10 minutes. Let them cool, peel, and chop into pieces. Transfer to a salad bowl. Remove the chicken from the oven and add to the salad bowl. Include the tomatoes and Greek yogurt and mix them. Layer 2 lettuce leaves each as cups and fill with 2 tbsp of egg salad each. Serve.

470.   Arugula Prawn Salad with Mayo Dressing

Ready in about: 15 minutes | Serves: 4 Per serving: Kcal 215, Fat 20.3g, Net Carbs 2g, Protein 8g

Ingredients

4 cups baby arugula ½ cup mayonnaise 3 tbsp olive oil 1 lb prawns, peeled and deveined 1 tsp Dijon mustard Salt to taste ½ tsp chili pepper 2 tbsp lemon juice ½ tsp garlic powder

Directions

Mix the mayonnaise, lemon juice, garlic, powder, and mustard in a small bowl until smooth and creamy. Set aside until ready to use. Heat 2 tbsp of olive oil in a skillet over medium heat. Add the prawns, season with salt and chili pepper, and fry for 3 minutes on each side until prawns are pink. Set aside to a plate. Place the arugula in a serving bowl and pour the mayo dressing over the salad. Toss with 2 spoons until mixed. Divide the salad between 4 plates and top with prawns. Serve immediately.

471.   Mozzarella & Tomato Salad with Anchovies & Olives

Ready in about: 10 minutes | Serves: 2 Per serving: Kcal 430, Fat: 26.8g, Net Carbs: 2.4g, Protein:38.8g

Ingredients

1 large tomato, sliced 4 basil leaves 8 mozzarella cheese slices 2 tsp olive oil 2 canned anchovies, chopped 1 tsp balsamic vinegar 4 black olives, pitted and sliced Salt to taste

Directions

Arrange the tomato slices on a serving plate. Place the mozzarella slices over and top with the basil. Add the anchovies and olives on top. Drizzle with olive oil and vinegar. Sprinkle with salt and serve.

472.   Spring Salad with Cheese Balls

Ready in about: 20 minutes | Serves: 6 Per serving: Kcal: 234; Fat 16.7g, Net Carbs 7.9g, Protein 12.4g

Ingredients

Cheese balls 3 eggs 1 cup feta cheese, crumbled ½ cup Pecorino cheese, shredded 1 cup almond flour 1 tbsp flax meal Salt and black pepper to taste Salad 1 head Iceberg lettuce, leaves separated ½ cup cucumber, thinly sliced 2 tomatoes, seeded and chopped ½ cup red onion, thinly sliced ½ cup radishes, thinly sliced ⅓ cup mayonnaise 1 tsp mustard 1 tsp paprika 1 tsp oregano Salt to taste Preheat oven to 390°F.

Directions

In a mixing dish, mix all ingredients for the cheese balls. Form balls out of the mixture. Set the balls on a lined baking sheet. Bake for 10 minutes until crisp. Arrange lettuce leaves on a large salad platter. Add in radishes, tomatoes, cucumbers, and red onion. In a small mixing bowl, mix the mayonnaise, paprika, salt, oregano, and mustard. Sprinkle the mixture over the vegetables. Add cheese balls on top and serve.

473. Shrimp & Avocado Cauliflower Salad

Ready in about: 30 minutes | Serves: 6 Per serving: Kcal 214, Fat: 17g, Net Carbs: 5g, Protein: 15g

Ingredients

1 cauliflower head, florets only 1 lb medium shrimp, peeled ¼ cup + 1 tbsp olive oil 1 avocado, chopped 2 tbsp fresh dill, chopped ¼ cup lemon juice 2 tbsp lemon zest Salt and black pepper to taste

Directions

Heat 1 tbsp olive oil in a skillet and cook shrimp for 8 minutes. Microwave cauliflower for 5 minutes. Place shrimp, cauliflower, and avocado in a bowl. Whisk the remaining olive oil, lemon zest, juice, dill, and salt, and pepper in another bowl. Pour the dressing over, toss to Combine, and serve immediately.

474. Bacon & Spinach Salad

Ready in about: 20 minutes | Serves: 4 Per serving: Kcal 350, Fat: 33g, Net Carbs: 3.4g, Protein: 7g

Ingredients

1 avocado, chopped 1 avocado, sliced 1 spring onion, sliced 4 bacon slices, chopped 2 cups spinach 2 small lettuce heads, chopped 2 eggs 3 tbsp olive oil 1 tsp Dijon mustard 1 tbsp apple cider vinegar Salt to taste

Directions

Place a skillet over medium heat and cook the bacon for 5 minutes until crispy. Remove to paper-towel lined plate to drain. Boil the eggs in boiling salted water for 10 minutes. Let them cool, peel, and chop. Combine the spinach, lettuce, eggs, chopped avocado, and spring onion in a large bowl. Whisk together the olive oil, mustard, apple cider vinegar, and salt in another bowl. Pour the dressing over the salad and toss to Combine. Top with the sliced avocado and bacon and serve.

475. Italian-Style Green Salad

Ready in about: 15 minutes | Serves: 4 Per serving: Kcal 205, Fat 20g, Net Carbs 2g, Protein 4g

Ingredients

2 (8 oz) pack mixed salad greens 8 pancetta strips 1 cup gorgonzola cheese, crumbled 1 tbsp white wine vinegar 3 tbsp extra virgin olive oil Salt and black pepper to taste

Directions

Fry the pancetta strips in a skillet over medium heat for 6 minutes, until browned and crispy. Remove to paper-towel lined plate to drain. Chop it when it is cooled. Pour the salad greens into a serving bowl. In a small bowl, whisk the white wine vinegar, olive oil, salt, and pepper. Drizzle the dressing over the salad and toss to coat. Top with gorgonzola cheese and pancetta. Divide salad into plates and serve.

476.   Warm Baby Artichoke Salad

Ready in about: 30 minutes | Serves: 4 Per serving: Kcal 170, Fat: 13g, Net Carbs: 5g, Protein: 1g

Ingredients

6 baby artichokes 6 cups water 1 tbsp lemon juice ¼ cup cherry peppers, halved ¼ cup pitted olives, sliced ¼ cup olive oil ¼ tsp lemon zest 2 tsp balsamic vinegar, sugar-free 1 tbsp chopped dill Salt and black pepper to taste 1 tbsp capers ¼ tsp caper brine

Directions

Combine the water and salt in a pot over medium heat. Trim and halve the artichokes. Add them to the pot and bring to a boil. Lower the heat and let simmer for 20 minutes until tender. Combine the rest of the ingredients, except for the olives, in a bowl. Drain and place the artichokes on a serving plate. Pour the prepared mixture over; toss to Combine well. Serve topped with the olives.

477.   Spinach & Turnip Salad with Bacon

Ready in about: 40 minutes | Serves: 4 Per serving: Kcal 193, Fat 18.3g, Net Carbs 3.1g, Protein 9.5g

Ingredients

2 turnips, cut into wedges 1 tsp olive oil 1 cup baby spinach, chopped 3 radishes, sliced 3 turkey bacon slices 4 tbsp sour cream 2 tsp mustard seeds 1 tsp Dijon mustard 1 tbsp red wine vinegar Salt and black pepper to taste 1 tbsp chopped chives Preheat oven to 400°F.

Directions

Line a baking sheet with parchment paper, toss the turnips with salt and black pepper, drizzle with the olive oil, and bake for 25 minutes, turning halfway. Let cool. Spread the baby spinach in the bottom of a salad bowl and top with the radishes. Remove the turnips to the salad bowl. Fry the bacon in a skillet over medium heat until crispy, about 5 minutes. Mix sour cream, mustard seeds, mustard, vinegar, and salt with the bacon. Add a little water to deglaze the bottom of the skillet. Pour the bacon mixture over the vegetables, scatter the chives over it. Serve.

478.   Cobb Salad with Blue Cheese Dressing

Ready in about: 30 minutes | Serves: 6 Per serving: Kcal 122, Fat 14g, Net Carbs 2g, Protein 23g

Ingredients

Dressing ½ cup buttermilk 1 cup mayonnaise 2 tbsp Worcestershire sauce ½ cup sour cream 1 cup blue cheese, crumbled 2 tbsp chives, chopped Salad 6 eggs 2 chicken breasts 5 strips bacon 1 iceberg lettuce, cut into chunks Salt and black pepper to taste 1 romaine lettuce, chopped 1 bibb lettuce, cored, leaves removed 2 avocado, pitted and diced 2 large tomatoes, chopped ½ cup blue cheese, crumbled 2 scallions, chopped

DirectionsIn a bowl, whisk the buttermilk, mayonnaise, Worcestershire sauce, and sour cream. Stir in the blue cheese and chives. Place in the refrigerator to chill until ready to use. Bring the eggs to boil in salted water over medium heat for 10 minutes. Transfer to an ice bath to cool. Peel and chop. Set aside. Preheat a grill pan over high heat. Season the chicken with salt and pepper. Grill for 3 minutes on each side. Remove to a plate to cool for 3 minutes and cut into bite-size chunks. Fry the bacon in the same pan until crispy, about 6 minutes. Remove, let cool for 2 minutes, and chop. Arrange the lettuce leaves in a salad bowl, and in single piles, add the avocado, tomatoes, eggs, bacon, and chicken. Sprinkle the blue cheese over the salad as well as the scallions and black pepper. Drizzle the blue cheese dressing on the salad and serve with low carb bread.

479.   Pancetta and Goat Cheese-Stuffed Mushrooms

(Ready in about 25 minutes | Servings 6) Per serving: 98 Calories; 5.8g Fat; 3.9g Carbs; 8.4g Protein; 0.6g Fiber

Ingredients

12 medium-sized button mushrooms, stems removed 3 slices of pancetta, chopped 2 ounces goat cheese, crumbled 2 tablespoons butter, melted 1 tablespoon oyster sauce Sea salt and black pepper, to taste 1 teaspoon basil 1 teaspoon fresh rosemary, minced

Directions

Brush your mushrooms with melted butter and oyster sauce. Season them with salt and pepper to taste. Mix the pancetta, basil, rosemary, and goat cheese. Spoon the mixture into the mushroom caps and arrange them on a parchment-lined baking sheet. Bake in the preheated oven at 360 degrees F for about 20 minutes or until tender.Enjoy!

480.   Roasted Autumn Vegetables

(Ready in about 35 minutes | Servings 6) Per serving: 137 Calories; 11.1g Fat; 3.1g Carbs; 1.2g Protein; 2.3g Fiber

Ingredients

3 tablespoons olive oil 1 onion, cut into wedges 1 fresh chili pepper, minced 1/2 pound celery, quartered 1/2 pound bell peppers, sliced 1/2 pound turnips, cut into wedges Sea salt and ground black pepper, to taste 1 teaspoon dried thyme 1 teaspoon dried basil 1 garlic clove, minced

Directions

Toss all ingredients in a roasting pan. Roast in the preheated oven at 410 degrees F for 30 minutes. Taste and adjust the seasoning.Bon appétit!

481.   Grilled Zucchini with Mediterranean Sauce

(Ready in about 15 minutes | Servings 4) Per serving: 132 Calories; 11.1g Fat; 4.1g Carbs; 3.1g Protein; 1.3g Fiber

Ingredients

1 pound zucchini, cut lengthwise into quarters 1/2 teaspoon red pepper flakes, crushed Salt, to season 1/4 cup extra-virgin olive oil 1 teaspoon garlic, minced For the Sauce: 1 tablespoon fresh scallions, minced 1 tablespoon fresh basil, chopped 1 teaspoon fresh rosemary, finely chopped 3/4 cup Greek-style yogurt

Directions

Begin by preheating your grill to a medium-low heat. Toss the zucchini slices with the olive oil, garlic, red pepper, and salt. Grill your zucchini on a lightly-oiled grill for about 10 minutes until tender and slightly charred. Make the sauce by whisking all of the sauce ingredients.Enjoy!

482.   Autumn Eggplant and Squash Stew

(Ready in about 35 minutes | Servings 6) Per serving: 113 Calories; 7.9g Fat; 3.7g Carbs; 2.8g Protein; 2.2g Fiber

Ingredients

2 tablespoons olive 2 garlic cloves, finely chopped 3 ounces acorn squash, chopped 1 celery, chopped 2 tablespoons fresh parsley, roughly chopped Sea salt and pepper, to taste 1/2 teaspoon ancho chili powder 2 tomatoes, pureed 2 tablespoons port wine 1 large onion, chopped 3 ounces eggplant, peeled and chopped

Directions

In a heavy-bottomed pot, heat olive oil over a moderately-high heat. Sauté the onion and garlic about 5 minutes. Add in the acorn squash, eggplant, celery and parsley; continue to cook for 5 to 6 minutes. Add in the other ingredients; turn the heat to a simmer. Continue to cook for about 25 minutes.Enjoy!

483.   Cheesy Italian Pepper Casserole

(Ready in about 1 hour | Servings 4) Per serving: 408 Calories; 28.9g Fat; 4.6g Carbs; 24.9g Protein; 3.5g Fiber

Ingredients

8 Italian sweet peppers, deveined and cut into fourths lengthwise 6 whole eggs 1/2 cup Greek-style yogurt 3/4 pound Asiago cheese, shredded 1 leek, thinly sliced 1/2 teaspoon garlic, crushed Sea salt and ground black pepper, to taste 1 teaspoon oregano

Directions

Arrange the peppers in a lightly greased baking dish. Top with half of the shredded cheese; add a layer of sliced leeks and garlic. Repeat the layers. After that, beat the eggs with the yogurt, salt, pepper, and oregano. Pour the egg/yogurt mixture over the peppers. Cover with a piece of foil and bake for about 30 minutes. Remove the foil and bake for a further 10 to 15 minutes.Bon appétit!

484.   Easy Vegetable Ratatouille

(Ready in about 1 hour | Servings 4) Per serving: 159 Calories; 10.4g Fat; 5.7g Carbs; 6.4g Protein; 5g Fiber

Ingredients

1 large onion, sliced 1/3 cup Parmesan cheese, shredded 1 celery, peeled and diced 1 poblano pepper, minced 1 eggplant, cut into thick slices 1 cup grape tomatoes, halved 1/2 garlic head, minced 2 tablespoons extra-virgin olive oil 1 tablespoon fresh basil leaves, snipped

Directions

Sprinkle the eggplant with 1 teaspoon of salt and let it stand for about 30 minutes; drain and rinse under running water. Place the eggplant slices in the bottom of a lightly-oiled casserole dish. Add in the remaining vegetable. Add in the olive oil and basil leaves. Bake in the preheated oven at 350 degrees F for about 30 minute or until thoroughly cooked.Bon appétit!

485.   Spring Mixed Greens Salad

(Ready in about 10 minutes | Servings 4) Per serving: 190 Calories; 17.6g Fat; 7.6g Carbs; 4.3g Protein; 3.9g Fiber

Ingredients

1 cup romaine lettuce 1 cup lollo rosso 1/3 cup goat cheese, crumbled 2 tablespoons fresh parsley, chopped 2 tablespoons extra-virgin olive oil 1/2 lime, freshly squeezed 2 cups baby spinach 1/2 cup blueberries 1 cup avocado, pitted, peeled and sliced Sea salt and white pepper, to taste

Directions

Toss all ingredients in a mixing bowl. Taste and adjust seasonings. Place in your refrigerator until ready to use.

486.   Cream of Thyme Tomato Soup

Ready in about: 20 minutes | Serves: 4 Per serving: Kcal 310, Fat 27g, Net Carbs 3g, Protein 11g

Ingredients

2 tbsp ghee 2 large red onions, diced ½ cup raw cashew nuts, diced 2 (28 oz) cans tomatoes 2 tsp fresh thyme leaves 1 ½ cups water Salt and black pepper to taste 1 cup heavy cream

Directions

Melt ghee in a pot over medium heat and sauté the onions for 4 minutes until softened. Stir in the tomatoes, thyme, water, and cashews and season with salt and black pepper. Cover and bring to a boil. Simmer for 10 minutes until thoroughly cooked. Open, turn the heat off, and puree the ingredients with an immersion blender. Adjust the taste and stir in the heavy cream. Spoon into soup bowls and serve.

487.   Green Minestrone Soup

Ready in about: 25 minutes | Serves: 4 Per serving: Kcal 227, Fat 20.3g, Net Carbs 2g, Protein 8g

Ingredients

2 tbsp ghee 2 tbsp onion-garlic puree 2 heads broccoli, cut into florets 2 celery stalks, chopped 4 cups vegetable broth 1 cup baby spinach Salt and black pepper to taste 2 tbsp Gruyere cheese, grated

Directions

Melt the ghee in a saucepan over medium heat and sauté the onion-garlic puree for 3 minutes until softened. Mix in the broccoli and celery, and cook for 4 minutes until slightly tender. Pour in the broth, bring to a boil, then reduce the heat to medium-low and simmer covered for about 5 minutes. Drop in the spinach to wilt, adjust the seasonings, and cook for 4 minutes. Ladle soup into serving bowls. Serve with a sprinkle of grated Gruyere cheese.

488. Buffalo Chicken Soup

Ready in about: 40 minutes | Serves: 4 Per serving: Kcal 215, Fat: 11.3g, Net Carbs: 2.4g, Protein: 7.5g

Ingredients

2 chicken legs 2 tbsp butter, melted 1 onion, chopped 2 garlic cloves, minced 1 carrot, chopped 1 bay leaf 2 tbsp fresh cilantro, chopped ⅓ cup buffalo sauce Salt and black pepper to taste

Directions

Add the chicken in a pot over medium heat and cover with water. Add in salt, pepper, and bay leaf. Boil for 15 minutes. Remove to a plate and let it cool slightly. Strain and reserve the broth. Melt the butter in a large saucepan over medium heat. Sauté the onion, garlic, and carrot for 5 minutes until tender, stirring occasionally. Remove skin and bones from chicken and discard. Chop the chicken and add it to the saucepan. Stir in the buffalo sauce for 1 minute and pour in the broth. Bring to a boil. Cook for 15 minutes. Adjust the taste with salt and pepper and top with cilantro. Serve.

489. Coconut Green Bean & Shrimp Curry Soup

Ready in about: 20 minutes | Serves: 4 Per serving: Kcal 375, Fat 35.4g, Net Carbs 2g, Protein 9g

Ingredients

1 lb jumbo shrimp, peeled and deveined 2 tbsp ghee 2 tsp ginger-garlic puree 2 tbsp red curry paste 6 oz coconut milk Salt and chili pepper to taste 1 lb green beans, trimmed, chopped

Directions

Melt the ghee in a medium saucepan over medium heat. Add the shrimp, season with salt and black pepper, and cook until opaque, about 2-3 minutes. Remove the shrimp to a plate. Add the ginger-garlic puree and red curry paste to the ghee and sauté for 2 more minutes until fragrant. Stir in the coconut milk. Add in the shrimp, salt, chili pepper, and green beans. Cook for 4 minutes. Reduce the heat to a simmer and cook for an additional 5-7 minutes, occasionally stirring. Adjust the taste with salt and fetch soup into serving bowls. Serve with cauli rice.

490. Creamy Cauliflower Soup with Chorizo Sausage

Ready in about: 40 minutes | Serves: 4 Per serving: Kcal 251, Fat: 19.1g, Net Carbs: 5.7g, Protein: 10g

Ingredients

1 cauliflower head, chopped 1 turnip, chopped 3 tbsp butter 1 chorizo sausage, sliced 2 cups chicken broth 1 small onion, chopped 2 cups water Salt and black pepper to taste

Directions

Melt 2 tbsp of the butter in a large pot over medium heat. Stir in the onion and cook until soft, 3-4 minutes. Add cauliflower and turnip and cook for another 5 minutes. Pour the broth and water over. Bring to a boil. Simmer covered for about 20 minutes until the vegetables are tender. Remove from heat. Melt the remaining butter in a skillet. Cook the chorizo for 5 minutes until crispy. Puree the soup with a hand blender until smooth. Adjust the seasonings. Serve the soup topped with the chorizo sausage.

491.   Pumpkin & Meat Peanut Stew

Ready in about: 45 minutes | Serves: 6 Per serving: Kcal 451, Fat: 33g, Net Carbs: 4g, Protein: 27.5g

Ingredients

1 cup pumpkin puree 2 lb chopped pork stew meat 1 tbsp peanut butter 4 tbsp peanuts, chopped 1 garlic clove, minced 1 onion, chopped ½ cup white wine 1 tbsp olive oil 1 tsp lemon juice ¼ cup granulated sweetener ¼ tsp cardamom powder ¼ tsp allspice 2 cups water 2 cups chicken stock

DirectionsHeat the olive oil in a large pot and sauté onion and garlic for 3 minutes until translucent. Add the pork and brown for about 5-6 minutes, stirring occasionally. Pour in the wine and cook for 1 minute. Add in the remaining ingredients, except for the lemon juice and peanuts. Bring the mixture to a boil and cook for 5 minutes. Reduce the heat to low, cover the pot, and let cook for about 30 minutes. Adjust seasonings and stir in the lemon juice before serving. Ladle into bowls and serve topped with peanuts.

492.   Mediterranean Salad

Ready in about: 10 minutes | Serves: 4 Per serving: Kcal 290, Fat: 25g, Net Carbs: 4.3g, Protein: 9g

Ingredients

3 tomatoes, sliced 1 large avocado, sliced 8 kalamata olives ¼ lb buffalo mozzarella, sliced 2 tbsp pesto sauce 1 tbsp olive oil

DirectionsArrange the tomato slices on a serving platter and place the avocado slices in the middle. Arrange the olives around the avocado slices and drop pieces of the mozzarella cheese on the platter. Drizzle the pesto sauce and olive oil all over and serve.

493.   Blue Cheese Chicken Salad

Ready in about: 15 minutes | Serves: 4 Per serving: Kcal 286, Fat 23g, Net Carbs 4g, Protein 14g

Ingredients

1 chicken breast, flattened Salt and black pepper to taste 4 tbsp olive oil 1 lb spinach and spring mix 1 tbsp red wine vinegar 1 cup blue cheese, crumbled

DirectionsSeason the chicken with salt and black pepper. Heat half of the olive oil in a pan over medium heat and fry the chicken for 4 minutes on both sides until golden brown. Remove and let cool before slicing. In a salad bowl, Combine the spinach and spring mix with the remaining olive oil, red wine vinegar, and salt and mix well. Top the salad with the chicken slices and sprinkle with blue cheese. Serve.

494.   Lobster Salad with Salsa Rosa

Ready in about: 10 minutes | Serves: 4 Per serving: Kcal 256, Fat: 15g, Net Carbs: 4.3g, Protein: 17.9g

Ingredients

2 hard-boiled eggs, sliced 1 cucumber, peeled and chopped ½ cup black olives 2 cups cooked lobster meat, diced 1 head Iceberg lettuce, shredded ½ cup mayonnaise ¼ tsp celery seeds Salt to taste 2 tbsp lemon juice ½ tsp sugar-free ketchup ¼ tsp dark rum

Directions

Combine the lettuce, cucumber, and lobster meat in a large bowl. Whisk together the mayonnaise, celery seeds, ketchup, rum, salt, and lemon juice in another bowl. Pour the dressing over the salad and gently toss to Combine. Top with olives and sliced eggs and serve.

495.   Strawberry Salad with Cheese & Almonds

Ready in about: 20 minutes | Serves: 2 Per serving: Kcal 445, Fat: 34.2g, Net Carbs: 5.3g, Protein: 33g

Ingredients

4 cups kale, chopped 4 strawberries, sliced ½ cup almonds, flaked 1 ½ cups hard goat cheese, grated 4 tbsp raspberry vinaigrette Salt and black pepper to taste Preheat oven to 400°F.

Directions

Arrange the grated goat cheese in two circles on two pieces of parchment paper. Place in the oven and bake for 10 minutes. Find two same bowls, place them upside down, and carefully put the parchment paper on top to give the cheese a bowl-like shape. Let cool that way for 15 minutes. Divide the kale among the bowls, sprinkle with salt and pepper and drizzle with vinaigrette. Toss to coat. Top with almonds and strawberries. Serve immediately.

496.   Green Mackerel Salad

Ready in about: 25 minutes | Serves: 4 Per serving: Kcal 356, Fat: 31.9g, Net Carbs: 0.8g, Protein: 1.3g

Ingredients

4 oz smoked mackerel, flaked 2 eggs 1 tbsp coconut oil 1 cup green beans, chopped 1 avocado, sliced 4 cups mixed salad greens 2 tbsp olive oil 1 tbsp lemon juice Salt and black pepper to taste

Directions

In a bowl, whisk together the lemon juice, olive oil, salt, and pepper. Set aside. Cook the green beans in boiling salted water over medium heat for about 3 minutes. Remove with a slotted spoon and let to cool. Add the eggs to the pot and cook for 8-10 minutes. Transfer the eggs to an ice water bath, peel the shells, and slice them. Place the mixed salad green in a serving bowl and add in the green beans and smoked mackerel. Pour the dressing over and toss to coat. Top with sliced eggs and avocado and serve.

497.   Caesar Salad with Smoked Salmon & Poached Eggs

Ready in about: 15 minutes | Serves: 4 Per serving: Kcal 260, Fat 21g, Net Carbs 5g, Protein 8g

Ingredients

8 eggs 2 cups torn romaine lettuce ½ cup smoked salmon, chopped 6 slices bacon 2 tbsp low carb Caesar dressing 1 tbsp white wine vinegar

Directions

Bring a pot of water to a boil and pour in the vinegar. Crack each egg into a small bowl and gently slide into the water. Poach for 2 to 3 minutes, remove with a perforated spoon, and transfer to a paper towel to remove any excess water, and plate. Poach the remaining 7 eggs. Put the bacon in a skillet and fry over medium heat until browned and crispy, about 6 minutes, turning once. Remove, allow cooling, and chop into small pieces. Toss the lettuce, smoked salmon, bacon, and Caesar dressing in a salad bowl. Top with two eggs each and serve immediately or chilled.

498.   Brussels Sprouts Salad with Pecorino Cheese

Ready in about: 35 minutes | Serves: 6 Per serving: Kcal 210, Fat 18g, Net Carbs 6g, Protein 4g

Ingredients

2 lb Brussels sprouts, halved 3 tbsp olive oil Salt and black pepper to taste 2 tbsp balsamic vinegar ¼ head red cabbage, shredded 1 cup Pecorino cheese, shaved Preheat oven to 400°F.

Directions

Toss the brussels sprouts with olive oil, salt, black pepper, and balsamic vinegar in a bowl. Spread on a baking sheet in an even layer. Bake until tender on the inside and crispy on the outside, about 20-25 minutes. Transfer to a salad bowl and add the red cabbage. Mix until well Combined. Sprinkle with the cheese, share the salad onto serving plates, and serve.

499.   Broccoli Slaw Salad with Mustard Vinaigrette

Ready in about: 10 minutes | Serves: 6 Per serving: Kcal 110, Fat: 10g, Net Carbs: 2g, Protein: 3g

Ingredients

½ tsp granulated swerve sugar 1 tbsp Dijon mustard 2 tbsp olive oil 4 cups broccoli slaw ⅓ cup mayonnaise 1 tsp celery seeds 2 tbsp slivered almonds 1 ½ tbsp apple cider vinegar Salt to taste

Directions

In a bowl, place the mayonnaise, Dijon mustard, swerve sugar, olive oil, celery seeds, vinegar, and salt and whisk until well Combined. Place broccoli slaw in a large salad bowl. Pour the vinaigrette over. Toss to coat. Sprinkle with the slivered almonds and serve immediately.

500.   Squid Salad with Cucumber & Chili Dressing

Ready in about: 30 minutes | Serves: 4 Per serving: Kcal 318, Fat 22.5g, Net Carbs 2.1g, Protein 24.6g

Ingredients

4 squid tubes, cut into strips ½ cup mint leaves 2 cucumbers, halved, cut into strips ½ cup cilantro, stems reserved ½ red onion, finely sliced Salt and black pepper to taste 1 tsp fish sauce 1 red chili, roughly chopped 1 clove garlic 2 limes, juiced 1 tbsp fresh parsley, chopped 1 tsp olive oil

Directions

In a salad bowl, mix mint leaves, cucumber strips, coriander leaves, and red onion. Season with salt, black pepper, and some olive oil; set aside. In the mortar, pound the cilantro stems and red chili to form a paste using the pestle. Add in the fish sauce and lime juice and mix with the pestle. Heat a skillet over medium heat. Sear the squid on both sides until lightly brown, about 5 minutes. Pour the squid on the salad and drizzle with the chili dressing. Toss to coat, garnish with parsley, and serve.

501.   Chicken Salad with Grapefruit & Cashews

Ready in about: 30 minutes + marinating time| Serves: 4 Per serving: Kcal 178, Fat: 13.5g, Net Carbs: 3.2g, Protein: 9.1g

Ingredients

1 grapefruit, peeled and segmented 1 chicken breast 4 green onions, sliced 10 oz baby spinach 2 tbsp cashews 1 red chili pepper, thinly sliced 1 lemon, juiced 3 tbsp olive oil Salt and black pepper to taste

Directions

Toast the cashews in a dry pan over high heat for 2 minutes, shaking often. Set aside to cool, then chop. Preheat the grill to medium heat. Season the chicken with salt and pepper and brush with some olive oil. Grill for 4 minutes per side. Remove to a plate and let it sit for a few minutes before slicing. Place the baby spinach and green onions on a serving platter. Season with salt, remaining olive oil, and lemon juice. Toss to coat. Top with chicken, chili pepper, and chicken. Sprinkle with cashews and serve.

502.   Tangy Cabbage Soup

(Ready in about 25 minutes | Servings 4) Per serving: 185 Calories; 16.6g Fat; 2.4g Carbs; 2.9g Protein; 1.9g Fiber

Ingredients

2 cups cabbage, shredded 1 cup sour cream 1 bell pepper, chopped 4 cups roasted vegetable broth 1 ½ tablespoons olive oil 1 yellow onion, chopped 2 garlic cloves, minced 1 celery, chopped

Directions

In a heavy-bottomed pot, heat olive oil over a moderate flame. Sauté the onion and garlic until just tender and aromatic. Add in the celery, cabbage, and pepper and continue to cook for about 6 minutes, stirring occasionally to ensure even cooking. Pour in the roasted vegetable broth and cook, partially covered, for 10 to 12 minutes longer. Puree the mixture with an immersion blender. Stir in the sour cream; and remove from heat; stir to combine well.Enjoy!

503.   Ground Chicken-Stuffed Tomatoes

(Ready in about 25 minutes | Servings 4) Per serving: 366 Calories; 23.2g Fat; 6.8g Carbs; 23.2g Protein; 2.1g Fiber

Ingredients

4 tomatoes, scoop out the pulp Seasoned salt and pepper, to taste 1/2 cup cream of celery soup 1 ½ cups Parmesan cheese, grated 1/2 cup onions, chopped 1 garlic clove, smashed 1 tablespoon canola oil 1/2 pound ground chicken 1 tablespoon fresh coriander, chopped 1 teaspoon oregano, chopped

Directions

In a frying pan, heat the oil over a moderately-high heat. Cook ground chicken, onion, and garlic for about 4 minutes, stirring periodically to ensure even cooking; set aside. Add in the tomato pulp, coriander, oregano, salt, and pepper. Divide this filling between tomatoes. Place the stuffed tomatoes in a lightly oiled casserole dish. Pour the cream of celery soup around stuffed tomatoes; bake in the preheated oven at 365 degrees F for about 20 until heated through.Enjoy!

504. Pasta with Alfredo Sauce

(Ready in about 30 minutes | Servings 4) Per serving: 614 Calories; 55.9g Fat; 3.6g Carbs; 25.6g Protein; 0g Fiber

Ingredients

1 stick butter 1 cup double cream 1 garlic clove, minced 2 cups Romano cheese, grated 2 ounces Ricotta cheese, room temperature 3 eggs, room temperature 1/2 teaspoon wheat gluten 1 teaspoon Italian spice mix

Directions

Mix the Ricotta cheese, eggs, and gluten until creamy. Press this mixture into a parchment-lined baking sheet. Bake at 310 degrees F for about 6 minutes. Let it cool for about 10 minutes and cut into strips using a sharp knife. Cook this the pasta in a lightly salted water for 3 to 4 minutes. In a saucepan, melt the butter over low heat. Cook the garlic and cream until warmed; stir in Romano cheese and Italian spice mix; heat off. Fold in the reserved pasta. Gently stir to combine.

505. Goat Cheese, Ham, and Spinach Muffins

(Ready in about 25 minutes | Servings 6) Per serving: 275 Calories; 15.8g Fat; 2.2g Carbs; 21.6g Protein; 1.2g Fiber

Ingredients

10 ounces baby spinach, cooked and drained 1/2 pound smoked ham, chopped 1 teaspoon Mediterranean seasoning mix 1 ½ cups goat cheese, crumbled 5 eggs 1/2 cup milk Salt and pepper, to taste

Directions

Thoroughly combine all ingredients in a mixing bowl. Spoon the batter into a lightly oiled muffin tin. Bake in the preheated oven at 350 degrees F for about 25 minutes.Enjoy!

506. Aromatic Prawns with Bok Choy

(Ready in about 15 minutes | Servings 4) Per serving: 171 Calories; 8.4g Fat; 5.8g Carbs; 18.9g Protein; 1.9g Fiber

Ingredients

10 ounces prawns, peeled and deveined 1 ½ pounds Bok choy, trimmed and thinly sliced 1 (1/2-inch) piece ginger, freshly grated 1 tablespoon fish sauce 2 tablespoons peanut oil 1 teaspoon garlic, minced Salt and pepper, to taste

Directions

Heat 1 tablespoon of the peanut oil in a frying pan over a moderately-high heat. Sauté the garlic until tender and aromatic. Stir in the Bok choy, ginger, fish sauce, salt, and pepper; cook for 5 to 6 minutes, stirring periodically to ensure even cooking. In the same pan, heat the remaining tablespoon of oil and cook the prawns until opaque, about 4 minutes. Serve your prawns with the reserved Bok choy.Enjoy!

507.   Brown Mushroom Stew

(Ready in about 30 minutes | Servings 4) Per serving: 133 Calories; 3.7g Fat; 5.7g Carbs; 14g Protein; 3.1g Fiber

Ingredients

1/2 pound brown mushrooms, chopped 1 tablespoon butter, room temperature 1 cup onions, chopped 1 bay laurel 1 celery, chopped 2 ½ cups vegetable broth 1/4 cup dry white wine 1 cup tomato puree Salt and ground black pepper, to taste 1/4 teaspoon ground allspice 1 teaspoon jalapeno pepper, deveined and minced 1 bell pepper, deveined and chopped 2 garlic cloves, pressed 1/4 cup fresh parsley, chopped

Directions

In Dutch oven, melt the butter over a moderate heat. Cook the onion, peppers, garlic, and celery for about 7 minutes. Add in the mushrooms and cook an additional 2 to 3 minutes. Add in the vegetable broth, wine, tomato puree, and seasonings; bring to a boil. Turn the heat to a simmer; let it simmer for about 20 minutes or until cooked through.Bon appétit!

508.   Roasted Tomatoes with Cheese

(Ready in about 25 minutes | Servings 4) Per serving: 247 Calories; 19.8g Fat; 5.3g Carbs; 11g Protein; 1.8g Fiber

Ingredients

1 ½ pounds tomatoes, sliced 1/4 cup extra-virgin olive oil 1 tablespoon balsamic vinegar 2 garlic cloves, pressed Sea salt and pepper, to taste 1 teaspoon Mediterranean spice mix 1 cup Caciocavallo cheese, shredded

Directions

Start by preheating your oven to 390 degrees F. Toss your tomatoes with olive oil, vinegar, garlic, salt, pepper, and Mediterranean spice mix. Place tomatoes on a lightly oiled baking sheet. Roast in the preheated oven for about 20 minutes until your tomatoes begin to caramelize.Enjoy!

509.   Mixed Greens with Caciocavallo Cheese

(Ready in about 25 minutes | Servings 5) Per serving: 160 Calories; 10g Fat; 5.1g Carbs; 11g Protein; 4.6g Fiber

Ingredients

2 pounds mixed greens, fresh or frozen, torn into pieces 1 tablespoon olive oil 1/4 cup cream of celery soup 1 tablespoon balsamic vinegar Sea salt and pepper, to taste 1 cup Caciocavallo cheese, shredded 1 teaspoon garlic, chopped 1/2 cup shallot

Directions

Het the olive oil in a Dutch oven over a moderately-high heat. Cook the garlic and shallot for 2 to 3 minutes or until tender and fragrant. Add in the mixed greens and cream of celery soup; continue to cook, partially covered, for about 15 minutes until greens are wilted. Add in the vinegar, salt, and pepper; heat off.Top with cheese and reheat in the saucepan until cheese melts completely. Enjoy!

510.   Cabbage Noodles with Meat Sauce

(Ready in about 20 minutes | Servings 4) Per serving: 236 Calories; 8.3g Fat; 5.1g Carbs; 29.9g Protein; 2.9g Fiber

Ingredients

1 pound green cabbage, spiralized 1/2 teaspoon garlic, chopped 3/4 pound ground chuck 1/2 teaspoon chili pepper, minced 2 slices pancetta, chopped 1/2 cup onion, thinly sliced 2 bay leaves Sea salt and black pepper, to taste

Directions

Parboil the cabbage in a pot of lightly salted water for 3 to 4 minutes; drain. Cook the pancetta over a moderately-high heat for about 4 minutes, breaking apart with a fork and reserve. Cook the onion and garlic in the bacon grease until they've softened. Add in the ground chuck, chili pepper, salt and black pepper; continue to cook until ground beef is no longer pink. Add the pancetta back to the pan. Top with the cabbage noodles.Bon appétit!

511. Roman-Style Chicory with Pine Nuts

(Ready in about 10 minutes | Servings 4) Per serving: 65 Calories; 4.7g Fat; 5.7g Carbs; 2.1g Protein; 1.5g Fiber

Ingredients

3 teaspoons butter 2 heads chicory, cut into chunks 1/4 cup pine nuts 2 garlic cloves, crushed 1 shallot, chopped Salt and pepper, to taste

Directions

Parboil the chicory in a pot of lightly salted water for 5 to 6 minutes; drain. Melt the butter over moderately-high heat and sauté the chicory with garlic and shallots. Season with salt and pepper. Top with pine nuts.Enjoy!

512.   Caciocavallo Cheese and Spinach Muffins

(Ready in about 30 minutes | Servings 6) Per serving: 252 Calories; 19.7g Fat; 3g Carbs; 16.1g Protein; 0.2g Fiber

Ingredients

1 cup spinach, chopped 2 tablespoons butter, melted Sea salt and black pepper, to taste 8 eggs 1 cup full-fat milk 1 ½ cups Caciocavallo cheese, shredded

Directions

Start by preheating your oven to 360 degrees F. Brush muffin cups with a nonstick spray. Whisk the eggs and milk until pale and frothy; add in the butter, salt, pepper, and spinach. Fold in the cheese. Bake in the preheated oven for 20 to 22 minutes or until a tester comes out dry and clean.Bon appétit!

513.   Kapusta (Polish Braised Cabbage)

(Ready in about 20 minutes | Servings 6) Per serving: 259 Calories; 18.1g Fat; 3.6g Carbs; 15.5g Protein; 1.8g Fiber

Ingredients

1 pound cabbage, shredded 1 bell pepper, finely chopped 1/2 cup vegetable broth 3 strips bacon, diced 1/2 teaspoon red pepper flakes, crushed

Directions

In a Dutch oven, fry the bacon for 5 to 6 minutes. Add in the cabbage and pepper and continue to cook until they've softened. Add in the broth and red pepper flakes and cover the pan. Turn the heat to medium-low and let it simmer for 10 to 13 minutes or until cooked through. Taste and adjust the seasonings.Bon appétit!

514.   Kohlrabi with Garlic-Mushroom Sauce

(Ready in about 15 minutes | Servings 4) Per serving: 220 Calories; 20g Fat; 5.3g Carbs; 4g Protein; 3.8g Fiber

Ingredients

3/4 pound kohlrabi, trimmed and thinly sliced 1/2 pound button mushrooms, sliced 1 ½ cups sour cream 3 tablespoons olive oil 1/2 cup white onions, chopped 1/2 teaspoon garlic, chopped Kosher salt and ground black pepper, to taste

Directions

In a large pot of salted water, place the kohlrabi and parboil over medium-high heat for about 8 minutes. Drain. In a saucepan, heat the oil over medium-high heat. Sauté the onions, mushrooms, and garlic until they've softened. Season with salt and pepper to taste. Add in the sour cream and stir to combine well.Bon appétit!

515.   Easy Keto Broccoli Pilaf

(Ready in about 20 minutes | Servings 4) Per serving: 126 Calories; 11.6g Fat; 5.4g Carbs; 1.3g Protein; 2.7g Fiber

Ingredients

1 head broccoli, broken into a rice-like chunks 1 Italian pepper, chopped 1 habanero pepper, minced 1/2 shallots, chopped 1/2 teaspoon garlic, smashed 1 celery rib, chopped 1/2 stick butter Salt and pepper, to your liking

Directions

In a saucepan, melt the butter over a moderately-high heat. Saute the shallot, garlic, and peppers for about 3 minutes. Stir in the broccoli and celery; continue to cook for 4 to 5 minutes or until tender and aromatic. Season with salt and pepper to taste. Continue to cook for 5 to 6 minutes or until everything is cooked through.Bon appétit!

516.   Chanterelle with Eggs and Enchilada Sauce

(Ready in about 15 minutes | Servings 4) Per serving: 290 Calories; 21.7g Fat; 6.5g Carbs; 10.6g Protein; 5.5g Fiber

Ingredients

1 pound Chanterelle mushroom, sliced 1/4 cup enchilada sauce 2 tablespoons butter, room temperature 1 yellow onion, chopped 4 eggs 1/2 teaspoon ginger-garlic paste Kosher salt and black pepper, to taste 2 tomatillos, chopped 1 medium-sized avocado, pitted and mashed

Directions

Melt the butter in a saucepan over a moderately-high flame. Cook the onion until tender and translucent. Add in the ginger-garlic paste, mushrooms, salt, black pepper, and chopped tomatillos. Add in the eggs and scramble them well.Enjoy!

517.Celery with Peppercorn Sauce

(Ready in about 40 minutes | Servings 6) Per serving: 183 Calories; 14.2g Fat; 6.5g Carbs; 2.6g Protein; 2.2g Fiber

Ingredients

Kosher salt and white pepper, to taste 2 tablespoons balsamic vinegar 1 ½ pounds celery, trimmed and halved lengthwise 2 tablespoons ghee, room temperature 1 teaspoon garlic, smashed For the Sauce: 1 ½ cups cream of celery soup 3 tablespoons rum 2 tablespoons ghee 1/2 cup onions, minced 1 cup double cream

Directions

Start by preheating your oven to 410 degrees F. Toss your celery with 2 tablespoons of ghee, salt, white pepper, balsamic vinegar, and garlic. Roast the celery in the preheated oven for about 30 minutes. In the meantime, melt the 2 tablespoons of ghee in a cast-iron skillet over a moderately-high heat. Once hot, cook the onions for 2 to 3 minutes until tender and translucent. Add the rum and cream of celery soup; bring it to a boil. Continue to cook for 4 to 5 minutes. Turn the heat to a simmer. Add in the double cream and continue to simmer until the sauce has thickened and reduced.Bon appétit!

518.   Oven-Baked Avocado

(Ready in about 25 minutes | Servings 6) Per serving: 255 Calories; 21g Fat; 3.3g Carbs; 10.8g Protein; 4.8g Fiber

Ingredients

3 medium-sized ripe avocados, halved and pitted 3 ounce Pancetta, chopped 2 eggs, beaten 3 ounces chive cream cheese Salt and pepper, to taste

Directions

Begin by preheating an oven to 380 degrees F. Place the avocado halves in a baking pan. Thoroughly combine the eggs, cheese, Pancetta, salt, and pepper. Spoon the mixture into avocado halves. Bake in the preheated oven for 18 to 20 minutes.

519. Cauliflower and Oyster Mushroom Medley

(Ready in about 20 minutes | Servings 4) Per serving: 300 Calories; 27.9g Fat; 8.6g Carbs; 5.2g Protein; 2.6g Fiber

Ingredients

1/2 head cauliflower, cut into small florets Salt and pepper, to taste 2 tablespoons Romano cheese, grated 10 ounces Oyster mushrooms, sliced 2 garlic cloves, minced 1/2 stick butter, room temperature 1/3 cup cream of celery soup 1/3 cup double cream 1/4 cup mayonnaise, preferably homemade

Directions

In a saucepan, melt the butter over a moderate heat. Once hot, sauté the cauliflower and mushrooms until softened. Add in the garlic and continue to sauté for a minute or so or until aromatic. Stir in the cream of celery soup, double cream, salt, and pepper. Continue to cook, covered, for 10 to 12 minutes, until most of the liquid has evaporated. Fold in the Romano cheese and stir to combine well.Serve with mayonnaise and enjoy!

520. Mediterranean Creamy Broccoli Casserole

(Ready in about 25 minutes | Servings 3) Per serving: 195 Calories; 12.7g Fat; 6.7g Carbs; 11.6g Protein; 3.2g Fiber

Ingredients

3/4 pound broccoli, cut into small florets 1 teaspoon Mediterranean spice mix 2 ounces Colby cheese, shredded 3 tablespoons sesame oil 1 red onion, minced 2 garlic cloves, minced 3 eggs, well-beaten 1/2 cup double cream

Directions

Begin by preheating your oven to 320 degrees F. Brush the sides and bottom of a casserole dish with a nonstick cooking spray. In a frying pan, heat the sesame oil over a moderately-high heat. Sauté the onion and garlic until just tender and fragrant. Add in the broccoli and continue to cook until crisp-tender for about 4 minutes. Spoon the mixture into the preparade casserole dish. Whisk the eggs with double cream and Mediterranean spice mix. Spoon this mixture over the broccoli layer. Bake in the preheated oven for 18 to 20 minutes.Bon appétit!

521. Greek Salad with Yogurt

(Ready in about 15 minutes + chilling time | Servings 4) Per serving: 318 Calories; 24.3g Fat; 4.1g Carbs; 15.4g Protein; 0.9g Fiber

Ingredients

1 cucumber, sliced 6 radishes, sliced 1 teaspoon basil 1 tablespoon fresh lemon juice 1/2 teaspoon oregano 1/4 cup fresh scallions, thinly sliced 1 cup Greek-style yogurt 2 tablespoons green garlic, minced Sea salt and ground black pepper, to taste 8 green oak lettuce leaves, torn into pieces

Directions

Whisk the yogurt with green garlic, lemon juice, basil, and oregano. Toss the remaining ingredients in a mixing bowl. Dress the salad and toss to combine well. Enjoy!

522. The Easiest Roasted Asparagus Ever

(Ready in about 20 minutes | Servings 4) Per serving: 48 Calories; 1.6g Fat; 4.4g Carbs; 5.5g Protein; 2.5g Fiber

Ingredients

1 pound asparagus spears 4 tablespoons pancetta, chopped 1/4 teaspoon caraway seeds 1/2 teaspoon dried rosemary Salt and freshly ground black pepper, to your liking 1 teaspoon shallot powder

Directions

Toss the asparagus spears with spices. Bake in the preheated oven at 450 degrees F for about 15 minutes. Top with the pancetta and continue to bake an additional 5 to 6 minutes.Enjoy!

523. Easy Keto Coleslaw

(Ready in about 10 minutes + chilling time | Servings 4) Per serving: 242 Calories; 20.5g Fat; 6.2g Carbs; 1g Protein; 3.1g Fiber

Ingredients

3/4 pound cabbage, cored and shredded 1/4 cup fresh cilantro, chopped 1/4 cup fresh chives, chopped 1 teaspoon fennel seeds Salt and pepper, to taste 1 large-sized celery, shredded 1 teaspoon deli mustard 2 tablespoons sesame seeds, lightly toasted 1 cup mayonnaise

Directions

Toss the cabbage, celery, mayonnaise, mustard, cilantro, chives, fennel seeds, salt, and pepper in a bowl. Sprinkle toasted sesame seeds over your salad.

524. Keto Noodles with Oyster Mushroom Sauce

(Ready in about 15 minutes | Servings 4) Per serving: 85 Calories; 3.5g Fat; 6.4g Carbs; 5.8g Protein; 3.3g Fiber

Ingredients

2 zucchinis, cut into thin strips 2 tablespoons olive oil 1 yellow onion, minced 2 garlic cloves, minced 1 pound oyster mushrooms, chopped 1 cup pureed tomatoes 1 cup vegetable broth 1 teaspoon Mediterranean sauce

Directions

Parboil the zucchini noodles for one minute or so. Reserve. Then, heat the oil in a saucepan over a moderately-high heat. Sauté the onion and garlic for 2 to 3 minutes. Add in the mushrooms and continue to cook for 2 to 3 minutes until they release liquid. Add in the remaining ingredients and cover the pan; let it simmer for 10 minutes longer until everything is cooked through. Top your zoodles with the prepared mushroom sauce.Enjoy!

525. Vegetables with Spicy Yogurt Sauce

(Ready in about 45 minutes | Servings 4) Per serving: 357 Calories; 35.8g Fat; 5.2g Carbs; 3.4g Protein; 2.5g Fiber

Ingredients

1/4 cup olive oil 1/2 teaspoon garlic, sliced 1/2 pound broccoli, cut into sticks 2 celery stalks, cut into sticks 2 bell peppers, deveined and sliced 1 red onion, sliced into wedges

For the Spicy Yogurt Sauce: 1 ½ cups Greek-Style yogurt Salt and pepper, to taste 2 tablespoons mayonnaise 1 poblano pepper, finely minced 1 tablespoon lemon juice

Directions

Toss the vegetables with olive oil and garlic. Arrange your vegetables on a parchment-lined baking sheet. Roast in the preheated oven at 380 degrees F for about 35 minutes, rotating the pan once or twice. Thoroughly combine all ingredients for the sauce.Bon appétit!

526. The Best Keto Pizza Ever

(Ready in about 25 minutes | Servings 4) Per serving: 234 Calories; 16.1g Fat; 6.3g Carbs; 13.6g Protein; 3.6g Fiber

Ingredients

For the Crust:

¼ cup double cream 1 tablespoon olive oil 1 pound cauliflower florets 1/2 cup Colby cheese 4 medium-sized eggs Salt and pepper, to taste For the Topping: 1 tomato, pureed 1/2 cup green mustard 1 tablespoon fresh basil 1/4 cup black olives, pitted and sliced 1 cup mozzarella cheese 1/2 cup romaine lettuce 1 cup lollo rosso

Directions

Parboil the cauliflower florets in a large pot of salted water until it is crisp-tender; add in the cheese, eggs, cream, olive oil, salt, and pepper. Press the crust mixture into the bottom of a lightly oiled baking pan. Bake in the middle of the oven at 385 degrees F. Bake for 13 to 15 minutes or until the crust is firm.Bon appétit!

527. Champinones Al Ajillo with Keto Naan

(Ready in about 20 minutes | Servings 6) Per serving: 281 Calories; 21.4g Fat; 6.1g Carbs; 6.4g Protein; 1.4g Fiber

Ingredients

1 pound button mushrooms, thinly sliced 1 teaspoon Spanish paprika 1/4 teaspoon flaky sea salt 8 tablespoons coconut oil, melted 1 egg plus 1 egg yolk, beaten 1/4 cup coconut flour 1/2 cup almond flour 1/2 teaspoon baking powder 2 tablespoons psyllium powder 1 tablespoon butter 1 teaspoon garlic, minced

Directions

Mix the flour with the baking powder, psyllium and salt until well combined. Add in 6 tablespoons of coconut oil, egg and egg yolk; pour in the water and stir to form a dough; let it stand for about 15 minutes. Divide the dough into 6 pieces and roll them out to form a disc. Use the remaining 2 tablespoons of coconut oil to bake naan bread. In a sauté pan, cook the mushrooms and garlic in hot butter until the mushrooms release liquid; season with Spanish paprika. Taste and adjust seasonings

528. Aromatic Chinese Cabbage

(Ready in about 15 minutes | Servings 4) Per serving: 142 Calories; 11.6g Fat; 5.7g Carbs; 2g Protein; 1.8g Fiber

Ingredients

4 tablespoons sesame oil 1 pound Chinese cabbage, outer leaves discarded, cored and shredded 1 tablespoon rice wine 1 celery rib, thinly sliced 1/4 teaspoon fresh ginger root, grated 1/2 teaspoon sea salt 1/2 cup onion, chopped 1 teaspoon garlic, pressed 1/2 teaspoon Sichuan pepper 1/4 cup vegetable stock

Directions

In a wok, heat the sesame oil over a medium-high flame. Stir fry the onion, and garlic for 1 minute or until just tender and fragrant. Add in the cabbage, celery, and ginger and continue to cook for 7 to 8 minutes more, stirring frequently to ensure even cooking. Stir in the remaining ingredients and continue to cook for a further 3 minutes.Bon appétit!

529. One-Pot Mushroom Stroganoff

(Ready in about 25 minutes | Servings 4) Per serving: 114 Calories; 7.3g Fat; 5.2g Carbs; 2.1g Protein; 3.1g Fiber

Ingredients

2 tablespoons canola oil 1 parsnip, chopped 1 cup fresh brown mushrooms, sliced 1 cup onions, chopped 2 garlic cloves, pressed 1/2 cup celery rib, chopped 1 teaspoon Hungarian paprika 3 ½ cups roasted vegetable broth 1 cup tomato puree 1 tablespoon flaxseed meal 2 tablespoons sherry wine 1 rosemary sprig, chopped 1/2 teaspoon dried basil 1/2 teaspoon dried oregano

Directions

In a heavy-bottomed pot, heat the oil over a moderately-high flame. Cook the onion and garlic for 2 minutes or until tender and aromatic. Add in the celery, parsnip, and mushrooms, and continue to cook until they've softened; reserve. Add in the sherry wine to deglaze the bottom of your pot. Add in the seasonings, vegetable broth, and tomato puree. Continue to simmer, partially covered, for 15 to 18 minutes. Add in the flaxseed meal and stir until the sauce has thickened.Bon appétit!

530. Zucchini Noodles with Famous Cashew Parmesan

(Ready in about 15 minutes | Servings 4) Per serving: 145 Calories; 10.6g Fat; 5.9g Carbs; 5.5g Protein; 1.6g Fiber

For Zoodles:

2 tablespoons canola oil 4 zucchinis, peeled and sliced into noodle-shape strands Salt and pepper, to taste

For Cashew Parmesan:

1/2 cup raw cashews 1/4 teaspoon onion powder 1 garlic clove, minced 2 tablespoons nutritional yeast Sea salt and pepper, to taste

Directions

In a saucepan, heat the canola oil over medium heat; once hot, cook your zoodles for 1 minute or so, stirring frequently to ensure even cooking. Season with salt and pepper to taste. In your food processor, process all ingredients for the cashew parmesan. Toss the cashew parmesan with the zoodles and enjoy!Enjoy!

531. Banana Blueberry Smoothie

(Ready in about 5 minutes | Servings 4) Per serving: 247 Calories; 21.7g Fat; 4.9g Carbs; 2.6g Protein; 3g Fiber

Ingredients

1/2 cup fresh blueberries 1/2 banana, peeled and sliced 1/2 cup water 1 ½ cups coconut milk 1 tablespoon vegan protein powder, zero carbs

Directions

Blend all ingredients until creamy and uniform.

532. Cajun Artichoke with Tofu

(Ready in about 30 minutes | Servings 4) Per serving: 138 Calories; 8.9g Fat; 6.8g Carbs; 6.4g Protein; 5g Fiber

Ingredients

1 pound artichokes, trimmed and cut into pieces 2 tablespoons coconut oil, room temperature 1 block tofu, pressed and cubed 1 teaspoon fresh garlic, minced 1 teaspoon Cajun spice mix 1 Spanish pepper, chopped 1/4 cup vegetable broth Salt and pepper, to taste

Directions Parboil your artichokes in a pot of lightly salted water for 13 to 15 minutes or until they're crisp-tender; drain. In a large saucepan, melt the coconut oil over medium-high heat; fry the tofu cubes for 5 to 6 minutes or until golden-brown. Add in the garlic, Cajun spice mix, Spanish pepper, broth, salt, and pepper. Add in the reserved artichokes and continue to cook until for 5 minutes more.

533. Colorful Creamy Soup

(Ready in about 25 minutes | Servings 6) Per serving: 142 Calories; 11.4g Fat; 5.6g Carbs; 2.9g Protein; 1.3g Fiber

Ingredients

2 cups Swiss chard, torn into pieces Sea salt and pepper, to taste 2 thyme sprigs, chopped 2 teaspoons sesame oil 1 onion, chopped 2 bay leaves 6 cups vegetable broth 1 cup grape tomatoes, chopped 1 cup almond milk, unflavored 1 teaspoon garlic, minced 2 celery stalks, chopped 1 zucchini, chopped 1/2 cup scallions, chopped

Directions In a heavy bottomed pot, heat the sesame oil in over a moderately-high heat. Sauté the onion, garlic, and celery, until they've softened. Add in the zucchini, Swiss chard, salt, pepper, thyme, bay leaves, broth, and tomatoes; bring to a rapid boil. Turn the heat to a simmer. Leave the lid slightly ajar and continue to simmer for about 13 minutes. Add in the almond milk and scallions; continue to cook for 4 minutes more or until thoroughly warmed. Enjoy!

534. Kadai Broccoli Masala

(Ready in about 15 minutes | Servings 4) Per serving: 100 Calories; 8.2g Fat; 4.7g Carbs; 3.7g Protein; 4g Fiber

Ingredients

1/4 cup sesame oil 1 pound broccoli florets 1/2 teaspoon Garam Masala 1 tablespoon Kasuri Methi (dried fenugreek leaves) 1 Badi Elaichi (black cardamom) 1 teaspoon garlic, pressed Salt and pepper, to taste

Directions

Parboil the broccoli for 6 to 7 minutes until it is crisp-tender. Heat the sesame oil in a wok or saucepan until sizzling. Once hot, cook your broccoli for 3 to 4 minutes. Add in the other ingredients and give it a quick stir. Adjust the spices to suit your taste.Bon appétit!

535. Broccoli Cheese Soup

Ready in about: 20 minutes | Serves: 4 Per serving: Kcal 561, Fat: 52.3g, Net Carbs: 7g, Protein: 23.8g

Ingredients

¾ cup heavy cream 1 onion, diced 1 garlic clove, minced 4 cups chopped broccoli 4 cups veggie broth 2 tbsp butter 1 ½ cups cheddar cheese, grated Salt and black pepper to taste 2 tbsp fresh mint, chopped

Directions

Melt the butter in a large pot over medium heat. Sauté onion and garlic for 3 minutes or until tender, stirring occasionally. Season with salt and black pepper. Add the broth and broccoli and bring to a boil. Reduce the heat and simmer for 10 minutes. Puree the soup with a hand blender until smooth. Add in 1 cup of the cheddar cheese and cook about 1 minute. Taste and adjust the seasoning. Stir in the heavy cream. Serve in bowls topped with the remaining cheddar cheese and sprinkled with fresh mint.

536. Tuna Salad with Lettuce & Olives

Ready in about: 5 minutes | Serves: 2 Per serving: Kcal 248, Fat: 20g, Net Carbs: 2g, Protein: 18.5g

Ingredients

1 cup canned tuna, drained 1 tsp onion flakes 3 tbsp mayonnaise 1 cup romaine lettuce, shredded 1 tbsp lime juice 6 black olives, pitted and sliced

DirectionsCombine the tuna, mayonnaise, and lime juice in a small bowl. Mix to Combine. In a salad platter, arrange the shredded lettuce and onion flakes. Spread the tuna mixture over. Top with black olives and serve.

537. Traditional Greek Salad

Ready in about: 10 minutes | Serves: 4 Per serving: Kcal 323, Fat: 28g, Net Carbs: 8g, Protein: 9.3g

Ingredients

5 tomatoes, chopped 1 large cucumber, chopped 1 green bell pepper, chopped 1 small red onion, chopped 10 Kalamata olives, chopped 4 tbsp capers 1 cup feta cheese, cubed 2 tbsp olive oil Salt to taste

DirectionsPlace tomatoes, bell pepper, cucumber, onion, feta cheese, salt, capers, and olive oil olives in a bowl. Mix to Combine well. Divide the salad between plates, top with the Kalamata olives, and serve.

538. Grilled Steak Salad with Pickled Peppers

Ready in about: 15 minutes | Serves: 4 Per serving: Kcal 315, Fat 26g, Net Carbs 2g, Protein 18g

Ingredients

½ lb skirt steak, sliced Salt and black pepper to taste 3 tsp olive oil 1 head Romaine lettuce, torn 3 chopped pickled peppers 2 tbsp red wine vinegar ½ cup queso fresco, crumbled 1 tbsp green olives, pitted, sliced

Directions

Brush the steak slices with some olive oil and season with salt and black pepper on both sides. Heat a grill pan over high heat and cook the steaks on each side for about 5-6 minutes. Remove to a bow. Mix the lettuce, pickled peppers, remaining olive oil, and vinegar in a salad bowl. Add the beef and sprinkle with queso fresco and green olives. Serve.

539. Pork Burger Salad with Yellow Cheddar

Ready in about: 25 minutes | Serves: 4 Per serving: Kcal 310, Fat 23g, Net Carbs 2g, Protein 22g

Ingredients

½ lb ground pork Salt and black pepper to taste 2 tbsp olive oil 2 hearts romaine lettuce, torn 2 firm tomatoes, sliced ¼ red onion, sliced 3 oz yellow cheddar cheese, grated 2 tbsp butter Season the pork with salt and black pepper, mix, and make medium-sized patties out of them.

Directions

Heat the butter in a skillet over medium heat and fry the patties on both sides for 10 minutes until browned and cook within. Transfer to a wire rack to drain oil. When cooled, cut into quarters. Mix the lettuce, tomatoes, and red onion in a salad bowl, season with olive oil and salt. Toss and add the pork on top. Top with the cheese and serve.

540. Italian-Style Tomato Crisps

(Ready in about 5 hours | Servings 6) Per serving: 161 Calories; 14g Fat; 6.2g Carbs; 4.6g Protein; 2.6g Fiber

Ingredients

1 tablespoon Italian spice mix 1 ½ pounds Romano tomatoes, sliced 1/4 cup extra-virgin olive oil

For Vegan Parmesan:

1/4 cup sunflower seeds Salt and pepper, to taste 1/4 teaspoon dried dill weed 1 teaspoon garlic powder 1/4 cup sesame seeds 1 tablespoon nutritional yeast

Directions

Process all ingredients for the vegan parmesan in your food processor. Toss the sliced tomatoes with the extra-virgin olive oil, Italian spice mix, and vegan parmesan. Arrange the tomato slices on a parchment-lined baking sheet in a single layer. Bake at 220 degrees F about 5 hours.

541. Greek-Style Spicy Tofu

(Ready in about 40 minutes | Servings 4) Per serving: 162 Calories; 10.9g Fat; 5.8g Carbs; 9.5g Protein; 3.3g Fiber

Ingredients

6 ounces tofu, pressed and cut into 1/4-inch thick slices 2 tablespoons balsamic vinegar 2 tablespoons olive oil 1 cup onions, chopped 1/2 teaspoon garlic, minced 1 tablespoon schug sauce For Vegan Tzatziki: 1 cup coconut yogurt 1/2 cucumber, shredded 1 teaspoon garlic, smashed 2 tablespoons fresh lime juice Sea salt and pepper, to taste 1 teaspoon dill weed, minced

Directions

Place the tofu, garlic, schug sauce, and balsamic vinegar in a ceramic bowl; let your tofu marinate for 30 minutes in your refrigerator. In a frying pan, heat the olive oil over a moderately-high heat. Cook the tofu with onions for 5 to 6 minutes until it is golden brown. Then, make the vegan tzatziki by whisking all ingredients in your bowl.Enjoy!

542.   Hungarian-Style Oyster Mushroom Stew

(Ready in about 50 minutes | Servings 4) Per serving: 65 Calories; 2.7g Fat; 6g Carbs; 2.7g Protein; 2.9g Fiber

Ingredients

2 teaspoons canola oil 2 ½ cups oyster mushrooms, chopped 1 tablespoon Hungarian paprika 2 thyme sprigs, chopped 1 bay laurel Salt and pepper, to taste 1 red onion, chopped 1/2 teaspoon garlic, finely minced 1 cup celery, chopped 2 bell peppers, chopped 1 ½ cups water 2 vegetable bouillon cubes 1 cup tomato puree

Directions

Heat canola oil in a soup pot over a moderately-high heat. Sauté the onion and garlic until they've softened. Stir in the celery, peppers, and mushrooms. Now, continue to cook for about 10 minutes, adding a splash of water to prevent sticking. Add in the remaining ingredients. Turn the heat to a simmer. Continue to cook, partially covered, for a further 30 minutes.Bon appétit!

543.   Vegetables with Crunchy Topping

(Ready in about 40 minutes | Servings 4) Per serving: 242 Calories; 16.3g Fat; 6.7g Carbs; 16.3g Protein; 3.2g Fiber

Ingredients

1/2 pound Brussels sprouts, quartered 2 tablespoons fresh parsley, chopped 1 cup vegetable broth 2 tablespoons sesame oil 1 cup onions, chopped 2 celery stalks, chopped Sea salt and pepper, to taste 1 teaspoon porcini powder 1 cup vegan parmesan

Directions

In a frying pan, heat the sesame oil over a moderately-high heat. Cook the onions, celery, and Brussels sprouts until they have softened. Spoon the vegetable mixture into a lightly greased baking dish. Whisk the vegetable broth with the salt, pepper, and porcini powder. Pour the mixture over the vegetables. Top with the vegan parmesan and parsley; bake in the preheated oven at 365 degrees F for 25 to 30 minutes.Bon appétit!

544.   Swiss Chard Dip

(Ready in about 25 minutes | Servings 6) Per serving: 75 Calories; 3g Fat; 6g Carbs; 2.9g Protein; 0.8g Fiber

Ingredients

2 cups Swiss chard 2 teaspoons sesame oil Salt and pepper, to taste 1 teaspoon dried Mediterranean spice mix 1 cup tofu, pressed and crumbled 1 teaspoon fresh garlic, smashed 1/2 cup almond milk 2 teaspoons nutritional yeast

Directions

Parboil the Swiss chard in a pot of lightly salted water for about 6 minutes. Transfer the mixture to the bowl of a food processor; add in the other ingredients. Process the ingredients until the mixture is homogeneous. Bake in the preheated oven at 390 degrees F for about 10 minutes.Enjoy!

545.   Cauliflower and Pepper Masala

(Ready in about 30 minutes | Servings 4) Per serving: 166 Calories; 13.9g Fat; 5.4g Carbs; 3g Protein; 3.1g Fiber

Ingredients

1 pound cauliflower florets 1/4 cup sesame oil 1 cup vegetable broth 2 bell peppers, halved 1 garlic clove, minced 2 sprigs curry leaves 1 teaspoon fennel seeds 1 tablespoon khus khus 1/2 of a star anise 1/2 teaspoon nigella seeds Salt and pepper, to taste

Directions

Parboil the cauliflower in a pot of a lightly-salted water for 5 to 6 minutes until crisp-tender. Dry roast all the apices on a low flame for about 3 minutes; reserve. In a wok, or a saucepan, heat the sesame oil until sizzling. Cook the cauliflower, peppers, and garlic for 5 to 6 minutes. Add in the salt, pepper, and broth and continue to cook for 10 minutes.Bon appétit!

546.   Pine Nut and Cauliflower Soup

(Ready in about 25 minutes | Servings 4) Per serving: 114 Calories; 6.5g Fat; 6.4g Carbs; 3.8g Protein; 3.5g Fiber

Ingredients

1/4 cup pine nuts, ground 1 pound cauliflower, broken into florets 4 cups vegetable broth 1 tablespoon sesame oil 1 cup onions, chopped 1 celery with leaves, chopped Salt and pepper, to taste 1 teaspoon garlic, smashed 1 tablespoon fresh coriander, minced

Directions

In a heavy-bottomed pot, heat sesame oil over a moderately-high flame. Sauté the onion, celery and garlic until tender and aromatic. Add in the cauliflower, vegetable broth, salt, pepper, and pine nuts. Bring to a boil. Immediately reduce the heat to simmer; continue to cook, partially covered, for about 18 minutes. Afterwards, add in the fresh coriander and puree your soup with an immersion blender.Enjoy!

547.   Keto "Oats" with Mixed Berries

(Ready in about 5 minutes + chilling time | Servings 4) Per serving: 176 Calories; 12.7g Fat; 6g Carbs; 9.7g Protein; 3.2g Fiber

Ingredients

1/2 cup hemp hearts 1/4 cup sunflower seeds 8 tablespoons granulated Swerve 1/2 teaspoon ground cinnamon 1/2 cup water 1/2 cup coconut milk, unsweetened 1 cup mixed berries

Directions

Thoroughly combine the water, milk, hemp hearts, sunflower seeds, Swerve, and cinnamon in an airtight container. Cover and let it stand in your refrigerator overnight.

548.   Chinese-Style Tofu in Spicy Sauce

(Ready in about 20 minutes | Servings 4) Per serving: 336 Calories; 22.2g Fat; 5.8g Carbs; 27.6g Protein; 3.4g Fiber

Ingredients

6 ounces smoked tofu, pressed, drained and cubed 1/2 teaspoon Chinese five-spice powder 2 tablespoons sesame oil 1 cup onions, chopped 2 garlic cloves, minced 1/2 cup vegetable broth For the Sauce: 1 teaspoon Sriracha sauce 1/2 tablespoon sesame oil 1/2 teaspoon cardamom 1 cup tomatoes, pureed 2 tablespoons Shaoxing rice wine

Directions

In a wok, heat 2 tablespoons of sesame oil over medium-high flame. Cook the tofu cubes until they are slightly browned or about 5 minutes. Add in the onions, garlic, vegetable broth, and Chinese five-spice powder. Stir fry for 5 to 7 minutes more until almost all liquid has evaporated. To make the Chinese sauce, heat 1/2 tablespoon of sesame oil over a moderate flame. Add in the pureed tomatoes and cook until thoroughly warmed. Add in the remaining ingredients and turn the heat to a simmer; continue to simmer for 8 to 10 minutes or until the sauce has reduced by half. Fold in tofu cubes and gently stir to combine.Enjoy!

549.   Cauliflower Slaw with Almonds

(Ready in about 15 minutes + chilling time | Servings 4) Per serving: 281 Calories; 26.8g Fat; 5.6g Carbs; 4.2g Protein; 3.4g Fiber

Ingredients

1 pound cauliflower florets 1/2 cup almonds, coarsely chopped 1 tablespoon balsamic vinegar 1 teaspoon deli mustard Salt and pepper, to taste 1/2 cup black olives, pitted and chopped 3/4 cup yellow onions, chopped 1 roasted pepper, chopped 1/4 cup olive oil

Directions

Parboil the cauliflower florets in a lightly-salted water for about 5 minutes until crisp-tender; transfer the cauliflower to a bowl.Bon appétit!

550.   Spicy Celery and Carrot Salad

(Ready in about 10 minutes | Servings 4) Per serving: 196 Calories; 17.2g Fat; 6g Carbs; 1.2g Protein; 2.2g Fiber

Ingredients

1/4 pound carrots, coarsely shredded 3/4 pound celery, shredded 1/4 cup fresh parsley, chopped For the Vinaigrette: 2 garlic cloves, smashed Sea salt and pepper, to taste 1/3 cup olive oil 1 lemon, freshly squeezed 2 tablespoons balsamic vinegar 1/2 teaspoon ground allspice 1/2 teaspoon Sriracha sauce

Directions

Toss the carrots, celery, and parsley in a bowl until everything is well combined. Mix all ingredients for a vinaigrette and dress your salad.

551.   Mushroom and Dijon Mustard-Stuffed Avocado

(Ready in about 10 minutes | Servings 8) Per serving: 245 Calories; 23.2g Fat; 6.2g Carbs; 2.4g Protein; 4g Fiber

Ingredients

4 avocados, halved 1 tablespoon Dijon mustard 1 shallot, chopped 2 garlic cloves, minced Salt and pepper, to taste 2 tablespoons sesame oil 2 cups brown mushrooms, chopped 1 cup grape tomatoes, diced 1/2 lemon, freshly squeezed

Directions

In a frying pan, heat sesame oil over a moderately-high heat. Sauté the mushrooms, shallot, and garlic until they are tender and fragrant. Scoop out about 1 tablespoon of the avocado flesh from each half. Add the avocado flash to the mushroom mixture along with the salt, pepper, Dijon mustard, and tomatoes. Divide the mushroom mixture among the avocado halves. Drizzle each avocado with lemon juice.

552.   Mediterranean Crunchy Salad with Seeds

(Ready in about 15 minutes | Servings 4) Per serving: 208 Calories; 15.6g Fat; 6.2g Carbs; 7.6g Protein; 6g Fiber

Ingredients

For Dressing:

2 tablespoons onions, chopped 1/2 teaspoon garlic, chopped 1 cup sunflower seeds, soaked overnight 1/2 cup almond milk 1 lemon, freshly squeezed 1/2 teaspoon Mediterranean herb mix Salt and pepper, to taste 1/2 teaspoon paprika

For the Salad:

2 tablespoons black olives, pitted 1 cup cherry tomatoes, halved 1 Lebanese cucumbers, sliced 1 head Romaine lettuce, separated into leaves 1 tablespoon cilantro leaves, coarsely chopped

Directions

Process all of the dressing ingredients until creamy and smooth. Toss all of the salad ingredients in a bowl. Dress your salad.

553.   Eggplant and Cashew Soup

(Ready in about 1 hour 20 minutes | Servings 4) Per serving: 159 Calories; 9.4g Fat; 7.1g Carbs; 4.2g Protein; 4g Fiber

Ingredients

1 pound eggplant, sliced 1/3 cup raw cashews, soaked overnight 1 teaspoon garlic, chopped 1/2 teaspoon Mediterranean herb mix 3 cups vegetable broth 1 tablespoon peanut oil 1 cup tomato puree 1 medium onion, chopped Salt and pepper, to season

Directions

Brush the eggplant slices with peanut oil. Roast in the preheated oven at 380 degrees F for about 35 minutes. Thoroughly combine the eggplant flesh with tomato, onion, garlic, Mediterranean herb mix, and vegetable broth in a heavy-bottomed pot. Leave the lid slightly ajar and continue to simmer for 35 to 40 minutes or until heated through. Puree the soup in your food processor or blender. Blend the soaked cashews with 1 cup of water until creamy and smooth. Spoon the cashew cream into the soup and stir until well combined. Season with salt and pepper to taste.Enjoy!

554.   Paprika Cauliflower Soup

(Ready in about 20 minutes | Servings 4) Per serving: 94 Calories; 7.2g Fat; 7g Carbs; 2.7g Protein; 2.8g Fiber

Ingredients

1/2 teaspoon paprika 2 heads of cauliflower, broken into florets 1/4 teaspoon mustard powder 1/2 teaspoon fenugreek 1/4 teaspoon ground cloves 1 ½ tablespoons vegetable broth 2 tablespoons extra-virgin olive oil

Directions

Parboil the cauliflower florets for about 12 minutes until crisp-tender. Add in the remaining ingredients and stir to combine. Let it simmer, partially covered, for about 10 minutes or until cooked through. Puree the mixture using your immersion blender.Enjoy!

555.   Fennel with Light Mediterranean Sauce

(Ready in about 20 minutes | Servings 4) Per serving: 135 Calories; 13.6g Fat; 3g Carbs; 0.9g Protein; 1.9g Fiber

Ingredients

1 fennel, thinly sliced 1/4 cup vegetable broth 2 tablespoons olive oil 1/2 teaspoon garlic, minced Salt and pepper, to taste 1 bay laurel For the Sauce: 1 cloves garlic, minced 1 cayenne pepper, minced 1 bunch fresh basil, leaves picked 1 teaspoon oregano 1 cup cherry tomatoes 2 tablespoons olive oil 1 teaspoon rosemary 1/2 cup red onion, chopped Sat and pepper, to taste

Directions

Heat 2 tablespoons of olive oil in a frying pan over a moderate flame. Sauté the garlic until aromatic. Add in the fennel, broth, salt, pepper, and bay laurel. Continue to cook until the fennel is just tender. Puree the sauce ingredients in your food processor until smooth and creamy. Heat the sauce over-medium low flame. Add in the fennel mixture and continue to cook for 5 to 6 minutes more or until everything is cooked through.Bon appétit!

556.   Vegetable Noodles with Classic Avocado Sauce

(Ready in about 15 minutes | Servings 4) Per serving: 233 Calories; 20.2g Fat; 6g Carbs; 1.9g Protein; 4g Fiber

Ingredients

3 tablespoons olive oil 1 yellow onion, chopped 1 poblano pepper, deveined and minced Salt and pepper, to season 1 avocado, peeled and pitted 1 lime, juiced and zested 2 tablespoons parsley, chopped 1/2 pound zucchini, spiralized 1/2 pound bell peppers, spiralized

Directions

In a saucepan, heat 1 tablespoon of olive oil over a moderately-high heat. Sauté the zucchini and peppers until crisp-tender or about 5 minutes. In your blender or food processor, pulse the other ingredients until well combined. Pour the avocado sauce over the vegetable noodles and toss to combine.Enjoy!

557.   Keto Crunch Cereal

(Ready in about 10 minutes | Servings 4) Per serving: 279 Calories; 23.6g Fat; 5.9g Carbs; 7.2g Protein; 2.2g Fiber

Ingredients

16 almonds, roughly chopped 1/3 cup coconut shreds 2 ½ cups almond milk, full-fat 1/2 cup water 2 tablespoons coconut oil, melted 4 tablespoons Swerve 1/2 cup hemp hearts A pinch of sea salt A pinch of grated nutmeg 1/2 teaspoon ground cinnamon

Directions

Place all ingredients, except for the almonds, in a deep saucepan over medium-low heat. Let it simmer, partially covered, for 5 to 6 minutes or until slightly thickened. Top each serving with slivered almonds.

558.   Easy Antipasto Skewers

(Ready in about 10 minutes | Servings 6) Per serving: 249 Calories; 19.3g Fat; 6g Carbs; 9.7g Protein; 1.4g Fiber

Ingredients

1 cup bacon, diced 4 ounces feta cheese, cubed 1/2 cup olives, pitted 6 ounces pickled cornichons, no sugar added 2 bell peppers, sliced 1/3 cup balsamic vinegar 1/3 cup olive oil 1/2 teaspoon cumin seeds

Directions

Toss all ingredients in a mixing bowl. Thread the pickled cornichons, bell peppers, feta cheese, bacon, and olives onto long wooden skewers, alternating the ingredients.

559.   Bell Pepper Bites

(Ready in about 20 minutes | Servings 4) Per serving: 252 Calories; 13.7g Fat; 5.6g Carbs; 26g Protein; 1.4g Fiber

Ingredients

4 bell peppers, deveined and quartered 2 tablespoons ghee, softened 2 ounces chorizo, chopped 1 yellow onion, minced 2 garlic cloves, minced 1 tablespoon fresh cilantro, finely chopped Salt and pepper, to taste 1/2

pound ground turkey 6 ounces cream cheese, softened

Directions

In a frying pan, melt the ghee over a moderately high flame. Once hot, sauté the onion until tender and translucent. Add in the ground turkey and continue to cook for a further 5 minutes or until no longer pink. Remove from the heat. Add in the cheese, garlic, cilantro, salt, and pepper. Divide the meat/cheese mixture between your peppers. Top with the chorizo and arrange your peppers on a parchment-lined baking sheet. Bake in the preheated oven at 370 degrees F for about 15 minutes or until the peppers are tender.

560.   Easy Bacon Chips

(Ready in about 15 minutes | Servings 6) Per serving: 409 Calories; 31.6g Fat; 1.1g Carbs; 28g Protein; 0.4g Fiber

Ingredients

1 pound bacon, cut into 1-inch squares 1 teaspoon Sriracha sauce 1 teaspoon lime juice 1 teaspoon lime zest 1 tablespoon smoked paprika

Directions Toss all ingredients in a mixing dish. Bake in the preheated oven at 365 degrees F approximately 15 minutes.Enjoy!

561.   Cheesy Carrot Sticks

(Ready in about 35 minutes | Servings 6) Per serving: 216 Calories; 18.7g Fat; 5.4g Carbs; 3.5g Protein; 3.6g Fiber

Ingredients

1 ½ pounds carrot, cuti into sticks 1/4 teaspoon mustard seeds 1 tablespoon Swerve 1 teaspoon basil 1/2 cup Colby cheese, grated 1 stick butter, melted Salt and pepper, to taste

Directions

Preheat your oven to 390 degrees F. Toss the carrot sticks with the melted butter, salt, pepper, mustard seeds, Swerve, and basil. Roast the carrot sticks in the preheated oven for 25 to 30 minutes, stirring every 10 minutes. Bon appétit!

562.   Spicy Double Cheese Chips

(Ready in about 20 minutes | Servings 6) Per serving: 225 Calories; 19.3g Fat; 0.6g Carbs; 12.1g Protein; 0.2g Fiber

Ingredients

4 slices prosciutto, crumbled 1 poblano pepper, finely chopped 1 cup Parmesan cheese, finely shredded 1 cup Cheddar cheese, shredded 1/2 teaspoon cayenne pepper 1/2 teaspoon allspice Salt and pepper, to taste

Directions Start by preheating your oven to 390 degrees F. Coat a baking sheet with a sheet of parchment paper. Mix all ingredients until well combined. Add the mixture in small heaps on the prepared baking sheet; be sure to leave enough room in between your crisps. Bake in the preheated oven approximately 10 minutes. Let them cool on a cooling rack.Enjoy!

563.   Cherry Tomatoes with Creamy Chive Sauce

(Ready in about 25 minutes | Servings 6) Per serving: 230 Calories; 21g Fat; 6g Carbs; 5.1g Protein; 2.5g Fiber

Ingredients

1 Adobo spice mix 1/4 cup extra-virgin olive oil 1 ½ pounds cherry tomatoes For the Sauce: 1/2 cup aïoli 1/2 cup fresh chives, chopped 1 cup cream cheese

Directions Toss your tomatoes with the Adobo spice mix and olive oil. Roast in the preheated oven at 420 degrees F for about 20 minutes. In the meantime, make the sauce by whisking all the sauce ingredients.Enjoy!

564.   Chives Cheese Bites

(Ready in about 10 minutes + chilling time | Servings 6) Per serving: 108 Calories; 9g Fat; 2.2g Carbs; 4.8g Protein; 0.2g Fiber

Ingredients

1/2 cup fresh chives, finely chopped 1/4 teaspoon champagne vinegar Salt and pepper, to taste 1 cup Cottage cheese 3 tablespoons butter

Directions Thoroughly combine the cheese, butter, and vinegar. Season with salt and pepper to taste. Place the cheese mixture in the refrigerator to chill for 2 to 3 hours. Roll the mixture into bite-sized balls and roll them in the chopped chives.Serve well chilled!

565. Garlic Romano Chicken Wings

(Ready in about 1 hour 10 minutes | Servings 6) Per serving: 312 Calories; 23g Fat; 0.9g Carbs; 24.6g Protein; 0.3g Fiber

Ingredients

2 pounds chicken wings, bone-in 1 teaspoon hot sauce 1 cup Romano cheese, grated Salt and black pepper, to taste 2 cloves garlic, smashed 1 stick butter 1 tablespoon champagne vinegar 1/2 cup Italian parsley, chopped

Directions

Line a large rimmed baking sheet with a metal rack. Preheat an oven to 420 degrees F. Set a metal rack on top of a baking sheet. Toss the wings with salt and black pepper. Bake in the preheated oven at 410 degrees F until golden and crispy, for 45 to 50 minutes. Place the garlic, butter, vinegar and hot sauce in a saucepan; cook over low heat until the sauce has thickened slightly. Remove from the heat and fold in the cheese; toss the wings with the cheese mixture until well coated. Bake an additional 8 minutes and top with parsley.Enjoy!

566. Cheese and Ground Meat Sauce

(Ready in about 15 minutes | Servings 10) Per serving: 195 Calories; 12g Fat; 1.5g Carbs; 19.5g Protein; 0g Fiber

Ingredients

8 ounces cream cheese, at room temperature 6 ounces Cheddar cheese, grated 1/2 pound ground pork 1/2 pound ground turkey 1 teaspoon shallot powder 1/2 teaspoon mustard powder 1/2 teaspoon porcini powder 1 tablespoon olive oil 1/2 teaspoon granulated garlic 1/2 teaspoon cayenne pepper Salt and black pepper, to taste

Directions

Heat the oil in a saucepan over a moderately-high flame. Cook the ground meat for about 5 minutes until no longer pink. Add in the remaining ingredients and continue to simmer over low heat for about 4 minutes. Enjoy!

567. Sesame Shrimp Bites

(Ready in about 15 minutes | Servings 6) Per serving: 107 Calories; 4.9g Fat; 1g Carbs; 15.3g Protein; 0.8g Fiber

Ingredients

1 pound shrimp, deveined and shelled 2 tablespoons sesame seeds 1/4 cup fish stock 2 garlic cloves, pressed 2 tablespoons sesame oil 1/2 cup onions, chopped 1 teaspoon chili powder 2 tablespoons dry white wine Salt and ground black pepper, to taste

Directions

Heat the oil in a saucepan over a moderately-high heat. Cook the shrimp, garlic and onions for about 3 minutes. Add in the remaining ingredients and cook for 10 minutes more until cooked through.Enjoy!

568.   Spicy Parm Meatballs

(Ready in about 15 minutes | Servings 10) Per serving: 158 Calories; 7.9g Fat; 0.4g Carbs; 20.4g Protein; 0.1g Fiber

Ingredients

1 egg, beaten 1/3 cup double cream 3/4 pound ground turkey 1/2 pound ground pork 2 garlic cloves, finely minced 1 teaspoon shallot powder 1/2 teaspoon mustard seeds 1 teaspoon hot sauce 1/4 cup pork rinds, crushed 1/3 cup Parmesan cheese, grated Sea salt and black pepper, to taste 1 teaspoon fresh basil, minced

Directions

In a mixing bowl, combine all ingredients until everything is well incorporated. Roll the mixture into small balls and arrange them on a parchment-lined baking sheet. Bake in the preheated oven at 390 degrees F for 8 to 10 minutes. Then, flip them over and cook another 8 minutes until they are browned and slightly crisp on top.Bon appétit!

569.   Sardine Stuffed-Eggs

(Ready in about 20 minutes | Servings 6) Per serving: 216 Calories; 17.3g Fat; 1.8g Carbs; 12.2g Protein; 0.2g Fiber

Ingredients

1 can sardines, drained 1/2 teaspoon smoked paprika 1 teaspoon fresh or dried basil 1 tablespoon fresh chives, chopped 1 poblano pepper, minced 12 eggs 1/3 cup aioli Salt and pepper, to taste

Directions

Place the eggs in a saucepan and cover them with water by 1 inch. Cover and bring the water to a boil over high heat. Boil for 6 to 7 minutes over medium-high heat. Peel the eggs and slice them in half lengthwise; mix the yolks with the remaining ingredients. Divide the mixture among the egg whites.Enjoy!

570.   Celery Fries with Pecans

(Ready in about 35 minutes | Servings 6) Per serving: 96 Calories; 8.5g Fat; 4.1g Carbs; 1.5g Protein; 2.6g Fiber

Ingredients

1 ½ pounds celery root, cut into sticks 2 tablespoons sesame oil 1/4 cup pecans, coarsely ground 1 tablespoon Adobo seasoning mix Salt and pepper, to taste 1/2 teaspoon smoked paprika

Directions

Start by preheating your oven to 395 degrees F. Coat a baking sheet with a Silpat mat. Toss the celery root with the sesame oil, salt, pepper, paprika, and Adobo seasoning mix. Place the celery stick on the prepared baking sheet and bake in the preheated oven for 30 to 35 minutes, turning them over once or twice. Sprinkle with pecans.Bon appétit!

571.Cheesy Cauliflower Florets

(Ready in about 40 minutes | Servings 6) Per serving: 167 Calories; 13.4g Fat; 2.4g Carbs; 7.5g Protein; 2.4g Fiber

Ingredients

1 ½ pounds cauliflower florets 1 cup Parmigiano-Reggiano cheese, grated 1 teaspoon hot sauce Sea salt and pepper, to your liking 1 teaspoon lemongrass, grated 1/4 cup butter, melted

Directions

Toss the cauliflower with melted butter, salt, pepper, lemongrass, and hot sauce. Place the cauliflower florets on a parchment-lined baking pan and roast them in the preheated oven at 420 degrees F. Roast the cauliflower florets for about 35 minutes. Toss with Parmigiano-Reggiano and roast an additional 5 to 7 minutes or until the top is crispy.

572.   Seafood Stuffed Mushrooms

(Ready in about 25 minutes | Servings 4) Per serving: 221 Calories; 13.5g Fat; 6g Carbs; 19.8g Protein; 1.9g Fiber

Ingredients

1 teaspoon Old Bay seasoning blend 1 cup Neufchâtel cheese 1/4 cup mayonnaise 1 pound button mushrooms, stems removed Salt and pepper, to taste 1/2 teaspoon mustard seeds 1/2 pound mixed seafood 1 teaspoon garlic, pressed 1 tablespoon scallions, minced

Directions

Start by preheating your oven to 395 degrees F. Brush a baking pan with a nonstick cooking spray. Sprinkle the mushrooms with salt, pepper, mustard seeds, and Old Bay seasoning blend. Mix the remaining ingredients to prepare the filling. Divide the filling mixture between mushroom caps. Bake in the preheated oven for about 18 minutes or until cooked through.

573.   Chicken Drumettes with Tomatillo Dip

(Ready in about 50 minutes | Servings 4) Per serving: 161 Calories; 3.5g Fat; 8.4g Carbs; 20.6g Protein; 2g Fiber

Ingredients

12 chicken drumettes 1 teaspoon coarse sea salt 1/2 teaspoon ground black pepper, or more to taste

For the Tomatillo Dip:

1 teaspoon chili pepper, deveined and finely minced 2 tablespoons coriander, finely chopped 2 tablespoons red wine vinegar 4 medium tomatillos, crushed 1 onion, finely chopped 1 cup peppers, chopped

Directions

Toss the chicken drumettes with salt and black pepper. Bake them in the preheated oven at 390 degrees F for about 40 minutes or until they are golden and crispy. In a mixing bowl, thoroughly combine all ingredients for the dip.Enjoy!

574. Italian Stuffed Mushrooms

(Ready in about 35 minutes | Servings 4) Per serving: 206 Calories; 13.4g Fat; 5.6g Carbs; 12.7g Protein; 4g Fiber

Ingredients

1 pound button mushrooms, stems removed 2 tablespoons coconut oil, melted 1 pound broccoli florets 1 Italian pepper, chopped 1 teaspoon Italian herb mix Salt and pepper, to taste 1 shallot, finely chopped 2 garlic cloves, minced 1 cup vegan parmesan

Directions

Parboil the broccoli in a large pot of salted water until crisp-tender, about 6 minutes. Mash the broccoli florets with a potato masher. In a saucepan, melt the coconut oil over a moderately-high heat. Once hot, cook the shallot, garlic, and pepper until tender and fragrant. Season with the spices and add in the broccoli. Fill the mushroom cups with the broccoli mixture and bake in the preheated oven at 365 degrees F for about 10 minutes. Top with the vegan parmesan and bake for 10 minutes more or until it melts. Enjoy!

575. Avocado with Pine Nuts

(Ready in about 10 minutes | Servings 4) Per serving: 263 Calories; 24.8g Fat; 6.5g Carbs; 3.5g Protein; 6.1g Fiber

Ingredients

2 avocados, pitted and halved 1 tablespoon coconut aminos 1/2 teaspoon garlic, minced 1 teaspoon fresh lime juice Salt and pepper, to taste 5 ounces pine nuts, ground 1 celery stalk, chopped

Directions

Thoroughly combine the avocado pulp with the pine nuts, celery, garlic, fresh lime juice, and coconut aminos. Season with salt and pepper to taste. Spoon the filling into the avocado halves.

576. Cream of Broccoli Soup

(Ready in about 15 minutes | Servings 4) Per serving: 252 Calories; 20.3g Fat; 5.8g Carbs; 8.1g Protein; 4.5g Fiber

Ingredients

1 pound broccoli, cut into small florets 8 ounces baby spinach 4 cups roasted vegetable broth 2 tablespoons olive oil 1 yellow onion, chopped 2 garlic cloves, minced 1/2 cup coconut milk Salt and pepper, to taste 2 tablespoons parsley, chopped

Directions

Heat the oil in a soup pot over a moderately-high flame. Then, sauté the onion and garlic until they're tender and fragrant. Add in the broccoli, spinach, and broth; bring to a rolling boil. Immediately turn the heat to a simmer. Pour in the coconut milk, salt, pepper, and parsley; continue to simmer, partially covered, until cooked through. Puree your soup with an immersion blender.Enjoy!

577. Mushroom and Cauliflower Medley

(Ready in about 30 minutes | Servings 4) Per serving: 113 Calories; 6.7g Fat; 6.6g Carbs; 5g Protein; 2.7g Fiber

Ingredients

8 ounces brown mushrooms, halved 1 head cauliflower, cut into florets 1/4 cup olive oil   1/2 teaspoon turmeric powder 1 teaspoon garlic, smashed 1 cup tomato, pureed Salt and pepper, to taste

Directions

Toss all ingredients in a lightly oiled baking pan. Roast the vegetable in the preheated oven at 380 degrees F for 25 to 30 minutes.Enjoy!

578. Tofu Stuffed Zucchini

(Ready in about 50 minutes | Servings 4) Per serving: 208 Calories; 14.4g Fat; 8.8g Carbs; 6.5g Protein; 4.3g Fiber

Ingredients

4 zucchinis, cut into halves lengthwise and scoop out the pulp 6 ounces firm tofu, drained and crumbled 2 garlic cloves, pressed 1/2 cup onions, chopped 1 tablespoon olive oil 1 cup tomato puree 1 tablespoon nutritional yeast 2 ounces pecans, chopped 1/4 teaspoon curry powder Sea salt and pepper, to taste

Directions

In a saucepan, heat the olive oil over a moderately-high heat; cook the tofu, garlic, and onion for about 5 minutes. Stir in the tomato puree and scooped zucchini pulp; add all seasonings and continue to cook for a further 5 to 6 minutes. Spoon the filling into the zucchini "shells" and arrange them in a lightly greased baking dish. Bake in the preheated oven at 365 degrees F for 25 to 30 minutes. Top with nutritional yeast and pecans nuts; bake for a further 5 minutes.Enjoy!

579. Lebanese Asparagus with Baba Ghanoush

(Ready in about 45 minutes | Servings 6) Per serving: 149 Calories; 12.1g Fat; 6.3g Carbs; 3.6g Protein; 4.6g Fiber

Ingredients

1/4 cup sesame oil 1 ½ pounds asparagus spears, med 1/2 teaspoon red pepper flakes Salt and pepper, to taste

For Baba Ghanoush:

2 tablespoons fresh lime juice 2 teaspoons olive oil 1/2 cup onion, chopped 3/4 pound eggplant 1 teaspoon garlic, minced 1 tablespoon sesame paste 1/2 teaspoon allspice 1/4 teaspoon ground nutmeg 1/4 cup fresh parsley leaves, chopped Salt and ground black pepper, to taste

Directions Toss the asparagus spears with sesame oil, salt, and pepper. Arrange the asparagus spears on a foil-lined baking pan. Roast in the preheated oven at 380 degrees F for 8 to 10 minutes. Meanwhile, make your Baba Ghanoush. Bake eggplants in the preheated oven at 420 degrees F for 25 to 30 minutes; discard the skin and stems. In a saucepan, heat 2 the olive oil over a moderately-high heat. Cook the onion and garlic until tender and fragrant; heat off. Add the roasted eggplant, sautéed onion mixture, sesame paste, lime juice, and spices to your blender or food processor. Pulse until creamy and smooth.

580.   Walnut-Stuffed Mushrooms

(Ready in about 30 minutes | Servings 4) Per serving: 139 Calories; 11.2g Fat; 5.4g Carbs; 4.8g Protein; 1.8g Fiber

Ingredients

1 pound button mushrooms, stems removed and chopped Salt and pepper, to taste 1/4 cup walnuts, chopped 2 tablespoons parsley, chopped 2

tablespoons olive oil 1 cup shallots, chopped 1/2 teaspoon garlic, minced

Directions

Preheat your oven to 365 degrees F. Line a baking pan with a parchment paper. In a saucepan, heat the olive oil over medium-high flame. Now, sauté the shallot and garlic until tender and aromatic. Add in the mushrooms stems and continue to cook until they've softened. Remove from the heat and season with salt and pepper. Stir in the chopped walnuts and parsley; stuff the mushroom caps with the prepared filling. Place your mushrooms on the prepared baking pan. Bake for 20 to 25 minutes until heated through.

581.   Zuppa Toscana with Zucchini

(Ready in about 45 minutes | Servings 4) Per serving: 165 Calories; 13.4g Fat; 6.7g Carbs; 2.2g Protein; 6g Fiber

Ingredients

3 cups zucchini, peeled and chopped 1 tomato, pureed 1 avocado pitted, peeled and mashed 1 cup scallions, chopped 1 celery, sliced 1 parsnip, sliced 3 teaspoons olive oil Salt and black pepper, to taste 4 cups vegetable broth

Directions

In a soup pot, heat the oil over a moderately-high heat. Sauté the scallion, celery, parsnip, and zucchini until they've softened. Add in the salt, pepper, vegetable broth, and pureed tomato; bring it to a boil. Turn the heat to a simmer. Continue to simmer for about 25 minutes. Remove from the heat and fold in the mashed avocado. Puree your soup with an immersion blender.Enjoy!

582.   Peanut Butter Berry Smoothie

(Ready in about 5 minutes | Servings 1) Per serving: 114 Calories; 8.2g Fat; 5.9g Carbs; 4.2g Protein; 1.8g Fiber

Ingredients

1 tablespoon peanut butter 1/3 cup mixed berries 3/4 cup coconut milk, unsweetened 1 teaspoon Swerve 1/2 cup lettuce

Directions

583.   Blend all ingredients until creamy and smooth.

Dark Chocolate Smoothie

(Ready in about 10 minutes | Servings 2) Per serving: 335 Calories; 31.7g Fat; 5.7g Carbs; 7g Protein; 1.9g Fiber

Ingredients

1 tablespoon chia seeds 1 tablespoon unsweetened cocoa powder 2 tablespoons Swerve 8 almonds 1/2 cup coconut milk 1/2 cup water 1 ½ cups baby spinach

Directions

Process all ingredients until smooth and creamy.

584.   Savoy Cabbage with Tempeh

(Ready in about 20 minutes | Servings 4) Per serving: 179 Calories; 11.7g Fat; 2.1g Carbs; 10.5g Protein; 2.3g Fiber

Ingredients

1/2 pound savoy cabbage, shredded 2 tablespoons sesame oil 6 ounces tempeh, crumbled 1 teaspoon garlic, minced 1/2 cup white onion, chopped 2 tablespoons vegetable broth 2 tablespoons coconut aminos Sea salt and pepper, to season

Directions

In a wok, heat the sesame oil over a moderately-high heat. Sauté the garlic and onion until tender and fragrant. Now, add in the remaining ingredients and cook for 15 minutes or until thoroughly cooked.Bon appétit!

585.   Easy Vegan Granola

(Ready in about 1 hour | Servings 8) Per serving: 262 Calories; 24.3g Fat; 5.2g Carbs; 5.1g Protein; 2.2g Fiber

Ingredients

1/2 cup pine nuts, chopped 1/2 cup almonds, slivered 2 tablespoons sunflower seeds 2 tablespoons sesame seeds 1/4 cup flax seeds 2 tablespoons granulated Swerve 2 tablespoons coconut oil, melted A pinch of Himalayan salt 1 teaspoon grated orange peel 1/8 teaspoon allspice, freshly grated 1 teaspoon ground cinnamon 1/3 cup shredded coconut flakes 1 ½ cups almond milk, unsweetened

Directions

Toss all ingredients in a parchment-lined baking pan. Roast in the preheated oven at 290 degrees F for about 70 minutes; check and stir every 20 minutes.

586.   Hemp and Chia Pudding

(Ready in about 5 minutes + prep time | Servings 3) Per serving: 153 Calories; 8g Fat; 6.7g Carbs; 6.7g Protein; 2.6g Fiber

Ingredients

2 cups coconut milk, unsweetened 9 blackberries, fresh or frozen 1/4 cup hemp hearts 1/4 cup chia seeds 1/4 teaspoon ground cloves 1/4 teaspoon grated nutmeg 1/4 teaspoon ground cinnamon 1/8 teaspoon coarse sea salt A few drops of liquid Stevia

Directions

Thoroughly combine the coconut milk, hemp hearts, chia seeds, ground cloves, nutmeg, cinnamon, salt, and Stevia in an airtight container. Cover and let it stand in your refrigerator overnight.Top with blackberries and serve.

587.   Easy Authentic Guacamole

(Ready in about 10 minutes + chilling time | Servings 8) Per serving: 112 Calories; 9.9g Fat; 6.5g Carbs; 1.3g Protein; 2.4g Fiber

Ingredients

2 tomatoes, pureed 2 avocados, peeled, pitted, and mashed 1 teaspoon garlic, smashed 1 ancho chili pepper, deveined and minced Sea salt and pepper, to taste 1 shallot, chopped 2 tablespoons cilantro, chopped 2 tablespoons fresh lemon juice

Directions

Thoroughly combine all ingredients Keep in your refrigerator until ready to serve. Bon appétit!

588. Chocolate and Berry Shake

(Ready in about 5 minutes | Servings 2) Per serving: 103 Calories; 5.9g Fat; 6.1g Carbs; 4.1g Protein; 2.4g Fiber

Ingredients

1 cup mixed berries 1 tablespoon cocoa, unsweetened 1 tablespoon peanut butter 1 tablespoon flax seeds, ground 1/4 teaspoon ground cloves 1/2 teaspoon ground cinnamon 2 tablespoons Swerve 1 cup water

Directions

Blend all ingredients until smooth, creamy, and uniform.

589. Traditional Ethiopian-Style Peppers

(Ready in about 40 minutes | Servings 4) Per serving: 77 Calories; 4.8g Fat; 5.4g Carbs; 1.6g Protein; 3.1g Fiber

Ingredients

4 bell peppers, seeds removed, and halved 1 cup tomato puree 1 ½ tablespoons avocado oil 1 teaspoon ancho chili powder 1 teaspoon Berbere 1 shallot, chopped 1/2 teaspoon garlic, smashed 1/2 pound cauliflower rice Kosher salt and red pepper, to season

Directions

Start by preheating your oven to 365 degrees F. Roast the peppers for about 15 minutes until the skin is slightly charred. In a saucepan, heat the avocado oil over medium-high flame. Sauté the shallot and garlic until they are just tender. Stir in the cauliflower rice, ancho chili powder, and Berbere spice and cook for 5 to 6 minutes. Spoon the cauliflower mixture into pepper halves. Place the peppers in a lightly greased casserole dish. Add the tomato, salt and pepper around to the casserole dish and bake for about 15 minutes.

590. Tofu Cubes with Pine Nuts

(Ready in about 13 minutes | Servings 4) Per serving: 232 Calories; 21.6g Fat; 5.3g Carbs; 8.3g Protein; 2.4g Fiber

Ingredients

1 cup extra firm tofu, pressed and cubed 1/4 cup pine nuts, coarsely chopped 2 teaspoons lightly toasted sesame seeds 3 teaspoons avocado oil 1 ½ tablespoons coconut aminos 3 tablespoons vegetable broth 1/2 teaspoon porcini powder 1/2 teaspoon ground cumin Salt and pepper, to season 2 garlic cloves, minced 1 teaspoon red pepper flakes

Directions In a wok, heat the avocado oil over a moderately-high heat. Now, fry the tofu cubes for 5 to 6 minutes until golden brown on all sides. Stir in the pecans, coconut aminos, broth, garlic, red pepper, porcini powder, cumin, salt, and pepper and continue to stir for about 8 minutes. Top with toasted sesame seeds.Bon appétit!

591. Thai-Style Braised Cabbage

(Ready in about 15 minutes | Servings 6) Per serving: 186 Calories; 17g Fat; 5.3g Carbs; 2.1g Protein; 2g Fiber

Ingredients

2 pounds Chinese cabbage, cut into wedges 1 Thai bird chili, minced 1 teaspoon sesame seeds 1/4 teaspoon cinnamon 1/2 cup vegetable broth 2 tablespoons fresh chives, chopped 4 tablespoons sesame oil 1/4 teaspoon cardamom Salt and black pepper, to taste

Directions

In a wok or a large saucepan, heat the sesame oil over medium-high heat. Then, fry the cabbage until crisp-tender. Stir in the remaining ingredients and continue to cook for 10 minutes more or until heated through.Bon appétit!

592. Garlicky Brussels Sprouts

(Ready in about 25 minutes | Servings 4) Per serving: 118 Calories; 7g Fat; 3.4g Carbs; 2.9g Protein; 4g Fiber

Ingredients

1/2 teaspoon Sichuan peppercorns, crushed 1/2 teaspoon Cassia 1/2 teaspoon jiāng (ginger) 1 pound Brussels sprouts, torn into pieces 2 tablespoons sesame oil 1/2 head garlic, smashed Salt and ground black pepper, to the taste

Directions

Parboil the Brussels sprouts in a pot of a lightly salted water for 15 to 17 minutes over a moderately-high heat. Drain. In a wok, heat the sesame oil over a moderately-high heat. Then, sauté the garlic for a minute or so. Add in the reserved Brussels sprouts and spices; continue to cook until everything is cooked through.

593. Spanish-Style Roasted Vegetables

(Ready in about 45 minutes | Servings 4) Per serving: 165 Calories; 14.3g Fat; 5.6g Carbs; 2.1g Protein; 1.9g Fiber

Ingredients

4 tablespoons olive oil 4 tablespoons cream of mushroom soup 1 teaspoon Ñora 1 teaspoon saffron 2 zucchinis, cut into thick slices 1 onion, quartered 4 garlic cloves, halved 3 Spanish peppers, deveined and sliced 1/2 head of cauliflower, broken into large florets 1 teaspoon dried sage, crushed Salt and pepper, to taste

Directions

Toss all ingredients in a parchment-lined roasting pan. Roast in the preheated oven at 420 degrees F for 35 to 40 minutes. Toss your vegetables halfway through the cook time. Taste and adjust the seasonings.

594. Rich and Easy Granola

(Ready in about 1 hour | Servings 6) Per serving: 449 Calories; 44.9g Fat; 6.9g Carbs; 9.3g Protein; 2.3g Fiber

Ingredients

1/3 cup coconut oil, melted 1/2 cup almonds, chopped 1 teaspoon lime zest 1/3 cup water 1 cup pecans, chopped 1/3 cup chia seeds 1/3 cup pumpkin seeds A few drops of Stevia 1/3 cup flax meal 1/3 cup almond milk 1 teaspoon ground cinnamon 1 teaspoon freshly grated nutmeg

Directions

Preheat an oven to 310 degrees F. Coat a cookie sheet with parchment paper. Toss all ingredients together and spread the mixture out in an even layer onto the prepared cookie sheet. Bake about for 50 to 55 minutes, stirring every 15 to 20 minutes.

595.   Vegan Skillet with Tofu and Cabbage

(Ready in about 25 minutes | Servings 4) Per serving: 128 Calories; 8.3g Fat; 6.5g Carbs; 5.1g Protein; 3.2g Fiber

Ingredients

1 pound cabbage, trimmed and quartered 8 ounces tofu, pressed, drained and cubed 1 celery stalk, chopped 1/2 cup onions, chopped 2 tablespoons sesame oil 1 teaspoon red pepper flakes, crushed Salt and pepper, to taste 1/2 teaspoon curry paste 1/4 teaspoon dried oregano 2 garlic cloves, pressed 2 tablespoons coconut aminos

Directions

Heat the sesame oil in a nonstick skillet over a moderately-high heat. Then, fry the tofu cubes for about 7 minutes or until golden brown on all sides. Add in the celery and onions, and continue to cook for a further 5 minutes until they are just tender. Add in the other ingredients and continue to cook, partially covered, for 7 to 8 minutes longer. Fold in the tofu cubes and gently stir to combine.Bon appétit!

596.   Pancetta and Chives Deviled Eggs

(Ready in about 20 minutes | Servings 10) Per serving: 128 Calories; 9.7g Fat; 3.3g Carbs; 6.8g Protein; 0.1g Fiber

Ingredients

10 eggs 1/4 cup pancetta, chopped 1 tablespoon deli mustard 1/4 teaspoon Sriracha sauce 1/2 cup mayonnaise 1 tablespoon fresh basil, finely chopped 2 teaspoons champagne vinegar

Directions

Place the eggs in a saucepan and cover them with water by 1 inch. Cover and bring the water to a boil over high heat. Boil for 6 to 7 minutes over medium-high heat. Peel the eggs and slice them in half lengthwise; mix the yolks with the remaining ingredients. Divide the mixture between the egg whites and arrange the deviled eggs on a nice serving platter.Enjoy!

597.   Cheese Cucumber Rounds

(Ready in about 10 minutes | Servings 10) Per serving: 63 Calories; 4.3g Fat; 2.7g Carbs; 4g Protein; 0.1g Fiber

Ingredients

2 cucumbers, cut into thick slices 2 tablespoons ham, chopped 1/4 cup chives, chopped 1 teaspoon ancho chili powder 1 cup goat cheese

Directions

Mix the cheese, ham, chives, and ancho chili powder until well combined. Divide the mixture between cucumber slices.

598.   Sour Cream and Bacon Dip

(Ready in about 5 minutes | Servings 6) Per serving: 147 Calories; 10.6g Fat; 2.7g Carbs; 10.2g Protein; 0.4g Fiber

Ingredients

5 ounces sour cream 1/2 cup Canadian bacon, crumbled 2 tablespoons fresh parsley, chopped 1 cup mozzarella cheese, shredded 5 ounces cream cheese, at room temperature

Directions

Mix all ingredients until well combined.Enjoy!

599.　Swiss Cheese and Salami Cups

(Ready in about 20 minutes | Servings 6) Per serving: 162 Calories; 13.1g Fat; 2.5g Carbs; 8.7g Protein; 1.7g Fiber

Ingredients

12 winter salami slices 1/2 cup spicy tomato sauce 1 teaspoon Italian spice mix 1 cup Swiss cheese, shredded 1/2 cup black olives, pitted and chopped

Directions

Spritz 12-cup muffin tin with a nonstick cooking spray. Place a salami slice in each muffin cup. Add in the cheese, tomato sauce, Italian spice mix, and olives. Bake in the preheated oven at 365 degrees F approximately 16 minutes.Enjoy!

600.　Keto Paprika Crackers

(Ready in about 30 minutes | Servings 12) Per serving: 119 Calories; 8g Fat; 4.7g Carbs; 2.6g Protein; 1.1g Fiber

Ingredients

1/2 cup sesame seeds 1/4 tablespoons sunflower seeds 2 tablespoons flax seeds 1 tablespoon pine nuts, ground 1/3 cup pumpkin seeds, ground 1/4 cup psyllium husks Coarse sea salt, to taste 1 teaspoon paprika

Directions

Mix all the above ingredients in a bowl. Add in the warm water to form a smooth dough ball. Then, roll the dough out as thin as possible. Use a pizza cutter to cut dough into 1-inch squares. Bake in the preheated oven at 365 degrees F for about 12 minutes or until golden and crispy. Turn your crackers over and bake for further 8 to 10 minutes.

601.　Italian Fried Cheese Sticks

(Ready in about 15 minutes | Servings 5) Per serving: 338 Calories; 26.5g Fat; 3.4g Carbs; 21g Protein; 2.3g Fiber

Ingredients

1 teaspoon Italian spice mix 1/4 cup almond meal 1/4 cup flaxseed meal 1/3 cup Romano cheese, grated 2 tablespoons buttermilk 2 eggs 10 pieces mozzarella cheese sticks Vegetable oil for frying

Directions

Mix the Italian spice mix, almond meal, flaxseed meal, and Romano cheese in a shallow bowl. In another dish, whisk buttermilk with eggs. Dip each cheese stick into the egg mixture; then, dredge them into the almond meal mixture, then quickly again in the egg mixture and again in the almond meal mixture. Fill a frying pan with about 2 inches of oil. Heat the oil over high heat. Deep fry the cheese sticks for 2 minutes per side until the crust is golden brown. Place the fried cheese sticks on paper towels to drain excess oil.Enjoy!

602. Saucy Cocktail Weenies

(Ready in about 2 hours 30 minutes | Servings 6) Per serving: 271 Calories; 22.2g Fat; 4.5g Carbs; 12.3g Protein; 3.2g Fiber

Ingredients

1 ½ pounds mini cocktail sausages 1 bottle barbecue sauce, no sugar added 1 tablespoon Erythritol 1 teaspoon granulated garlic 3 tablespoons deli mustard 1 teaspoon shallot powder 1 teaspoon porcini powder

Directions

Sear the sausage in a preheated nonstick skillet for 3 to 4 minutes. Place all ingredients in your slow cooker. Cook on the Lowest setting for 2 hours. Serve with cocktail sticks or toothpicks.Enjoy!

603. Hungarian Paprika Bacon Crisps

(Ready in about 20 minutes | Servings 4) Per serving: 118 Calories; 10g Fat; 1.9g Carbs; 5g Protein; 0.4g Fiber

Ingredients

1 tablespoon Hungarian paprika 12 bacon strips, cut into small squares 2 tablespoons Erythritol

Directions

Start by preheating your oven to 365 degrees F Toss the bacon strips with Erythritol and Hungarian paprika. Place the bacon squares on a parchment lined baking sheet and bake for 13 to 15 minutes.Enjoy!

604. Bacon and Broccoli Mini Frittatas

(Ready in about 30 minutes | Servings 6) Per serving: 375 Calories; 27.6g Fat; 6g Carbs; 24.8g Protein; 1.6g Fiber

Ingredients

6 eggs, whisked 5 ounces cooked bacon, chopped 1 ½ cups cheddar cheese, freshly grated 1 head broccoli, grated 1 cup onions, chopped Sea salt and

pepper, to taste 1/2 teaspoon Adobo seasoning mix

For the Dipping Sauce:

1 Spanish pepper, chopped 2 vine-ripened tomatoes, chopped 1/2 teaspoon garlic, chopped 1/2 shallot, minced 2 tablespoons sesame oil 1 teaspoon basil

Directions

In a mixing bowl, combine the eggs, bacon, cheese, broccoli, onions, salt, pepper, and Adobo seasoning mix. Preheat your oven to 385 degrees F. Spoon the mixture into lightly buttered muffin cups and bake for 20 to 30 minutes, or until golden brown. In the meantime, place all the sauce ingredients in a saucepan over medium-low heat. Let it simmer until reduced by half.

605.   Rich and Easy Ground Meat Pie

(Ready in about 25 minutes | Servings 6) Per serving: 231 Calories; 16.4g Fat; 3.5g Carbs; 17.3g Protein; 0.7g Fiber

Ingredients

1 ½ cups ground turkey 1 shallot, chopped 1 teaspoon garlic, crushed 1 cup sharp Cheddar cheese, shredded 1 cup Monterey-Jack cheese, shredded 1 cup Colby cheese, shredded Salt and black pepper, to your liking 1/2 teaspoon mustard powder 2 tomatoes, crushed

Directions

Preheat your oven to 395 degrees F. Coat a baking sheet with a piece of parchment paper. Spread the shredded cheese on the bottom of your baking sheet. Bake for 11 to 13 minutes or until golden-browned on top. Meanwhile, preheat a lightly oiled skillet over a moderately-high heat and cook the shallot until just tender and translucent. Add in the garlic and continue to sauté until aromatic. Stir in the ground turkey and spices and continue to cook, breaking it up in the pan to cook through. Top the cheese "crust" with the meat mixture; return it to the oven and bake an additional 7 minutes. Top with the tomatoes.

606.   Easy Turkey Bites with Spicy Sauce

(Ready in about 30 minutes | Servings 8) Per serving: 153 Calories; 6.7g Fat; 4.6g Carbs; 21.8g Protein; 0.7g Fiber

Ingredients

1/3 cup flax meal 3/4 cup almond flour 2 eggs, whisked 1 ¼ pounds turkey tenderloin, cut into 20 pieces Salt and black pepper, to season

For the Sauce:

1/2 tablespoon Sriracha sauce 1/2 teaspoon cayenne pepper 1 teaspoon deli mustard 1 teaspoon garlic powder 1/3 cup tomato paste 1/3 teaspoon cumin

Directions

Start by preheating your oven to 365 degrees F. Brush the bottom of a baking pan with cooking spray. Toss the turkey pieces with salt and pepper. Mix the flax meal with the almond meal. Dip the turkey pieces in the whisked egg, then, coat them with the meal mixture. Bake for 25 to 28 minutes. Whisk all the sauce ingredients and reserve.Bon appétit!

607.   Classic Cheese and Artichoke Dip

(Ready in about 5 minutes | Servings 8) Per serving: 157 Calories; 11g Fat; 5.9g Carbs; 6.5g Protein; 2.7g Fiber

Ingredients

12 ounces canned artichoke hearts, drained 1/2 pound cream cheese 1/2 cup Cheddar cheese, shredded 1/2 cup mayonnaise 1 teaspoon garlic, minced 4 tablespoons chives 2 tablespoons spring onions Salt and black pepper, to taste 1 teaspoon cayenne pepper

Directions

In a deep saucepan, combine artichoke hearts and cream cheese over the lowest heat. Let the cheese melt for a couple of minutes. Remove from the heat and add in the remaining ingredients. Taste and adjust the seasonings. Enjoy!

608.   Chicken Wings with Cheese Dip

(Ready in about 1 hour 15 minutes | Servings 10) Per serving: 227 Calories; 10.2g Fat; 0.4g Carbs; 31.5g Protein; 0.2g Fiber

Ingredients

3 pounds chicken wings Salt and red pepper, to taste 1 teaspoon mustard seeds 1 teaspoon olive oil

For Feta Cheese Dip:

2 tablespoons sour cream 1/4 cup fresh parsley leaves, finely chopped 2 cloves garlic, smashed 1 teaspoon porcini powder 1/2 teaspoon ground cumin 1 cup feta cheese, shredded 1/3 cup mayonnaise

Directions

Toss the chicken wings with the olive oil, salt, red pepper, and mustard seeds. Roast in the preheated oven at 380 degrees F approximately 35 minutes. Turn the oven up to 410 degrees F and bake for a further 35 minutes on the higher shelf until crispy. In the meantime, mix all ingredients for the cheese sauce.Enjoy!

609.   Chicharrones with Cream Cheese Dip

(Ready in about 3 hours 10 minutes | Servings 10) Per serving: 420 Calories; 43g Fat; 3.1g Carbs; 5g Protein; 0.8g Fiber

Ingredients

1 tablespoon olive oil 1 ½ pounds pork skin, trimmed of excess fat Sea salt and pepper, to taste 12 ounces cream cheese 1/2 cup mayonnaise 2 cups mustard greens, torn into pieces and steamed 1 tablespoon chili paste (sambal) 1 teaspoon onion powder 1 teaspoon granulated garlic 1/4 teaspoon mustard powder

Directions

Toss the pork skin with salt until well coated. Place them on a wire rack over a baking sheet. Bake in the preheated oven at 350 degrees F for about 3 hours, until skin is completely dried out. Heat the olive oil in a nonstick skillet and can cook your chicharrónes in batches until they puff up, about 5 minutes. Place on a paper towel-lined plate. Meanwhile, parboil the mustard greens for about 7 minutes. Add in the remaining ingredients and mix to combine well.Bon appétit!

610.   Roasted Zucchini Bites

(Ready in about 40 minutes | Servings 4) Per serving: 91 Calories; 6.1g Fat; 6g Carbs; 4.2g Protein; 0.4g Fiber

Ingredients

2 tablespoons olive oil 2 egg whites Salt and pepper, to taste 1/2 teaspoon basil 1/2 teaspoon oregano 4 zucchinis, cut into thick slices

Directions

Toss the zucchini with the remaining ingredients. Roast in the preheated oven at 410 degrees F for about 30 minutes until the slices are crispy and golden.Enjoy!

611. Glazed Oyster Mushrooms

(Ready in about 10 minutes | Servings 4) Per serving: 75 Calories; 5.2g Fat; 3.3g Carbs; 2.9g Protein; 1.1g Fiber

Ingredients

1 pound oyster mushrooms, sliced 3 tablespoons butter 1 teaspoon garlic, minced 1 tablespoon coconut aminos 1 tablespoons Swerve Salt and white pepper, to taste

Directions

Melt the butter in a saucepan over a moderately-high heat. Now, sauté the garlic for a minute or so. Stir in the mushrooms and continue to cook them for 3 to 4 minutes, until they release the liquid. Add in the other ingredients and continue to cook until the mushrooms are caramelized.

612. Chunky Ground Meat Dip

(Ready in about 10 minutes | Servings 24) Per serving: 153 Calories; 11.2g Fat; 2.2g Carbs; 10.8g Protein; 0.4g Fiber

Ingredients

3 cups cream cheese 1 cup feta cheese 1/2 cup tomato paste 1 pound ground beef 1/2 pound ground turkey 1 teaspoon garlic, minced 1 cup black olives, pitted and chopped 1 teaspoon Greek seasoning mix

Directions

Preheat a lightly oiled nonstick pan over a moderately-high heat. Cook ground meat for 5 to 6 minutes until no longer pink, breaking apart with a fork. Thoroughly combine the cheese, tomato paste, garlic, and spices. Place 1/2 of meat mixture in a bowl. Top with 1/2 of the cheese mixture; repeat the layers and top with olives.

613. Cauliflower Bites with Greek Dip

(Ready in about 30 minutes | Servings 6) Per serving: 182 Calories; 13.1g Fat; 5.9g Carbs; 11.5g Protein; 1.7g Fiber

Ingredients

1 ½ cups cheddar cheese, grated 1 pound cauliflower florets 1 shallot, finely chopped 1/2 teaspoon garlic, minced Salt and pepper, to taste 3 eggs, whisked

For Greek Dip:

1/2 cup feta cheese 1 teaspoon lime juice 1/2 teaspoon garlic, minced 2 tablespoons mayonnaise 1/2 cup Greek yogurt

Directions

Parboil the cauliflower in a pot of a lightly-salted water until crisp-tender, for 5 to 6 minutes. Then, place the cauliflower florets, cheese, eggs, shallot, garlic, salt, and pepper in your food processor. Pulse until well blended. Roll the cauliflower mixture into bite-sized balls and arrange them in a parchment-lined baking pan. Bake in the preheated oven at 395 degrees F for about 20 minutes. Meanwhile, make the sauce by whisking the remaining ingredients.

614. Winter Cheese and Kulen Roll-Ups

(**Ready in about 10 minutes | Servings 5**) Per serving: 381 Calories; 31.2g Fat; 4.8g Carbs; 17.6g Protein; 0.4g Fiber

Ingredients

10 slices Kulen salami 10 slices Cheddar cheese 4 ounces mayonnaise 10 slices bacon 10 olives, pitted

Directions

Spread a thin layer of mayo onto each slice of Cheddar cheese. Add a slice of bacon on top of the mayo. Top with a slice of salami. Roll them up, garnish with olives and secure with toothpicks.Enjoy!

615. Ciauscolo and Cheese Fat Bombs

(**Ready in about 10 minutes | Servings 5**) Per serving: 341 Calories; 30.6g Fat; 3.4g Carbs; 12.8g Protein; 1g Fiber

Ingredients

5 ounces mozzarella cheese 5 ounces Ciauscolo salami, chopped 1 teaspoon Roman mustard 1/2 teaspoon smoked paprika 4 large egg yolks, hard-boiled 2 tablespoons sesame seeds, lightly toasted 2 tablespoons extra-virgin olive oil

Directions

Thoroughly combine all ingredients, except for the sesame seeds, in a mixing dish. Now, roll your mixture into 10 small balls. Roll each ball over the toasted sesame seeds until well coated on all sides.Serve well chilled!

616. The Ultimate Ranch Cheese Ball

(**Ready in about 10 minutes | Servings 6**) Per serving: 182 Calories; 15.5g Fat; 3g Carbs; 7.6g Protein; 1.1g Fiber

Ingredients

6 slices of ham, chopped 1/4 cup mayonnaise 6 black olives, pitted and sliced 1 teaspoon poppy seeds 1 tablespoon ketchup 6 ounces cream cheese 1 ounce package Ranch seasoning Salt and pepper, to taste

Directions

Thoroughly combine the cream cheese, Ranch seasoning, mayonnaise, ketchup, chopped ham, salt, pepper, and poppy seeds. Shape the mixture into a ball. Garnish with black olives.Enjoy!

617. Mascarpone Fat Bombs

(**Ready in about 10 minutes + chilling time | Servings 6**) Per serving: 214 Calories; 20.4g Fat; 1.2g Carbs; 5.6g Protein; 0.3g Fiber

Ingredients

1 cup Mascarpone cheese Salt and pepper, to season 1/2 cup fresh parsley, finely chopped 3 ounces bacon, chopped 1/4 teaspoon champagne vinegar

Directions

In a mixing bowl, thoroughly combine the cheese, bacon, vinegar, salt, and pepper. Cover the bowl and place in your refrigerator for 2 to 3 hours to help firm it up. Roll the mixture into balls. Roll the fat bombs over chopped parsley until well coated.Serve well chilled!

618.   Mediterranean Broccoli Dip

(Ready in about 10 minutes | Servings 8) Per serving: 134 Calories; 10.2g Fat; 6.5g Carbs; 5.1g Protein; 1.6g Fiber

Ingredients

1/3 cup mayonnaise 1 pound broccoli florets Salt and pepper, to taste 1/2 cup Greek-style yogurt 1/2 cup blue cheese 1 teaspoon Mediterranean seasoning mix

Directions

Parboil broccoli florets for about 7 minutes or until crisp-tender. Place the broccoli florets in a bowl of your food processor. Add in the yogurt, cheese, and spices and blend briefly to combine. Fold in the well-chilled mayonnaise and continue to blend until everything is well incorporated.

619.   Pepperoni and Ricotta Balls

(Ready in about 15 minutes + chilling time | Servings 5) Per serving: 323 Calories; 28.4g Fat; 2.6g Carbs; 13.1g Protein; 0.3g Fiber

Ingredients

5 ounces pepperoni, chopped 1 teaspoon brown mustard 2 teaspoons tomato paste 10 ounces Ricotta cheese, room temperature 1/4 cup mayonnaise 1 teaspoon tequila 1 teaspoon lime juice, freshly squeezed 8 black olives, pitted and chopped

Directions

Mix all ingredients in a bowl until well combined. Place in your refrigerator for 2 hours. Roll the mixture into balls.Serve well chilled!

620.   Swiss Chard Chips with Avocado Dip

(Ready in about 20 minutes | Servings 6) Per serving: 269 Calories; 26.7g Fat; 3.4g Carbs; 2.3g Protein; 4.1g Fiber

Ingredients

1 tablespoon coconut oil Sea salt and pepper, to taste 2 cups Swiss chard, cleaned

Avocado Dip:

3 ripe avocados, pitted and mashed 2 garlic cloves, finely minced 2 tablespoons extra-virgin olive oil 2 teaspoons lemon juice Salt and pepper, to taste

Directions

Toss the Swiss chard with the coconut oil, salt, and pepper. Bake the Swiss chard leaves in the preheated oven at 310 degrees F for about 10 minutes until the edges brown but are not burnt. Thoroughly combine the ingredients for the avocado dip.Enjoy!

621. Spicy and Peppery Fried Tofu

(Ready in about 20 minutes | Servings 2) Per serving: 223 Calories; 15.9g Fat; 5.1g Carbs; 15.6g Protein; 3.3g Fiber

Ingredients

2 bell peppers, deveined and sliced 1 chili pepper, deveined and sliced 1 ½ tablespoons almond meal Salt and pepper, to taste 1 teaspoon ginger-garlic paste 1 teaspoon onion powder 6 ounces extra-firm tofu, pressed and cubed 1/2 teaspoon ground bay leaf 1 tablespoon sesame oil

Directions

Toss your tofu, with almond meal, salt, pepper, ginger-garlic paste, onion powder, ground bay leaf. In a sauté pan, heat the sesame oil over medium-high heat. Fry the tofu cubes along with the peppers for about 6 minutes. Enjoy!

622. Autumn Squash Smoothie Bowl

(Ready in about 5 minutes | Servings 2) Per serving: 71 Calories; 2.3g Fat; 4.1g Carbs; 4.3g Protein; 2.4g Fiber

Ingredients

1/2 cup butternut squash, roasted 1/2 teaspoon pumpkin spice mix 2 tablespoons cocoa powder, unsweetened 1 ½ cups almond milk, unsweetened 1/2 cup butterhead lettuce

Directions

Blend all ingredients until well combined.

623. Genoa Salami and Egg Balls

(Ready in about 5 minutes + chilling time | Servings 6) Per serving: 327 Calories; 25.7g Fat; 6.4g Carbs; 17g Protein; 0.4g Fiber

Ingredients

1/2 cup Ricotta cheese, softened 1/3 cup mayonnaise 6 hard-boiled eggs, peeled and chopped 1/2 teaspoon Italian seasoning mix Sea salt and pepper, to taste 1/2 teaspoon paprika 6 slices genoa salami, chopped Directions Thoroughly combine all ingredients until well combined. Roll the mixture into balls.Bon appétit!

624. Nacho Cheese Chips

(Ready in about 15 minutes | Servings 6) Per serving: 268 Calories; 20.4g Fat; 3.4g Carbs; 18.1g Protein; 0g Fiber

Ingredients

3 cups Mexican blend cheese, shredded 1 tablespoon Taco seasoning mix

Directions

Toss the shredded cheese with Taco seasoning mix. Drop tablespoons of this mixture into small piles. Roast in the preheated oven at 410 degrees F for about 12 minutes.Enjoy!

625.   Celery Bites with Crab and Cheese

(Ready in about 10 minutes | Servings 16) Per serving: 29 Calories; 1.9g Fat; 0.7g Carbs; 2.5g Protein; 1.9g Fiber

Ingredients

8 celery sticks, cut into halves 6 ounces crab meat 1 teaspoon Mediterranean spice mix 2 tablespoons apple cider vinegar 1 cup cream cheese Salt and pepper, to taste

Directions

In a mixing bowl, combine the crab meat, apple cider vinegar, cream cheese, salt, pepper, and Mediterranean spice mix. Divide the crab mixture between celery sticks.Bon appétit!

626.   Homemade Tortilla Chips

(Ready in about 20 minutes | Servings 10) Per serving: 109 Calories; 8.4g Fat; 5.3g Carbs; 2.2g Protein; 3.1g Fiber

Ingredients

For the chips:

1 tablespoon coconut oil 1/4 teaspoon baking powder 1/4 cup psyllium husk powder 2 tablespoons canola oil 3/4 cup almond meal 2 tablespoons

flax seed meal

For the Guacamole:

1 serrano jalapeno pepper, stems and seeds removed, minced 1/2 cup green onions, chopped 1 cup tomatoes, chopped 2 ripe avocados, seeded and peeled Juice of 1 fresh lemon Salt and pepper, to taste 2 tablespoons fresh cilantro, chopped 2 garlic cloves, finely minced

Directions

Mix all ingredients for the tortilla chips. Pour in hot water to form a dough. Place the dough in between two large pieces of parchment pepper; roll it out as thin as possible. Cut the dough into triangles. Bake your tortilla chips in the preheated oven at 360 degrees F for about 12 minutes until the chips are crisp, but not too browned. Make your guacamole by mixing the remaining ingredients in your blender or food processor.

627.   Provençal-Style Mini Muffins

(Ready in about 20 minutes | Servings 6) Per serving: 269 Calories; 20.7g Fat; 5g Carbs; 15.5g Protein; 2.4g Fiber

Ingredients

2 eggs 1/2 cup Greek-style yogurt 10 slices hunter salami, chopped 1/3 cup almond meal 1/3 cup flaxseed meal 1/3cup coconut flour 2 tablespoons granulated Swerve 1/2 teaspoon baking powder 2 teaspoons psyllium Salt and pepper, to taste 1 teaspoon herbes de Provence

Directions Preheat your oven to 365 degrees F. Brush a muffin tin with a nonstick spray. Thoroughly combine the almond meal, flaxseed meal, coconut flour, Swerve, baking powder, psyllium, salt, pepper, and herbes de Provence. Fold in the eggs, Greek-style yogurt, and chopped hunter salami. Spoon the mixture into the prepared muffin tin. Bake in the preheated oven for 13 to 15 minutes until golden brown. Place on a wire rack to cool slightly before unmolding.Bon appétit!

628.   Classic Cajun Shrimp Skewers

(Ready in about 15 minutes | Servings 4) Per serving: 218 Calories; 11g Fat; 5.1g Carbs; 23.5g Protein; 1.4g Fiber

Ingredients

3 tablespoons olive oil 1 pound large shrimp, peeled and deveined 2 tablespoons fresh scallions, chopped 1 teaspoon garlic, minced 1 tablespoon Cajun seasoning mix 1 tablespoon fresh lemon juice 1 tablespoon white vinegar 2 tablespoons minced coriander 2 Italian peppers, diced 1 cup cherry tomatoes

Directions

In a saucepan, heat olive oil over a moderately-high flame. Cook the shrimp and scallions for about 4 minutes. Stir in the garlic and Cajun seasoning mix and continue to sauté for a minute or so, until aromatic. Heat off; toss your shrimp with lemon juice, vinegar and coriander. Tread the prawns onto bamboo skewers, alternating them with Italian peppers and cherry tomatoes.Enjoy!

629.   Pork Rinds with Mexican Sauce

(Ready in about 2 hours 30 minutes | Servings 6) Per serving: 199 Calories; 16.1g Fat; 6.5g Carbs; 7.5g Protein; 3.8g Fiber

Ingredients

1 whole pork skin from a pork belly Salt, to taste

For Mexican Sauce:

1 Anaheim pepper, deveined and minced 2 tablespoons fresh-squeezed lemon juice 1 cup tomatillo, chopped 2 tablespoons cilantro, chopped 1 teaspoon garlic, smashed 2 avocados, seeded, peeled and chopped 1/4 teaspoon ground mustard seeds 1/2 cup scallions, finely chopped

Directions

Toss the pork skin with salt until well coated. Bake in the preheated oven at 350 degrees F for 2 hours 30 minutes, until skin is completely dried out. Meanwhile, make the Mexican sauce by whisking all of the ingredients in the order listed above.

630.   Rich and Easy Cocktail Meatballs

(Ready in about 40 minutes | Servings 5) Per serving: 244 Calories; 13.3g Fat; 3.7g Carbs; 28.1g Protein; 1.1g Fiber

Ingredients

1/3 pound ground chicken 2/3 pound ground pork 1/2 cup ground pine nuts 2 ounces Pecorino cheese, grated 1/2 cup green onions, chopped 2 tablespoons green garlic, minced 1 tablespoon deli mustard 2 tablespoons buttermilk 2 eggs, whisked 1 poblano pepper, deveined and minced Salt and black pepper, to taste

Directions

In a mixing bowl, combine all of the above ingredients, except for the ground nuts. Shape the mixture into small balls. Roll these balls over the ground nuts until they're coated on all sides. Preheat a lightly greased skillet over a moderately-high heat. Fry your meatballs in batches until the juice is clear.Bon appétit!

631. Mozzarella-Stuffed Meatballs

(Ready in about 25 minutes | Servings 10) Per serving: 214 Calories; 12.6g Fat; 1.6g Carbs; 21.9g Protein; 0.4g Fiber

Ingredients

1/3 cup Pecorino-Romano cheese, grated 2 eggs 1 cup Mozzarella cheese, cubed Sea salt and pepper, to taste 1 teaspoon paprika 1 teaspoon fish sauce 1/2 cup shallots, finely chopped 1/2 pound ground chuck 1 pound ground pork 1 teaspoon garlic, smashed

Directions

In a mixing dish, combine all ingredients, except for the Mozzarella cheese. Roll this mixture into golf ball sized meatballs using your hands. Press a Mozzarella cheese cube into the middle of each meatball, fully enclosing it. Bake in the preheated oven at 395 degrees F for 18 to 22 minutes until they are fully cooked.Bon appétit!

Dessert

632.   Mini Brownies with Almonds

(Ready in about 25 minutes | Servings 12) Per serving: 251 Calories; 21.5g Fat; 4.6g Carbs; 6.4g Protein; 0.8g Fiber

Ingredients

4 ounces cocoa powder 1/2 cup almonds, ground 5 eggs 1/2 teaspoon ground cinnamon 6 ounces sour cream 2 tablespoons Swerve 2/3 cup coconut oil, melted 1 teaspoon rum extract 3/4 teaspoon baking powder

Directions

Begin by preheating your oven to 365 degrees F. Brush a muffin tin with a nonstick spray. Mix all ingredients in a bowl and scrape the batter into the muffin cups. Bake for about 20 minutes; let it cool slightly before unmolding and storing.Enjoy!

633.   Rum Chocolate Pralines

(Ready in about 10 minutes + chilling time | Servings 8) Per serving: 70 Calories; 3.4g Fat; 5.1g Carbs; 2.4g Protein; 1.6g Fiber

Ingredients

1 cup bakers' chocolate, sugar-free 2 tablespoons dark rum 1/8 teaspoon ground cloves 1/8 teaspoon cinnamon powder 1/2 teaspoon almond extract 1/2 teaspoon rum extract 3 tablespoons cocoa powder 1/4 cup almond butter 1 cup almond milk

Directions

Microwave the chocolate, cocoa and almond butter until they have completely melted. Add in the other ingredients and mix to combine well. Pour the mixture into silicone molds and place in your refrigerator until set. Bon appétit!

634.   Vanilla Berry Meringues

(Ready in about 2 hours | Servings 10) Per serving: 51 Calories; 0g Fat; 4g Carbs; 12g Protein; 0.1g Fiber

Ingredients

1 teaspoon vanilla extract   3 tablespoons freeze-dried mixed berries, crushed 3 large egg whites, at room temperature 1/3 cup Erythritol 1 teaspoon lemon rind

Directions

In a mixing bowl, beat the egg whites until foamy. Add in vanilla extract, lemon rind, and Erythritol; continue to mix, using an electric mixer until stiff and glossy. Add the crushed berries and mix again until well combined. Use two teaspoons to spoon meringue onto parchment-lined cookie sheets. Bake at 220 degrees F for about 1 hour 45 minutes.Bon appétit!

635.   Mother's Day Pecan Truffles

(Ready in about 25 minutes + chilling time | Servings 6) Per serving: 113 Calories; 8.5g Fat; 5.9g Carbs; 1.7g Protein; 3.3g Fiber

Ingredients

1/2 cup toasted pecans, finely chopped 1/2 cup double cream 1 teaspoon vanilla paste 3 bars chocolate, sugar-free 1/4 teaspoon ground cardamom 1/4 teaspoon ground cinnamon 1/4 teaspoon coarse salt

Directions

In a medium stainless steel bowl set over a pot of gently simmering water, melt the chocolate and cream. Add in the vanilla, cardamom, cinnamon, and salt and place in your refrigerator for 7 to 8 hours or until firm. Shape the mixture into balls and roll the balls into the chopped pecans.Bon appétit!

636.   Blueberry and Coconut Protein Shake

(Ready in about 10 minutes | Servings 4) Per serving: 274 Calories; 26.8g Fat; 7.5g Carbs; 3.9g Protein; 1.3g Fiber

Ingredients

1/2 cup blueberries, frozen 1/2 teaspoon vanilla essence 1/2 teaspoon Monk fruit powder 2 tablespoons collagen protein 2 tablespoons coconut cream 1/4 cup coconut shreds 1 cup coconut milk

Directions

Pulse the frozen blueberries in your blender. Add in the other ingredients and mix until creamy, smooth and uniform.

637.   Classic Chocolate Bars

(Ready in about 25 minutes + chilling time | Servings 10) Per serving: 119 Calories; 11.7g Fat; 5.2g Carbs; 1.1g Protein; 5g Fiber

Ingredients

1/2 stick butter, cold 1 ½ cups whipped cream A pinch of coarse salt 8 ounces chocolate chunks, sugar-free 1/4 teaspoon cinnamon 1/2 teaspoon rum extract 1 teaspoon vanilla extract 1/4 cup coconut flour 1/4 cup flaxseed meal 1 cup almond meal 2 packets stevia

Directions

Start by preheating your oven to 340 degrees F. Coat a baking dish with a piece of parchment paper. Add the coconut flour, flaxseed meal, almond meal, stevia, cinnamon, rum extract, vanilla, and salt to your blender. Blend until everything is well incorporated. Cut in the cold butter and continue to blend until well combined. Spoon the batter into the bottom of the prepared baking pan. Bake for 12 to 15 minutes and place on a wire rack to cool slightly. Bring the whipped cream to a simmer; add in the chocolate chunks and whisk to combine. Spread the chocolate filling over the crust and place in your refrigerator until set. Cut into bars.Bon appétit!

638.   The Best Chocolate Cake Ever

(Ready in about 50 minutes + chilling time | Servings 10) Per serving: 313 Calories; 30.7g Fat; 7.5g Carbs; 7.3g Protein; 1.9g Fiber

Ingredients

5 eggs 1/2 teaspoon ground cinnamon A pinch of coarse salt 1/2 cup water 3/4 cup erythritol 14 ounces chocolate, unsweetened 2 sticks butter, cold

For Peanut-Choc Ganache:

9 ounces chocolate, unsweetened 1/4 cup smooth peanut butter A pinch of coarse salt 3/4 cups whipped cream

Directions

In a medium-sized pan, bring the water to a boil; add in the erythritol and let it simmer until it has dissolved. Melt the chocolate and butter; beat the mixture with an electric mixer. Add the chocolate mixture to the hot water mixture. Fold in the eggs, one at a time, beating continuously. Add in the cinnamon and salt, and stir well to combine. Spoon the mixture into a parchment-lined baking pan and wrap with foil. Lower the baking pan into a larger pan that is filled with hot water about 1 inch deep. Bake in the preheated oven at 365 degrees F for about 45 minutes. Meanwhile, place the whipped cream in a pan over a moderately-high heat and bring to a boil. Pour the hot cream over the chocolate and whisk to combine. Add in the peanut butter and salt; continue to mix until creamy and smooth. Glaze your cake and place in the refrigerator until set.Enjoy!

639.   Creamsicle Pudding with Coconut

(Ready in about 1 hour 5 minutes | Servings 4) Per serving: 226 Calories; 17.9g Fat; 7g Carbs; 5.9g Protein; 4.6g Fiber

Ingredients

1 cup unsweetened coconut milk 1 cup water 1/4 cup coconut flakes 2 tablespoons Swerve 1/2 teaspoon ground star anise 1 cup double cream 1 teaspoon coconut extract 1 cup chia seeds

Directions

Mix the ingredients until everything is well incorporated. Place in your refrigerator for about 1 hour.Enjoy!

640.   Father's Day Ice Cream

(Ready in about 15 minutes + chilling time | Servings 8) Per serving: 89 Calories; 9.3g Fat; 1.5g Carbs; 0.8g Protein; 0g Fiber

Ingredients

3/4 cup double cream 1/2 cup coconut milk 1 tablespoon rum flavoring 24 packets of stevia A pinch of grated nutmeg A pinch of salt 1/4 cup Greek-style yogurt

Directions

Melt the double cream and coconut milk in a saucepan over a medium-low heat. Stir until there are no lumps. Allow it to cool and add in the other ingredients. Beat the ingredients using an electric mixer until creamy and uniform.Bon appétit!

641. Classic Chocolate Fudge

(Ready in about 15 minutes + chilling time | Servings 8) Per serving: 220 Calories; 20g Fat; 7g Carbs; 1.7g Protein; 2.1g Fiber

Ingredients

3/4 cup chocolate chunks, unsweetened 2 tablespoons coconut oil 4-5 drops Monk fruit sweetener 1/2 cup double cream 1/2 cup butter, at room temperature 1 cup full-fat milk

Directions

Microwave the chocolate and milk until they've completely melted; spoon into a foil-lined pie pan and freeze until firm. Then, melt the butter, coconut oil, Monk fruit sweetener, and double cream; mix with a wire whisk to combine well. Spoon the cream mixture over the chocolate layer and freeze until solid.Enjoy!

642. Butterscotch Pudding Popsicles

(Ready in about 1 hour | Servings 6) Per serving: 248 Calories; 20.8g Fat; 7g Carbs; 4.6g Protein; 4.1g Fiber

Ingredients

1 teaspoon orange juice 1 cup buttermilk 1 cup coconut milk 1 tablespoon butterscotch extract 1 cup Swerve 1/8 teaspoon xanthan gum 3 avocados, pitted, peeled and mashed

Directions

Place all ingredients in your blender. Process until well combined.Enjoy!

643. American-Style Mini Cheesecakes

(Ready in about 25 minutes | Servings 12) Per serving: 134 Calories; 12.5g Fat; 3.3g Carbs; 4.6g Protein; 0.4g Fiber

Ingredients

6 ounces Neufchatel cheese, at room temperature 7 tablespoons coconut oil, melted 5 eggs 1/4 teaspoon ground cinnamon 1/4 cup Swerve 2 ounces cocoa powder, unsweetened 1 teaspoon vanilla paste 1 teaspoon rum extract 1/3 teaspoon baking powder

Directions Beat the ingredients using your electric mixer on high speed. Line a mini muffin pan with 12 liners. Spoon the mixture into prepared muffins cups. Bake in the preheated oven at 350 degrees F for about 20 minutes.Bon appétit!

644. Peanut Butter Cupcakes

(Ready in about 10 minutes + chilling time | Servings 10) Per serving: 266 Calories; 28.1g Fat; 2.6g Carbs; 3.3g Protein; 0.5g Fiber

Ingredients

1 stick butter 4 tablespoons heavy cream 1 tablespoon Erythritol 1 cup peanut butter

Directions

Place a bowl over a saucepan of simmering water. Add in all of the above ingredients and stir continuously until well melted and blended. Spoon the batter into muffin cups lined with cupcake wrappers. Allow them to harden for about 1 hour in your freezer.Enjoy!

645.   Old-Fashioned Walnut Candy

(Ready in about 1 hour | Servings 10) Per serving: 162 Calories; 14.6g Fat; 5.9g Carbs; 2.3g Protein; 1.7g Fiber

Ingredients

4 tablespoons walnuts, coarsely chopped 1 tablespoon rum 1/2 teaspoon pure vanilla extract 1/2 cup lightly toasted walnuts, chopped 1/2 cup chocolate, sugar-free 1/2 coconut oil, room temperature 4 ounces coconut cream 1/4 cup confectioners' Swerve

Directions

Melt the coconut oil in a double boiler and fold in the coconut cream and confectioners' Swerve; stir to combine well. Remove from the heat and add in the rum, vanilla extract and chopped walnuts. Let it cool to room temperature. Roll into 20 balls and chill for about 50 minutes. Then, melt the chocolate and dip each ball into the chocolate glaze. Roll your candies in the chopped walnuts until well coated.Bon appétit!

646.   Cashew and Pecan Fat Bombs

(Ready in about 40 minutes | Servings 12) Per serving: 114 Calories; 10.6g Fat; 3.4g Carbs; 3.1g Protein; 1g Fiber

Ingredients

2/3 cup pecans, chopped 10 drops Monk fruit powder 1 teaspoon vanilla essence 1/4 cup almond flour 2 tablespoons cocoa powder, unsweetened 1/2 cup cashew butter 1/2 cup coconut oil

Directions

Mix all ingredients in a bowl until well combined. Drop by teaspoonfuls onto foil-lined baking sheets. Chill in your refrigerator until firm.Bon appétit!

647.   Easy Coconut Mousse

(Ready in about 15 minutes+ chilling time | Servings 6) Per serving: 303 Calories; 30g Fat; 3.1g Carbs; 3.5g Protein; 2.7g Fiber

Ingredients

1/2 cup coconut milk A pinch of grated nutmeg 1 cup double cream 1/2 cup panela cheese 2 tablespoons powdered Erythritol 1/2 cup coconut creamer 1 ½ cups avocado, pitted, peeled and mashed

Directions

Warm the coconut milk and creamer over low heat. Remove from the heat. Stir in the avocado and nutmeg; continue to stir until everything is well incorporated. Add in the remaining ingredients. Beat using an electric mixer on medium-high speed. Place in your refrigerator until firm.Enjoy!

648. Cheesecake Squares with Berry Topping

(Ready in about 30 minutes | Servings 6) Per serving: 333 Calories; 28.4g Fat; 6.3g Carbs; 11.7g Protein; 0.1g Fiber

Ingredients

For the Cheesecake Squares:

1 cup soft cheese 1 teaspoon vanilla essence 3 tablespoons Swerve 1/2 cup butter, melted 4 eggs

For the Berry Topping:

1/2 teaspoon lime juice 1 ½ tablespoons coconut milk 3/4 cup, frozen mixed berries 2 tablespoons Swerve

Directions

Start by preheating your oven to 340 degrees F. Line a baking pan with a Silpat mat. In a mixing bowl, combine all ingredients for the cheesecake squares using an electric mixer. Press the crust into the baking pan. Bake in the preheated oven for about 23 minutes. Warm all of the topping ingredients in a saucepan over a moderate flame. Reduce the heat to a simmer and continue to cook until the sauce has reduced by half. Spoon the berry topping over the chilled cheesecake.Bon appétit!

649. Greek-Style Coconut Cheesecake

(Ready in about 30 minutes | Servings 12) Per serving: 246 Calories; 22.2g Fat; 5.7g Carbs; 8.1g Protein; 1.9g Fiber

Ingredients

5 ounces Greek-style yogurt 1 ounce coconut flakes 10 ounces almond meal 1/4 teaspoon grated nutmeg 1 teaspoon lemon zest 5 ounces soft cheese 1 teaspoon baking powder 4 eggs, lightly beaten 4 ounces Swerve 1/4 coconut oil

Directions Brush two spring form pans with a nonstick spray. Mix the almond meal, coconut flakes, nutmeg, and baking powder. Add in the eggs, one at a time, whisking constantly; add in 2 ounces of Swerve. Spoon the mixture into spring form pans and bake at 360 degrees F for 23 minutes. In another bowl, combine the coconut oil, lemon zest, yogurt, soft cheese, and the remaining 2 ounces of Swerve. Mix to combine and spoon the filling over the first crust. Spread half of the filling over it. Top with another crust and spread the rest of the filling over the top.Bon appétit!

650. The Best Keto Birthday Cake

(Ready in about 40 minutes + chilling time | Servings 10) Per serving: 241 Calories; 22.6g Fat; 4.2g Carbs; 6.6g Protein; 0.7g Fiber

Ingredients

For the Cake Base: 2/3 cup coconut flour 2 ½ tablespoons butter 4 eggs 1 cup full-fat milk 1 teaspoon vanilla extract 1 ½ cups almond meal 1/2 teaspoon baking powder A pinch of coarse salt 1 cup erythritol

For the Frosting: 1/3 cup erythritol 3 ounces coconut oil, at room temperature A few drops coconut flavor 10 ounces soft cheese

Directions

Mix all ingredients for the cake base until well combined. Press the crust into a parchment-lined springform pan. Bake at 365 degrees F for 30 minutes or until a toothpick comes out clean; allow it to cool to room temperature. Meanwhile, beat the cheese using your electric mixer until creamy. Stir in the remaining ingredients and continue to mix until well combined. Frost your cake and serve well-chilled.Bon appétit!

651.   Decadent Macchiato Penuche

(Ready in about 10 minutes + chilling time | Servings 8) Per serving: 145 Calories; 12.8g Fat; 6.2g Carbs; 0.9g Protein; 1.2g Fiber

Ingredients

1 teaspoon warm coffee 1 teaspoon caramel flavor 6 tablespoons butter 1 tablespoon peanut butter 3 ounces dark chocolate, unsweetened 1 teaspoon liquid Monk fruit

Directions

Microwave the butter and chocolate until they are completely melted. Fold in the remaining ingredients. Spoon the batter into a foil-lined baking pan, smoothing out the top. Place in your refrigerator for 30 minutes before cutting. Enjoy!

652.   Coconut and Peanut Bark

(Ready in about 10 minutes + chilling time | Servings 12) Per serving: 316 Calories; 31.6g Fat; 4.6g Carbs; 6.6g Protein; 2.6g Fiber

Ingredients

3/4 cup coconut oil 1/2 teaspoon pure almond extract 1/2 cup coconut, shredded 3/4 cup peanut butter 1 cup powdered Erythritol

Directions

Melt all ingredients in a double boiler over medium-low heat. Scrape the batter into a parchment-lined baking pan. Place in your freezer for about 1 hour; break your bark into pieces.Bon appétit!

653.   Orange Crème Brûlée

(Ready in about 45 minutes + chilling time | Servings 5) Per serving: 205 Calories; 16.4g Fat; 6.5g Carbs; 7.4g Protein; 0g Fiber

Ingredients

3/4 cup Erythritol 6 eggs 1 ½ cups double cream 1 teaspoon orange rind, grated 1 teaspoon orange juice 1/2 teaspoon star anise, ground 3/4 cup water

Directions

In a saute pan, melt Erythritol until it has caramelized. Spoon the caramelized Erythritol into 5 ramekins. Bring the cream along with water to a boil. Whisk the eggs until pale and frothy; add in the remaining ingredients and stir to combine well. Add the mixture to the warm cream mixture and stir to combine well. Spoon the egg/cream mixture over the caramelized Erythritol. Lower the ramekins into a large cake pan. Pour hot water into the pan to come halfway up the sides of your ramekins. Bake at 325 degrees F for about 45 minutes. Refrigerate for at least 2 hours.Enjoy!

654. Chocolate Marshmallows

Ready in about: 30 minutes | Serves: 4 Per serving: Kcal 55, Fat 2.2g, Net Carbs 5.1g, Protein 0.5g

Ingredients

2 tbsp unsweetened cocoa powder ½ tsp vanilla extract ½ cup swerve sugar 1 tbsp xanthan gum A pinch Salt 2 ½ tsp gelatin powder

Directions

Dusting 1 tbsp unsweetened cocoa powder 1 tbsp swerve confectioner's sugar Line the loaf pan with parchment paper and grease with cooking spray. Mix the xanthan gum with 1 tbsp water and pour it into a saucepan. Stir in the swerve sugar, 2 tbsp of water, and salt. Place the pan over medium heat and bring the mixture to a boil. Reduce the heat and simmer for 7 minutes. Cover the gelatin with cold water in a small bowl. Let sit there without stirring to dissolve for 5 minutes. While the gelatin dissolves, pour the remaining water into a small bowl and heat in the microwave for 30 seconds. Stir in cocoa powder and mix it into the gelatin. When the sugar solution has hit the right temperature, gradually pour it directly into the gelatin mixture while continuously whisking. Beat for 10 minutes to get a light and fluffy consistency. Next, stir in the vanilla and pour the blend into the loaf pan. Let the marshmallows set for 3 hours and then use an oiled knife to cut them it into cubes; place them on a plate. Mix the remaining cocoa powder and confectioner's sugar together. Sift it over the marshmallows.

655. Coconut Cheesecake

Ready in about: 30 minutes + freezing time | Serves: 12 Per serving: Kcal 256, Fat: 25g, Net Carbs: 3g, Protein: 5g

Ingredients

Crust 2 egg whites ¼ cup erythritol 3 cups desiccated coconut 1 tsp coconut oil ¼ cup melted butter Filling 3 tbsp lemon juice 6 oz raspberries 2 cups erythritol 1 cup whipped cream Zest of 1 lemon 24 oz cream cheese

Directions

Grease the bottom and sides of a cake pan with coconut oil. Line with parchment paper. Preheat oven to 350°F and mix all crust ingredients. Pour the crust into the pan. Bake for about 25 minutes; let cool. Meanwhile, beat the cream cheese with an electric mixer until soft. Add the lemon juice, zest, and erythritol. Fold the whipped cream into the cheese cream mixture. Fold in the raspberries gently. Spoon the filling into the baked and cooled crust. Place in the fridge for 4 hours.

656. Berry Tart

Ready in about: 45 minutes | Serves: 4 Per serving: Kcal 305, Fat: 26.5g, Net Carbs: 4.9g, Protein: 15g

Ingredients

4 eggs 2 tsp coconut oil 2 cups berries 1 cup coconut milk 1 cup almond flour ¼ cup sweetener ½ tsp vanilla powder 1 tbsp powdered sweetener A pinch of salt Preheat oven to 350°F.

Directions

Place all ingredients except coconut oil, berries, and powdered sweetener, in a blender; blend until smooth. Gently fold in the berries. Grease a baking dish with the oil. Pour the mixture into the prepared pan and bake for 35 minutes. Sprinkle with powdered sugar to serve.

657.   Passion Fruit Cheesecake Slices

Ready in about: 15 minutes + cooling time | Serves: 6 Per serving: Kcal 287, Fat 18g, Net Carbs 6.1g, Protein 4.4g

Ingredients

1 cup crushed almond biscuits ½ cup melted butter Filling 1 ½ cups cream cheese ¾ cup swerve sugar 1 ½ whipping cream 1 tsp vanilla bean paste 4-6 tbsp cold water 1 tbsp gelatin powder Passionfruit jelly 1 cup passion fruit pulp ¼ cup swerve confectioner's sugar 1 tsp gelatin powder ¼ cup water, room temperature

Directions

Mix the crushed biscuits and butter in a bowl, spoon into a spring-form pan, and use the back of the spoon to level at the bottom. Set aside in the fridge. Put the cream cheese, swerve sugar, and vanilla paste into a bowl, and use the hand mixer to whisk until smooth; set aside. Cover the gelatin with cold water in small bowl. Let dissolve for 5 minutes. Pour the gelatin liquid along with the whipping cream in the cheese mixture and fold gently. Remove the spring-form pan from the refrigerator and pour over the mixture. Return to the fridge. For the passionfruit jelly: add 2 tbsp of cold water and sprinkle 1 tsp of gelatin powder. Let dissolve for 5 minutes. Pour confectioner's sugar and ¼ cup of water into it. Mix and stir in passion fruit pulp. Remove the cake again and pour the jelly over it. Swirl the pan to make the jelly level up. Place the pan back into the fridge to cool for 2 hours. When completely set, remove, and unlock the spring-pan. Lift the pan from the cake and slice the dessert.

658.   Granny Smith Apple Tart

Ready in about: 65 minutes | Serves: 6 Per serving: Kcal 302, Fat: 26g, Net Carbs: 6.7g, Protein: 7g

Ingredients

6 tbsp butter 2 cups almond flour 1 tsp cinnamon ⅓ cup sweetener Filling 2 cups sliced Granny Smith ¼ cup butter ¼ cup sweetener ½ tsp cinnamon ½ tsp lemon juice Topping ¼ tsp cinnamon 2 tbsp sweetener

Directions

Preheat oven to 370°F and combine all crust ingredients in a bowl. Press this mixture into the bottom of a greased pan. Bake for 5 minutes. Remove and let it cool slightly. Combine the apples and lemon juice in a bowl and arrange them on top of the cooled crust. Combine the rest of the filling ingredients and brush the mixture over the apples. Bake for about 30 minutes. Press the apples down with a spatula, return to oven, and bake for 20 more minutes. Combine the cinnamon and sweetener in a bowl and sprinkle over the tart. Note: Granny Smith apples have just 9.5g of net carbs per 100g. Still high for you? Substitute with Chayote squash, which has the same texture and rich nutrients, and just around 4g of net carbs.

659.   Chocolate Chip Cookies

Ready in about: 20 minutes | Serves: 4 Per serving: Kcal 317, Fat 27g, Net Carbs 8.9g, Protein 6.3g

Ingredients

1 cup butter, softened 2 cups swerve brown sugar 3 eggs 2 cups almond flour 2 cups unsweetened chocolate chips Preheat oven to 350°F.

Directions Line a baking sheet with parchment paper. Whisk the butter and sugar with a hand mixer for 3 minutes or until light and fluffy. Add the eggs one at a time, and scrape the sides as you whisk. Mix in almond flour at low speed until well combined. Fold in the chocolate chips. Scoop 3 tablespoons each on the baking sheet, creating spaces between each mound, and bake for 15 minutes to swell and harden. Remove, cool, and serve.

660.   Lemon Cheesecake Mousse

Ready in about: 5 minutes + cooling time | Serves: 4 Per serving: Kcal 223, Fat 18g, Net Carbs 3g, Protein 12g

Ingredients

24 oz cream cheese, softened 2 cups swerve confectioner's sugar 2 lemons, juiced and zested ¼ tsp salt 1 ¼ cups whipped cream

Directions

Whip the cream cheese in a bowl with a hand mixer until light and fluffy. Mix in the swerve sugar, lemon juice, and salt. Fold in 1 cup of the whipped cream to evenly combine. Spoon the mousse into serving cups and refrigerate to thicken for 1 hour. Swirl with the remaining whipped cream and garnish lightly with lemon zest. Let sit in the fridge before serving.

661.   Chia & Blackberry Pudding

Ready in about: 10 minutes + chilling time | Serves: 2 Per serving: Kcal 169, Fat: 10g, Net Carbs: 4.7g, Protein: 7.5g

Ingredients

1 cup full-fat natural yogurt 2 tsp swerve sugar 2 tbsp chia seeds 1 cup fresh blackberries 1 tbsp lemon zest Mint leaves, to serve

Directions

In a bowl, mix the yogurt and swerve sugar. Stir in the chia seeds. Reserve 4 blackberries for garnish. Mash the remaining ones with a fork. Stir in the yogurt mixture. Put in the fridge for 30 minutes. Divide the mixture between 2 glasses. Top each with a couple of blackberries, mint, and lemon zest. Serve.

662.   Vanilla Chocolate Mousse

Ready in about: 30 minutes | Serves: 4 Per serving: Kcal 370, Fat: 25g, Net Carbs: 3.7g, Protein: 7.6g

Ingredients

3 eggs 1 cup dark chocolate chips 1 cup heavy cream 1 cup fresh strawberries, sliced 1 vanilla extract 1 tbsp swerve sugar

DirectionsMelt the chocolate in a bowl, in your microwave for a minute on high, and let it cool for 10 minutes. Meanwhile, in a medium-sized mixing bowl, whip the cream until very soft. Add the eggs, vanilla extract, and swerve; whisk to combine. Fold in the cooled chocolate. Divide the mousse between four glasses, top with the strawberry slices, and chill in the fridge for at least 30 minutes before serving.

663.   Blueberry Ice Pops

Ready in about: 5 minutes + cooling time | Serves: 6 Per serving: Kcal 48, Fat 1.2g, Net Carbs 7.9g, Protein 2.3g

Ingredients

3 cups blueberries ½ tbsp lemon juice ¼ cup swerve sugar Pour the blueberries, lemon juice, swerve sugar, and ¼ cup water in a blender, and puree on high speed for 2 minutes until smooth.

Directions

Strain through a sieve into a bowl, discard the solids. Mix in more water if too thick. Divide the mixture into ice pop molds, insert stick cover, and freeze for 4 hours to 1 week. When ready to serve, dip in warm water and remove the pops.

664. Blackcurrant Iced Tea

Ready in about: 10 minutes | Serves: 4 Per serving: Kcal 22, Fat 0g, Net Carbs 5g, Protein 0g

Ingredients

½ cup sugar-free blackcurrant extract 6 unflavored tea bags Swerve to taste

Directions

Ice cubes for serving Lemon slices to garnish Pour the ice cubes in a pitcher and place it in the fridge. Bring 2 cups of water to boil in a saucepan over medium heat for 3 minutes and turn the heat off. Stir in the sugar to dissolve and steep the tea bags in the water for 2 minutes. Remove the bags after and let the tea cool down. Stir in the blackcurrant extract until well incorporated, remove the pitcher from the fridge, and pour the mixture over the ice cubes. Let sit for 3 minutes to cool and after, pour the mixture into tall glasses. Add some more ice cubes, place the lemon slices on the rim of the glasses, and serve the tea cold.

665. Almond Butter Fat Bombs

Ready in about: 3 minutes + cooling time | Serves: 4 Per serving: Kcal 193, Fat 18.3g, Net Carbs 2g, Protein 4g

Ingredients

½ cup almond butter ½ cup coconut oil 4 tbsp unsweetened cocoa powder ½ cup erythritol

Directions

Melt butter and coconut oil in the microwave for 45 seconds, stirring twice until properly melted and mixed. Mix in cocoa powder and erythritol until thoroughly combined. Pour into muffin molds and refrigerate for 3 hours to harden.

666. Berry Merry

Ready in about: 6 minutes | Serves: 4 Per serving: Kcal 83, Fat 3g, Net Carbs 8g, Protein 2.7g

Ingredients

1 cup strawberries + extra for garnishing 1 ½ cups blackberries 1 cup blueberries 2 small beets, peeled and chopped 2/3 cup ice cubes 1 lime, juiced

Directions

For the extra strawberries for garnishing, make a single deep cut on their sides; set aside. Add the blackberries, strawberries, blueberries, beet, and ice cubes into the smoothie maker. Blend the ingredients at high speed until smooth and frothy, for about 60 seconds. Add the lime juice, and puree further for 30 seconds. Pour the drink into tall smoothie glasses, fix the reserved strawberries on each glass rim, stick a straw in, and serve the drink immediately.

667.   Peanut Butter Pecan Ice Cream

Ready in about: 36 minutes + chilling time | Serves: 4 Per serving: Kcal 302, Fat 32g, Net Carbs 2g, Protein 5g

Ingredients

½ cup swerve sweetener confectioners 2 cups heavy cream 1 tbsp erythritol ½ cup smooth peanut butter 1 tbsp olive oil 2 eggs yolks ½ cup pecans, chopped

Directions

Warm heavy cream with peanut butter, olive oil, and erythritol in a small pan over low heat without boiling for about 3 minutes. Remove from the heat. In a bowl, beat the egg yolks until creamy in color. Stir the eggs into the cream mixture. Continue stirring until a thick batter has formed, about 3 minutes. Pour the cream mixture into a bowl. Refrigerate for 30 minutes. Stir in sweetener confectioners. Pour the mixture into the ice cream machine and churn it according to the manufacturer's instructions. Stir in the pecans after and spoon the mixture into a loaf pan. Freeze for 2 hours before serving.

668.   Mixed Berry Trifle

Ready in about: 3 minutes + cooling time | Serves: 4 Per serving: Kcal 321, Fat 28.5g, Net Carbs 8.3g, Protein 9.8g

Ingredients

½ cup walnuts, toasted 1 avocado, chopped 1 cup mascarpone cheese, softened 1 cup fresh blueberries 1 cup fresh raspberries 1 cup fresh blackberries

Directions

In four dessert glasses, share half of the mascarpone, half of the berries (mixed), half of the walnuts, and half of the avocado, and repeat the layering process for a second time to finish the ingredients. Cover the glasses with plastic wrap and refrigerate for 45 minutes until quite firm

669.   Chocolate Bark with Almonds

Ready in about: 5 minutes + cooling time | Serves: 12 Per serving: Kcal 161, Fat: 15.3g, Net Carbs: 1.9g, Protein: 1.9g

Ingredients

½ cup toasted almonds, chopped ½ cup butter 10 drops stevia ¼ tsp salt ½ cup unsweetened coconut flakes 4 oz dark chocolate

Directions

Melt together the butter and chocolate, in the microwave, for 90 seconds. Remove and stir in stevia. Line a cookie sheet with waxed paper and spread the chocolate evenly. Scatter the almonds on top, coconut flakes, and sprinkle with salt. Refrigerate for one hour.

670. Coconut Fat Bombs

Ready in about: 2 minutes +cooling time | Serves: 4 Per serving: Kcal 214, Fat 19g, Net Carbs 2g, Protein 4g

Ingredients

2/3 cup coconut oil, melted 1 (14 oz) can coconut milk 18 drops stevia liquid 1 cup unsweetened coconut flakes

Directions

Mix the coconut oil with the milk and stevia to combine. Stir in the coconut flakes until well distributed. Pour into silicone muffin molds and freeze for 1 hour to harden.

671. Chia Pudding with Coconut and Lemon

(Ready in about 1 hour | Servings 4) Per serving: 270 Calories; 24.7g Fat; 6.5g Carbs; 4.6g Protein; 4g Fiber

Ingredients

1/3 cup chia seeds 1/2 cup Greek-style yogurt 1/3 teaspoon vanilla extract 1/2 teaspoon ground cloves 1/4 teaspoon ground cinnamon 1/2 cup coconut milk 1 cup coconut cream 2 tablespoons Erythritol

Directions Place all ingredients in a glass jar and let it sit in your refrigerator for 1 hour.

672. Peanut Butter Fudge Cake

(Ready in about 3 hours | Servings 8) Per serving: 180 Calories; 18.3g Fat; 4.5g Carbs; 1g Protein; 1.1g Fiber

Ingredients

3/4 cup peanut butter, sugar-free, preferably homemade 3 tablespoons cocoa nibs, unsweetened and melted 1/4 teaspoon baking powder 3 tablespoons coconut oil, at room temperature 1 teaspoon vanilla extract 1 stick butter 1/3 cup almond milk 1/3 cup Swerve A pinch of salt A pinch of grated nutmeg

Directions Melt the butter in your microwave. Stir in the milk, 1/4 cup of Swerve, salt, nutmeg, and baking powder. Spoon the batter into a parchment-lined baking dish. Refrigerate for about 3 hours or until set. Meanwhile, make the sauce by whisking the remaining ingredients until everything is well incorporated. Spoon the sauce over your fudge cake.Enjoy!

673. Mom's Coconut Tarts

(Ready in about 40 minutes + chilling time | Servings 4) Per serving: 304 Calories; 27.7g Fat; 6.6g Carbs; 11.6g Protein; 1.5g Fiber

Ingredients

1 cup coconut cream, unsweetened A pinch of nutmeg 1/4 teaspoon ground cinnamon 1/2 cup granulated Erythritol 1 teaspoon pure almond extract 4 eggs 1/2 cup almond butter A pinch of salt

Directions

Melt the coconut cream in a sauté pan over medium-low heat. Remove form heat. Mix the remaining ingredients until well combined. Now, gradually pour the egg mixture into the warm coconut cream, whisking to combine well. Spoon the mixture into small tart cases. Bake in the preheated oven at 350 degrees F for about 30 minutes until they are golden and firm.Bon appétit!

674.   Bourbon Vanilla Cheesecake

(Ready in about 30 minutes + chilling time | Servings 10) Per serving: 211 Calories; 19g Fat; 4.4g Carbs; 7g Protein; 0.5g Fiber

Ingredients

For the Crust:

2 tablespoons walnuts, chopped 4 tablespoons peanut butter, room temperature 1 cup coconut flour

For the Filling:

1/2 teaspoon vanilla essence 2 tablespoons bourbon 1 teaspoon fresh ginger, grated 10 ounces cream cheese, room temperature 2 eggs 1/2 teaspoon Monk fruit sweetener

Directions

Mix all of the crust ingredients. Press the crust into a parchment-lined springform pan and bake at 330 degrees F for about 10 minutes. Place the springform pan in a deep baking tray filled with 2 inches of warm water to help create steam during baking. Make the cheesecake filling by mixing all the ingredients using an electric mixer. Spread the filling onto the crusts and bake an additional 20 minutes.Bon appétit!

675.   Easy Lemon Panna Cotta

(Ready in about 10 minutes + chilling time | Servings 10) Per serving: 221 Calories; 21.5g Fat; 3.8g Carbs; 4.3g Protein; 0g Fiber

Ingredients

1 teaspoon lemon juice 1 teaspoon lemon rind, grated 1 teaspoon vanilla extract 1 ½ teaspoons gelatins powder, unsweetened 1/2 cup almond milk 1 cup double cream 1/4 cup erythritol

Directions

Place the gelatin and milk in a saucepan and let it sit for 2 minutes. Add in the other ingredients and stir to combine. Let it simmer for 3 to 4 minutes until the gelatin has dissolved completely. Pour the mixture into 4 ramekins and transfer to your refrigerator; cover and let it sit overnight or at least 6 hours. Enjoy!

676.   Frozen Walnut Dessert

(Ready in about 10 minutes + chilling time | Servings 6) Per serving: 84 Calories; 8.9g Fat; 1.5g Carbs; 0.8g Protein; 0.7g Fiber

Ingredients

1/2 stick butter, melted 1/2 teaspoon almond extract A few drops Monk fruit powder 2 tablespoons cocoa powder 2 tablespoons walnuts, chopped

Directions

Melt the butter in your microwave; add in the almond extract, Monk fruit powder, and cocoa powder. Spoon the mixture into a parchment-lined baking tray. Scatter the chopped walnuts on top and place in your freezer until set.Bon appétit!

677.   Coconut and Berry Ice Cream

(Ready in about 10 minutes + chilling time | Servings 4) Per serving: 305 Calories; 18.3g Fat; 4.5g Carbs; 1g Protein; 2.7g Fiber

Ingredients

1 ¼ cups coconut milk 1/2 teaspoon xanthan gum 1/3 cup double cream A few drops Monk fruit 1/2 cup coconut flakes

Directions

In a mixing bowl, combine coconut milk, double cream, Monk fruit, and coconut flakes. Add in the xanthan gum, whisking constantly, until the mixture has thickened. Then, prepare your ice cream in the ice cream maker according to manufacturer's instructions.Bon appétit!

678.   Mixed Berry Scones

(Ready in about 25 minutes | Servings 10) Per serving: 245 Calories; 21.6g Fat; 7.4g Carbs; 3.8g Protein; 0.6g Fiber

Ingredients

1 cup mixed berries 1 ½ sticks butter 1 cup double cream 1 cup Swerve A pinch of salt A pinch of grated nutmeg 1 cup almond meal 1 cup coconut flour 1 teaspoon baking powder 2 eggs 1 teaspoon vanilla paste

Directions

Thoroughly combine the almond meal, coconut flour, baking powder, salt, nutmeg, and berries. In another bowl, whisk the eggs with the butter and double cream. Stir in Swerve and vanilla paste; stir until everything is well combined. Add the egg mixture to the almond flour mixture; stir until a soft dough forms. Shape the dough into 16 triangles and place them on a foil-lined baking sheet. Bake in the preheated oven at 360 degrees F for about 20 minutes.

679.   Greek Frappé Coffee

(Ready in about 2 hours | Servings 2) Per serving: 222 Calories; 15.8g Fat; 7.1g Carbs; 5.9g Protein; 0.3g Fiber

Ingredients

1 tablespoon cacao butter 1 cup almond milk 1/2 cup prepared instant espresso, cooled 1/2 teaspoon Monk fruit powder 2 tablespoons coconut whipped cream

Directions

In your blender, mix the cacao butter, almond milk, instant espresso, and Monk fruit powder until well combined.Enjoy!

680. Old-Fashioned Walnut Cheesecake

(Ready in about 1 hour | Servings 14) Per serving: 393 Calories; 38g Fat; 4.1g Carbs; 9.8g Protein; 1.1g Fiber

Ingredients

The Crust: 1/3 cup Swerve 1/4 teaspoon ground cinnamon 8 ounces walnuts, chopped A pinch of salt 1 stick butter, melted 1/4 teaspoon ground cloves

For the Filling:

1 cup Swerve 1 teaspoon pure vanilla extract 4 eggs 14 ounces Greek-style yogurt 22 ounces Neufchâtel cheese, at room temperature

Directions

Mix all ingredients for the crust; press the mixture into a baking pan and set it aside Whip the Neufchâtel cheese using your electric mixer on low speed. Add in 1 cup of Swerve and vanilla. Fold in the eggs, one at a time, mixing constantly on low speed. Add in Greek-style yogurt and gently stir to combine. Bake in the preheated oven at 290 degrees F for 50 to 55 minutes. Bon appétit!

681. Chocolate Nut Clusters

(Ready in about 15 minutes + chilling time | Servings 8) Per serving: 166 Calories; 17.2g Fat; 2.2g Carbs; 1.2g Protein; 1.1g Fiber

Ingredients

1/2 cup walnuts, chopped 1/2 cup coconut oil, at room temperature 1/4 cup cocoa powder, unsweetened 1/4 cup Erythritol A pinch of coarse salt

Directions

Melt the coconut oil in your microwave; add in cocoa powder and Erythritol. Remove from the heat and stir well. Add in the ground walnuts and coarse salt and stir until everything is well combined.   Drop by teaspoonfuls onto foil-lined baking sheets. Chill in your refrigerator until firm.Bon appétit!

682. Hazelnut Cake Squares

(Ready in about 30 minutes | Servings 8) Per serving: 241 Calories; 23.6g Fat; 3.7g Carbs; 5.2g Protein; 1g Fiber

Ingredients

2 cups almond meal 3 eggs 1 teaspoon almond extract 3/4 cup heavy cream A pinch of sea salt 1/2 cup coconut oil, at room temperature 1/2 cup hazelnuts, chopped 3/4 teaspoon baking powder 1 cup Erythritol 1/2 teaspoon ground cinnamon 1/4 teaspoon ground cardamom

Directions

Start by preheating your oven to 365 degrees F. Coat the bottom of your baking pan with parchment paper. Thoroughly combine the almond meal, baking powder, Erythritol, cinnamon, cardamom, and salt. After that, stir in the coconut oil, eggs, almond extract, and heavy cream; whisk until everything is well incorporated. Stir in the chopped hazelnuts. Scrape the batter into the prepared baking pan. Bake in the preheated oven for about 25 minutes.Enjoy!

683.   Chocolate Jaffa Custard

(Ready in about 15 minutes | Servings 4) Per serving: 154 Calories; 13g Fat; 6.3g Carbs; 5.3g Protein; 1.7g Fiber

Ingredients

3 ounces cream cheese, at room temperature 2 egg yolks 1/4 teaspoon ground cardamom 1/4 teaspoon grated nutmeg 1/4 cup Swerve 1/4 cup cocoa powder, unsweetened 3/4 cup double cream 1 tablespoon orange juice, freshly squeezed

Directions

Whip the egg yolks using an electric mixer until pale and frothy. Warm the cream and gradually fold in the hot cream into the beaten eggs. Let it simmer for about 4 minutes, stirring continuously, until the mixture has reduced and thickened slightly. In another mixing bowl, beat the remaining ingredients until everything is creamy and uniform. Fold the avocado mixture into the egg/cream mixture; gently stir until well combined.Enjoy!

684.   Perfect Lemon Curd

(Ready in about 10 minutes + chilling time | Servings 6) Per serving: 180 Calories; 17.6g Fat; 5.2g Carbs; 2.8g Protein; 0.1g Fiber

Ingredients

4 ounces fresh lemon juice 1 ½ cups Erythritol A pinch of salt A pinch of nutmeg 2 eggs + 1 egg yolk, well whisked 1/2 cup butter, at room temperature

Directions

In a sauté pan, beat the eggs over a low heat. Add in the remaining ingredients and cook for about 5 minutes, whisking constantly. Turn the heat to the lowest setting and continue to stir with a wire whisk for 1 to 2 minutes longer. Cover with a plastic wrap.Enjoy!

685.   Autumn Pear Crumble

(Ready in about 30 minutes | Servings 8) Per serving: 152 Calories; 11.8g Fat; 6.2g Carbs; 2.5g Protein; 1.7g Fiber

Ingredients

2 ½ cups pears, cored and sliced 1/2 cup coconut flour 3/4 cup granulated Swerve 2 eggs, whisked 1/2 tablespoon fresh lime juice 1/3 teaspoon xanthan gum 3/4 cup almond meal 5 tablespoons butter

Directions

Preheat your oven to 365 degrees F. Brush the sides and bottom of a baking dish with a nonstick spray. Arrange your pears on the bottom of the baking dish. Drizzle the lime juice and xanthan gum over them. In a mixing dish, thoroughly combine the almond meal, coconut flour, and Swerve. Fold in the eggs, one at a time, mixing constantly until your mixture resembles coarse meal. Spread this mixture over the pear layer. Cut in the cold butter and bake in the preheated oven for 20 to 23 minutes or until golden brown on the top.Bon appétit!

686.   Espresso Pudding Shots

(Ready in about 10 minutes + chilling time | Servings 6) Per serving: 218 Calories; 24.7g Fat; 1.1g Carbs; 0.4g Protein; 0.7g Fiber

Ingredients

2 teaspoons butter, softened A pinch of grated nutmeg 1 teaspoon pure vanilla extract 4 ounces coconut oil 3 tablespoons powdered Erythritol 4 ounces coconut milk creamer 1 teaspoon espresso powder

Directions

Melt the butter and coconut oil in a double boiler over medium-low heat. Add in the remaining ingredients and stir to combine. Pour into silicone molds.Enjoy!

687.   Creamy Gelatin Dessert

(Ready in about 45 minutes | Servings 10) Per serving: 56 Calories; 5.5g Fat; 0.4g Carbs; 1.5g Protein; 0g Fiber

Ingredients

2 envelopes lemon gelatin 5 tablespoons powdered Erythritol 1 ¼ cups double cream 1/2 teaspoon ginger, minced 1 teaspoon vanilla extract 3/4 cup boiling water

Directions

Combine the gelatin, Erythritol, ginger, and vanilla in a heatproof dish. Pour in the boiling water. Stir until the gelatin has dissolved completely. Stir in the double cream; continue to stir with a wire whisk. Pour the mixture into molds and transfer to your refrigerator for 30 to 35 minutes or until they are solid.

688.   Chocolate Sheet Pan Cookie Cake

(Ready in about 30 minutes | Servings 10) Per serving: 157 Calories; 14.8g Fat; 3.5g Carbs; 4.5g Protein; 2.2g Fiber

Ingredients

1/2 cup coconut oil 2 eggs 5 drops liquid Monk fruit 1/4 teaspoon ground cinnamon 1/2 cup walnuts, chopped 1/3 cup baker's chocolate chunks, unsweetened 3/4 cup coconut flour 1 cup almond meal 1/2 teaspoon baking powder 1/4 teaspoon ground cardamom 1/2 teaspoon almond extract

Directions

Start by preheating your oven to 360 degrees F. Line a baking sheet with a parchment paper. Melt the coconut oil in a double over low heat. Thoroughly combine the almond extract, eggs, and Monk fruit. Add in the melted coconut oil along with the remaining ingredients. Stir to combine well. Scrape the mixture into the prepared baking sheet. Bake in the preheated oven for 25 to 30 minutes.Enjoy!

689.   Almond Fluff Fudge

(Ready in about 2 hours | Servings 8) Per serving: 167 Calories; 17.1g Fat; 6.8g Carbs; 2.4g Protein; 0.9g Fiber

Ingredients

2 ounces almonds, chopped 1/2 teaspoon vanilla extract 1/4 teaspoon orange zest 1 cup Swerve 1 cup coconut milk, unsweetened 1/2 cup butter, at room temperature

Directions

Combine the Swerve and coconut milk in a double boiler over low heat. Add in the butter and vanilla extract and beat the mixture using an electric mixer at low speed. Fold in the chopped almond and orange zest. Scrape the batter into a lightly greased baking dish and freeze until firm about 1 hour 50 minutes.Enjoy!

690.   Easy Cappuccino Creamsicles

(Ready in about 10 minutes + chilling time | Servings 8) Per serving: 117 Calories; 11.2g Fat; 5g Carbs; 1.3g Protein; 3g Fiber

Ingredients

1 ½ cups avocado, pitted, peeled and mashed 2 tablespoons cocoa powder 3 tablespoons Swerve 1/2 teaspoon cappuccino flavor extract 1 cup brewed coffee 1 cup double cream

Directions

Using a stand mixer with a whisk attachment, whip the double cream until soft peaks form. Process all ingredients in your blender or food processor until everything is creamy and smooth. Pour the mixture into popsicle molds and freeze overnight.Enjoy!

691.   Classic Coconut Truffles

(Ready in about 15 minutes + chilling time | Servings 16) Per serving: 90 Calories; 6.3g Fat; 4.9g Carbs; 3.7g Protein; 0.5g Fiber

Ingredients

4 tablespoons coconut flakes 1/4 cup unsweetened cocoa powder 1/4 cup coconut oil 1 cup whipped cream 1 ½ cups bakers' chocolate, unsweetened 3 tablespoons Swerve 1 teaspoon vanilla extract 1 tablespoon rum

Directions

Melt the chocolate in your microwave. Add in the coconut flakes, coconut oil, cream, Swerve, vanilla extract, and rum. Place in your refrigerator until the batter is well-chilled. Roll the mixture into balls and cover with cocoa powder on all sides.Bon appétit!

692.   Butterscotch Cheesecake Cupcakes

(Ready in about 30 minutes + chilling time | Servings 8) Per serving: 165 Calories; 15.6g Fat; 5.4g Carbs; 5.2g Protein; 1.7g Fiber

Ingredients

2 eggs 1 tablespoon whiskey 2 packets stevia 3 tablespoons butter, melted 10 ounces soft cheese, at room temperature 1/2 teaspoon ground cinnamon For the Frosting: 1 teaspoon butterscotch extract 1/2 stick butter, at room temperature 1/2 cup powdered erythritol 1 ½ tablespoons coconut milk, unsweetened

Directions

Start by preheating your oven to 365 degrees F. Mix 3 tablespoons of butter, soft cheese, whiskey, eggs, stevia, and cinnamon until well combined. Scrape the batter into the muffin pan and bake approximately 15 minutes; place the muffin pan in the freezer for 2 hours. In a mixing bowl, beat 1/2 stick of butter with powdered erythritol and butterscotch extract. Gradually pour in the milk and mix again. Afterwards, frost the chilled cupcakes.Bon appétit!

693.   Tangerine Chocolate Pudding

(Ready in about 15 minutes + chilling time | Servings 6) Per serving: 158 Calories; 15.7g Fat; 7.2g Carbs; 2.2g Protein; 1.6g Fiber

Ingredients

3 1/3 tablespoons Dutch-processed brown cocoa powder 2 cups whipped cream Fresh juice and zest of 1/2 tangerine 1/4 teaspoon ground cloves 1/2 teaspoon crystallized ginger 6 ounces chocolate, unsweetened 3 tablespoons powdered erythritol

Directions

Using a stand mixer with a whisk attachment, whip the cream until soft peaks form. Add in the powdered erythritol and cocoa powder and beat again. Add in the remaining ingredients and beat until everything is well incorporated.

694.   Peanut Butter Mousse

(Ready in about 15 minutes | Servings 4) Per serving: 288 Calories; 27.3g Fat; 6.9g Carbs; 6.2g Protein; 5.2g Fiber

Ingredients

1/2 cup peanut butter 1 ½ cups avocado, peeled, pitted, and diced 1 teaspoon vanilla extract 1 tablespoon lemon juice 1/2 cup coconut cream 1 teaspoon monk fruit powder 1/2 cup coconut milk

Directions

Place all ingredients in your blender or food processor. Process until well combined.

695. White Chocolate Fudge Squares

(Ready in about 15 minutes + chilling time | Servings 12) Per serving: 202 Calories; 21.3g Fat; 2.3g Carbs; 2.4g Protein; 2.2g Fiber

Ingredients

3 ounces white chocolate, unsweetened 3/4 cup coconut oil 1/3 cup almond milk 2 tablespoons Swerve 1/8 teaspoon coarse sea salt 1 ¼ cups almond butter

Directions

Microwave the coconut oil, almond butter, and white chocolate until they are melted. Add in the remaining ingredients and process in your blender. Scrape the mixture into a parchment-lined baking tray. Cut into squares and serve.Enjoy!

696. Homemade Mint Chocolate

(Ready in about 35 minutes | Servings 8) Per serving: 140 Calories; 14g Fat; 5.9g Carbs; 2g Protein; 2.4g Fiber

Ingredients

4 ounces cacao butter 1 teaspoon vanilla paste 1/4 teaspoon grated nutmeg 1/2 cup hazelnuts, chopped 1 tablespoon coconut oil 8 tablespoons

cocoa powder 1/4 cup Erythritol 1 teaspoon peppermint oil

Directions

Microwave the cacao butter and coconut oil for about 1 minute. Now, stir in the cocoa powder, Erythritol, peppermint oil, vanilla, and nutmeg. Spoon the mixture into an ice cube tray. Fold in the chopped hazelnuts and place in your freezer for about 30 minutes until set.Bon appétit!

697. Brazilian Berry Brigadeiro

(Ready in about 15 minutes + chilling time | Servings 10) Per serving: 334 Calories; 37g Fat; 5.3g Carbs; 1.6g Protein; 0.6g Fiber

Ingredients

4 ounces bakers' chocolate chunks, unsweetened 1/2 teaspoon vanilla extract 1/2 teaspoon coconut extract 1/4 cup butter 1/2 cup peanut butter 3/4 cup coconut oil 1 cup freeze-dried mixed berries, crushed

Directions

Melt the butter, peanut butter, and coconut oil in a double boiler over medium-low heat. Fold in the chocolate chunks, mixed berries, vanilla extract, and coconut extract. Shape the batter into small balls and let them harden in your refrigerator.Bon appétit!

698.   Dark Chocolate Mousse with Stewed Plums

Ready in about: 45 minutes + cooling time | Serves: 6 Per serving: Kcal 288, Fat 23g, Net Carbs 6.9g, Protein 9.5g

Ingredients

8 eggs, separated into yolks and whites 12 oz unsweetened chocolate 2 tbsp salt ¾ cup swerve sugar ½ cup olive oil 3 tbsp brewed coffee Stewed plums 6 plums, pitted and halved ½ stick cinnamon ½ cup swerve sugar ½ cup water ½ lemon, juiced

Directions

Melt the chocolate in the microwave for 1 ½ minutes. In a separate bowl, whisk the yolks with half of the swerve until a pale yellow has formed, then beat in salt, olive oil, and coffee. Mix in the melted chocolate until smooth. In a third bowl, whisk the whites with a hand mixer until a soft peak has formed. Sprinkle the remaining swerve over and gently fold in with a spatula. Fetch a tablespoon full of the chocolate mixture and fold in to combine. Pour in the remaining chocolate mixture and whisk to mix. Pour the mousse into 6 ramekins, cover with plastic wrap, and refrigerate overnight. The next morning, pour water, swerve sugar, cinnamon, and lemon juice in a saucepan and bring to a simmer for 3 minutes, occasionally stirring to ensure the swerve has dissolved and a syrup has formed. Add the plums and poach in the sweetened water for 18 minutes until soft. Turn the heat off and discard the cinnamon stick. Spoon a plum with syrup on each mousse ramekin and serve.

699.   Vanilla Ice Cream

Ready in about: 5 minutes + cooling time | Serves: 4 Per serving: Kcal 290, Fat 23g, Net Carbs 6g, Protein 13g

Ingredients

½ cup smooth peanut butter ½ cup swerve sugar 3 cups half and half 1 tsp vanilla extract 1 pinch of salt

Directions

Beat peanut butter and swerve in a bowl with a hand mixer until smooth. Gradually whisk in half and half until thoroughly combined. Mix in vanilla and salt. Pour mixture into a loaf pan and freeze for 45 minutes until firmed up. Scoop into glasses when ready to eat and serve.

700.   Vanilla Flan with Mint

Ready in about: 60 minutes + cooling time | Serves: 4 Per serving: Kcal 269, Fat: 26g, Net Carbs: 1.7g, Protein: 7.6g

Ingredients

⅓ cup erythritol, for caramel 2 cups almond milk 4 eggs 1 tbsp vanilla extract 1 tbsp lemon zest ½ cup erythritol, for custard 2 cup heavy whipping cream

Directions

Mint leaves, to serve Heat erythritol for the caramel in a deep pan. Add 2-3 tablespoons of water, and bring to a boil. Reduce the heat and cook until the caramel turns golden brown. Divide between 4-6 metal tins. Set aside to cool. In a bowl, mix eggs, remaining erythritol, lemon zest, and vanilla. Add almond milk and beat until well combined. Pour the custard into each caramel-lined ramekin and place it in a deep baking tin. Fill over the way with the remaining hot water. Bake at 345°F for 45-50 minutes. Take out the ramekins and let cool for at least 4 hours in the fridge. Run a knife slowly around the edges to invert onto a dish. Serve with dollops of whipped cream, scattered with mint leaves.

701.   Raspberry Nut Truffles

Ready in about: 6 minutes + cooling time | Serves: 4 Per serving: Kcal 251, Fat 18.3g, Net Carbs 3.5g, Protein 12g

Ingredients

1 ½ cups sugar-free raspberry preserves 2 cups raw cashews 2 tbsp flax seed 3 tbsp swerve 10 oz unsweetened chocolate chips 3 tbsp olive oil

Directions

Line a baking sheet with parchment paper. Grind the cashews and flax seeds in a blender for 45 seconds until smoothly crushed. Add the raspberry and 2 tbsp of swerve. Process for 1 minute until well combined. Form 1-inch balls of the mixture, place on the baking sheet, and freeze for 1 hour or until firmed up. Melt the chocolate chips, oil, and 1tbsp of swerve in a microwave for 1 ½ minutes. Toss the truffles to coat in the chocolate mixture, put on the baking sheet, and freeze further for at least 2 hours. Serve.

702.   Ice Cream Bars Covered with Chocolate

Ready in about: 20 minutes + freezing time | Serves: 15 Per serving: Kcal 345 Fat: 32g, Net Carbs: 5g, Protein: 4g

Ingredients

Ice cream 1 cup heavy whipping cream 1 tsp vanilla extract ¾ tsp xanthan gum ½ cup peanut butter 1 cup half and half 1 ½ cups almond milk ⅓ tsp stevia powder 1 tbsp vegetable glycerin 3 tbsp xylitol Chocolate ¾ cup coconut oil ¼ cup cocoa butter pieces, chopped 2 oz unsweetened chocolate 3 ½ tsp

Directions

THM super sweet blend Blend all ice cream ingredients until smooth. Place in an ice cream maker and follow the instructions. Spread the ice cream into a lined pan, and freezer for about 4 hours. Combine all chocolate ingredients in a microwave-safe bowl and heat until melted. Allow cooling. Remove the ice cream from the freezer and slice into bars. Dip them into the cooled chocolate mixture and return to the freezer for about 10 minutes before serving.

703.   Eggless Strawberry Mousse

Ready in about: 10 minutes + cooling time | Serves: 6 Per serving: Kcal 290, Fat 24g, Net Carbs 5g, Protein 5g

Ingredients

2 tbsp sugar-free strawberry preserves 2 cups chilled heavy cream 2 cups fresh strawberries, hulled 5 tbsp erythritol 2 tbsp lemon juice ¼ tsp strawberry extract

Directions

Beat the heavy cream in a bowl with a hand mixer at high speed until a stiff peak forms, about 1 minute. Refrigerate. Puree the strawberries in a blender and pour into a saucepan. Add erythritol and lemon juice, and cook on low heat for 3 minutes while stirring continuously. Stir in the strawberry extract evenly, turn off the heat and allow cooling. Fold in the whipped cream until evenly incorporated, and spoon into six ramekins. Refrigerate for 4 hours to solidify. Garnish with strawberry preserves and serve immediately.

704. Chocolate Cakes

Ready in about: 25 minutes | Serves: 6 Per serving: Kcal 218, Fat: 20g, Net Carbs: 10g, Protein: 4.8g

Ingredients

½ cup almond flour ¼ cup xylitol 1 tsp baking powder ½ tsp baking soda 1 tsp cinnamon, ground A pinch of salt A pinch of ground cloves ½ cup butter, melted ½ cup buttermilk 1 egg 1 tsp pure almond extract For the Frosting: 1 cup heavy cream 1 cup dark chocolate, flaked Preheat oven to 360°F.

Directions

In a bowl, mix the cloves, almond flour, baking powder, salt, baking soda, xylitol, and cinnamon. In a separate bowl, combine the almond extract, butter, egg, and buttermilk. Mix the wet mixture into the dry mix. Evenly spoon the batter into a greased donut pan. Bake for 17 minutes. Set a pan over medium heat and warm heavy cream; simmer for 2 minutes. Fold in the chocolate flakes; combine until all the chocolate melts; let cool. Spread the top of the cakes with the frosting.

705. Blueberry Tart with Lavender

Ready in about: 35 minutes + cooling time | Serves: 6 Per serving: Kcal 198, Fat 16.4g, Net Carbs 10.7g, Protein 3.3g

Ingredients

1 large low carb pie crust 1 ½ cups heavy cream 2 tbsp swerve sugar 1 tbsp culinary lavender 1 tsp vanilla extract 2 cups fresh blueberries Preheat oven to 400°F.

Directions

Place the pie crust with its pan on a baking tray and bake in the oven for 30 minutes, until golden brown; remove and let cool. Mix the heavy cream and lavender in a saucepan. Set the pan over medium heat and bring the mixture to a boil. Turn the heat off and let cool. Strain the cream through a colander into a bowl to remove the lavender pieces. Mix swerve and vanilla into the cream and pour into the cooled crust. Scatter with the blueberries. Refrigerate the pie. Serve.

706. Green Tea Brownies with Macadamia Nuts

Ready in about: 28 minutes | Serves: 4 Per serving: Kcal 248, Fat 23.1g, Net Carbs 2.2g, Protein 5.2g

Ingredients

1 tbsp green tea powder ¼ cup unsalted butter, melted 4 tbsp swerve confectioner's sugar A pinch of salt ¼ cup coconut flour ½ tsp baking powder 1 egg ¼ cup chopped macadamia nuts

Directions

Preheat oven to 350°F and line a square baking dish with parchment paper. Pour the melted butter into a bowl, add sugar and salt, and whisk to combine. Crack the egg into the bowl. Beat the mixture until the egg has incorporated. Pour coconut flour, green tea, and baking powder into a fine-mesh sieve, sift into the egg bowl, and stir. Add the nuts, stir again, and pour the mixture into the lined baking dish. Bake for 18 minutes, remove and slice into brownie cubes.

707. Lychee and Coconut Lassi

Ready in about: 30 minutes + cooling time | Serves: 4 Per serving: Kcal 285, Fat 26.1g, Net Carbs 1.5g, Protein 5.3g

Ingredients

2 cups lychee pulp, seeded 2 ½ cups coconut milk 4 tsp swerve sugar 2 limes, zested and juiced 1 ½ cups plain yogurt 1 lemongrass, white part only, torn 2 tbsp toasted coconut shavings A pinch of salt

Directions

In a saucepan, add the lychee pulp, coconut milk, swerve sugar, lemongrass, and lime zest. Stir and bring to boil on medium heat for 2 minutes, stirring continually. Then reduce the heat, and simmer for 1 minute. Turn the heat off and let the mixture sit for 15 minutes. Remove the lemongrass and pour the mixture into a smoothie maker or a blender. Add in the yogurt, salt, and lime juice and process the ingredients until smooth, about 60 seconds. Pour into a jug and refrigerate for 2 hours until cold; stir. Serve garnished with coconut shavings.

708. Mint Chocolate Protein Shake

Ready in about: 4 minutes | Serves: 4 Per serving: Kcal 191, Fat 14.5g, Net Carbs 4g, Protein 15g

Ingredients

3 cups flax milk, chilled 3 tsp unsweetened cocoa powder 1 avocado, pitted, peeled, sliced 1 cup coconut milk, chilled 3 mint leaves + extra to garnish 3 tbsp erythritol 1 tbsp low carb

Directions

Protein powder Whipping cream for topping Combine the milk, cocoa powder, avocado, coconut milk, mint leaves, erythritol, and protein powder into a blender, and blend for 1 minute until smooth. Pour into serving glasses, lightly add some whipping cream on top, and garnish with mint leaves.

709. Strawberry & Basil Lemonade

Ready in about: 3 minutes | Serves: 4 Per serving: Kcal 66, Fat 0.1g, Net Carbs 5.8g, Protein 0.7g

Ingredients

4 cups water 12 strawberries, leaves removed 1 cup fresh lemon juice ⅓ cup fresh basil ¾ cup swerve sugar

Directions

Crushed Ice Halved strawberries to garnish Basil leaves to garnish Spoon some crushed ice into 4 serving glasses and set aside. In a pitcher, add the water, strawberries, lemon juice, basil, and swerve. Insert the blender and process the ingredients for 30 seconds. The mixture should be pink, and the basil finely chopped. Adjust the taste. Drop 2 strawberry halves and some basil in each glass and serve immediately.

710. Cranberry Chocolate Barks

Ready in about: 5 minutes + cooling time | Serves: 6 Per serving: Kcal 225, Fat 21g, Net Carbs 3g, Protein 6g

Ingredients

10 oz unsweetened dark chocolate, chopped ½ cup erythritol ⅓ cup dried cranberries, chopped ⅓ cup toasted walnuts, chopped ¼ tsp dark run ¼ tsp salt

Directions

Line a baking sheet with parchment paper. Pour chocolate and erythritol into a bowl, and melt in the microwave for 25 seconds, stirring three times until fully melted. Stir in the cranberries, dark rum, walnuts, and salt, reserving a few cranberries and walnuts for garnishing. Pour the mixture on the baking sheet and spread out. Sprinkle with remaining cranberries and walnuts. Refrigerate for 2 hours to set. Break into bite-size pieces to serve.

711. Chocolate Cheesecake Bites

Ready in about: 4 minutes + cooling time | Serves: 12 Per serving: Kcal 241, Fat 22g, Net Carbs 3.1g, Protein 5g

Ingredients

10 oz unsweetened dark chocolate chips ½ half and half 20 oz cream cheese, softened 1 tsp vanilla extract

DirectionsIn a saucepan, melt the chocolate with half and a half on low heat for 1 minute. Turn the heat off. In a bowl, whisk the cream cheese, swerve sugar, and vanilla extract with a hand mixer until smooth. Stir into the chocolate mixture. Spoon into silicone muffin tins and freeze for 4 hours until firm.

712.Strawberry Vanilla Shake

Ready in about: 2 minutes | Serves: 4 Per serving: Kcal 285, Fat 22.6g, Net Carbs 3.1g, Protein 16g

Ingredients

2 cups strawberries, stemmed and halved 12 strawberries to garnish ½ cup unsweetened almond milk 2/3 tsp vanilla extract ½ cup heavy whipping cream 2 tbsp swerve sugar

DirectionsProcess the strawberries, milk, vanilla extract, whipping cream, and swerve in a large blender for 2 minutes; work in two batches if needed. The shake should be frosty. Pour into glasses, stick in straws, garnish with strawberry halves, and serve.

713.Cinnamon and Turmeric Latte

Ready in about: 7 minutes | Serves: 4 Per serving: Kcal 132, Fat 12g, Net Carbs 0.3g, Protein 3.9g

Ingredients

3 cups almond milk ⅓ tsp cinnamon powder 1 cup brewed coffee ½ tsp turmeric powder 1 ½ tsp erythritol Cinnamon sticks to garnish

Directions

In the blender, add the almond milk, cinnamon powder, coffee, turmeric, and erythritol. Blend the ingredients at medium speed for 45 seconds and pour the mixture into a saucepan. Set the pan over low heat and heat through for 5 minutes; do not boil. Keep swirling the pan to prevent boiling. Turn the heat off, and serve in latte cups, with a cinnamon stick in each one.

714.   Almond Milk Hot Chocolate

Ready in about: 7 minutes | Serves: 4 Per serving: Kcal 225, Fat 21.5g, Net Carbs 0.6g, Protein 4.5g

Ingredients

3 cups almond milk 4 tbsp unsweetened cocoa powder 2 tbsp swerve sugar 3 tbsp almond butter Finely chopped almonds to garnish

Directions

In a saucepan, add the almond milk, cocoa powder, and swerve sugar. Stir the mixture until the sugar dissolves. Set the pan over low to heat through for 5 minutes, without boiling. Swirl the mix occasionally. Turn the heat off and stir in the almond butter to be incorporated. Pour the hot chocolate into mugs and sprinkle with chopped almonds. Serve hot.

715.Raspberry Flax Seed Dessert

Ready in about: 5 minutes | Serves: 4 Per serving: Kcal 390, Fat 33.5g, Net Carbs 3g, Protein 13g

Ingredients

2 cups raspberries, reserve a few for topping 3 cups unsweetened vanilla almond milk 1 cup heavy cream ½ cup chia seeds ½ cup flaxseeds, ground 4 tsp liquid stevia Chopped mixed nuts for topping

DirectionsIn a medium bowl, crush the raspberries with a fork until pureed. Pour in the almond milk, heavy cream, chia seeds, and liquid stevia. Mix and refrigerate the pudding overnight. Spoon the pudding into serving glasses, top with raspberries, mixed nuts, and serve

716.   ⸲ Cinnamon Cookies

Ready in about: 25 minutes | Serves: 4 Per serving: Kcal 134, Fat: 13g, Net Carbs: 1.5g, Protein: 3g

Ingredients

Cookies 2 cups almond flour ½ tsp baking soda ¾ cup sweetener ½ cup butter, softened A pinch of salt Coating 2 tbsp erythritol sweetener 1 tsp cinnamon Preheat oven to 350°F.

DirectionsCombine all cookie ingredients in a bowl. Make 16 balls out of the mixture and flatten them with hands. Combine the cinnamon and erythritol. Dip the cookies in the cinnamon mixture and arrange them on a lined cookie sheet. Cook for 15 minutes, until crispy.

717.Vanilla Bean Frappuccino

Ready in about: 6 minutes | Serves: 4 Per serving: Kcal 193, Fat 14g, Net Carbs 6g, Protein 15g

Ingredients

3 cups unsweetened vanilla almond milk, chilled Unsweetened chocolate shavings to garnish 2 tsp swerve sugar 1 ½ cups heavy cream, cold 1 vanilla bean ¼ tsp xanthan gum

Directions

Combine the almond milk, swerve, heavy cream, vanilla bean, and xanthan gum in the blender and process on high speed for 1 minute until smooth. Pour into tall shake glasses, sprinkle with chocolate shavings, and serve immediately.

718. Coffee Fat Bombs

Ready in about: 3 minutes + cooling time | Serves: 6 Per serving: Kcal 145, Fat 14g, Net Carbs 2g, Protein 4g

Ingredients

6 tbsp brewed coffee, room temperature 1 ½ cups mascarpone cheese ½ cup melted butter 3 tbsp unsweetened cocoa powder ¼ cup erythritol

Directions

Whisk the mascarpone cheese, butter, cocoa powder, erythritol, and coffee with a hand mixer until creamy and fluffy, about 1 minute. Fill into muffin tins and freeze for 3 hours until firm.

719. Mixed Berry & Mascarpone Bowl

Ready in about: 8 minutes | Serves: 4 Per serving: Kcal 480, Fat 40g, Net Carbs 5g, Protein 20g

Ingredients

4 cups Greek yogurt Liquid stevia to taste 1 ½ cups mascarpone cheese 1 ½ cups blueberries and raspberries 1 cup toasted pecans

Directions

Mix the yogurt, stevia, and mascarpone in a bowl until evenly combined. Divide the mixture into 4 bowls, share the berries and pecans on top of the cream. Serve the dessert immediately.

720. Creamy Coconut Kiwi Drink

Ready in about: 3 minutes | Serves: 4 Per serving: Kcal 351, Fat 28g, Net Carbs 9.7g, Protein 16g

Ingredients

5 kiwis, pulp scooped 2 tbsp erythritol 2 cups unsweetened coconut milk 2 cups coconut cream 7 ice cubes Mint leaves to garnish

Directions

In a blender, process the kiwis, erythritol, milk, cream, and ice cubes until smooth, about 3 minutes. Pour into four serving glasses, garnish with mint leaves, and serve.

721. Walnut Cookies

Ready in about: 15 minutes | Serves: 12 Per serving: Kcal 101, Fat: 11g, Net Carbs: 0.6g, Protein: 1.6g

Ingredients

1 egg 2 cups ground pecans ¼ cup sweetener ½ tsp baking soda 1 tbsp butter 20 walnuts halves Preheat oven to 350°F.

Directions

Mix the ingredients, except the walnuts, until combined. Make 20 balls out of the mixture and press them with your thumb onto a lined cookie sheet. Top each cookie with a walnut half. Bake for about 12 minutes.

722.   Raspberry Sorbet

Ready in about: 10 minutes + cooling time | Serves: 1 Per serving: Kcal 173, Fat: 10g, Net Carbs: 3.7g, Protein: 4g

Ingredients

¼ tsp vanilla extract 1 packet gelatine, without sugar 1 tbsp heavy whipping cream 2 tbsp mashed raspberries 1 ½ cups crushed

Directions

Ice Cover the gelatin with cold water in small bowl. Let dissolve for 5 minutes. Transfer to a blender. Add the remaining ingredients and ⅓ cup of cold water. Blend until smooth and freeze for at least 2 hours.

723.   Dark Chocolate Mochaccino Ice Bombs

Ready in about: 5 minutes + cooling time | Serves: 4 Per serving: Kcal 127, Fat: 13g, Net Carbs: 1.4g, Protein: 1.9g

Ingredients

½ lb cream cheese 4 tbsp powdered sweetener 2 oz strong coffee 2 tbsp cocoa powder, unsweetened 1 tbsp cocoa butter, melted 2 ½ oz dark chocolate, melted

Directions

Combine cream cheese, sweetener, coffee, and cocoa powder, in a food processor. Roll 2 tbsp of the mixture and place on a lined tray. Mix the melted cocoa butter and chocolate, and coat the bombs with it. Freeze for 2 hours.

Other Keto Favorites

724.   Spanish Tortilla Pizza

(Ready in about 15 minutes | Servings 2) Per serving: 397 Calories; 31g Fat; 6.1g Carbs; 22g Protein; 1.4g Fiber

Ingredients

For the Crust:

4 eggs, beaten 1/2 teaspoon coriander, minced Salt and pepper, to taste 1 tablespoon extra-virgin olive oil 1/4 cup cream cheese 2 tablespoons flax seed meal 1 teaspoon chili pepper, deveined and minced

For the Toppings:

2 ounces Manchego cheese, shredded 2 tablespoons tomato paste

Directions

In a mixing bowl, combine ingredients for the crust. Divide the batter into two pieces. Cook in a frying pan for about 5 minutes; flip your tortilla and cook on the other side until crisp and golden-brown on their edges. Repeat with another tortilla. Spread the tomato paste and cheese over the top of each of the prepared tortillas. Place under the preheated broiler for about 5 minutes until the cheese is hot and bubbly.

725.   Rich Keto Grits with Hemp

(Ready in about 20 minutes | Servings 4) Per serving: 405 Calories; 37g Fat; 6.6g Carbs; 14.8g Protein; 2.3g Fiber

Ingredients

1/4 cup hemp hearts 2 tablespoons butter, softened 1 teaspoon coconut extract 1/4 teaspoon coarse salt 8 walnuts, chopped 4 eggs, lightly whisked 1/4 cup flax seed, freshly ground 2 teaspoons liquid Monk fruit 1/4 teaspoon pinch psyllium husk powder

Directions

Mel the butter in a sauté pan over medium-low heat. Add in the remaining ingredients and continue to cook until the mixture starts to boil. Remove from heat and stir in the chopped walnuts; stir to combine.Bon appétit!

726.   Nutty Breakfast Porridge

(Ready in about 25 minutes | Servings 2) Per serving: 430 Calories; 41.1g Fat; 5.8g Carbs; 11.4g Protein; 0.1g Fiber

Ingredients

3 eggs 3 tablespoons erythritol 1/2 cup sour cream 1 ½ tablespoons butter 1/2 teaspoon star anise 1/4 cup almonds

Directions

Whisk the eggs, erythritol, and sour cream until well combined. Melt the butter and add in the egg mixture along with star anise; continue to cook on medium-low heat until thoroughly warmed. Top with slivered almonds.Bon appétit!

727.   Keto Pancakes with Blueberry Topping

(Ready in about 20 minutes | Servings 4) Per serving: 237 Calories; 16.3g Fat; 5.5g Carbs; 14.5g Protein; 0.9g Fiber

Ingredients

For the Batter:

6 ounces soft cheese 1 teaspoon baking powder 5 eggs

For the Topping:

1 cup fresh blueberries 2 tablespoons Swerve 2 tablespoons canola oil 1/2 cup sour cream

Directions

In a mixing bowl, whisk all the batter ingredients. Brush your pan with a small amount of the oil. Once hot, spoon the batter onto the pan and form into circles. Cover and cook until bubbles start to form. Flip and cook on the other side until browned. Repeat with the rest of the batter.

728.   Authentic Greek Aioli

(Ready in about 10 minutes | Servings 8) Per serving: 116 Calories; 13.2g Fat; 0.2g Carbs; 0.4g Protein; 0.1g Fiber

Ingredients

1 tablespoon white vinegar 1 teaspoon dried dill weed Salt and pepper, to taste 1/2 cup olive oil 1 egg yolk, at room temperature 1/2 teaspoon garlic, crushed

Directions

In your blender, process the vinegar, egg yolk, garlic, salt, and pepper; pulse until smooth and uniform. Turn to low setting. Gradually drizzle in the olive oil and continue to mix until well blended. Add in the dried dill and place in your refrigerator.

729.   Autumn Nut and Seed Granola

(Ready in about 35 minutes | Servings 8) Per serving: 281 Calories; 26.6g Fat; 7.7g Carbs; 5.4g Protein; 3.3g Fiber

Ingredients

2 tablespoons hemp hearts 1/4 cup sunflower seeds 1 teaspoon pumpkin pie spice mix 3/4 cup almonds, chopped 1/2 cup cashews, chopped 1 tablespoon Monk fruit powder 1 cup coconut flakes 3 tablespoons coconut oil 1/4 cup pepitas seeds 1/4 cup flaxseeds

Directions

Toss all ingredients in a rimmed baking pan. Bake in the preheated oven 290 degrees F, tossing once or twice.

730.   Omelet with Spring Onions

(Ready in about 15 minutes | Servings 2) Per serving: 319 Calories; 25g Fat; 7.4g Carbs; 14.9g Protein; 2.7g Fiber

Ingredients 4 eggs, beaten 2 teaspoons olive oil 2 tomatoes, chopped 1 chili pepper, minced Salt and black pepper, to taste 2 spring onions, chopped 1 teaspoon spring garlic, minced 8 ounces Greek-style yogurt

Directions

In a frying pan, heat the olive oil over a moderate flame. Once hot, cook the spring onion and garlic until they've softened or about 2 minutes. Beat the eggs with the Greek-style yogurt. Pour the egg mixture into the pan; cook until the eggs are puffy and golden-brown. Place the tomatoes and pepper on one side of the omelet. Sprinkle with salt and pepper and fold the omelet in half.

731.Great-Grandma's Cheesy Meatballs

(Ready in about 35 minutes | Servings 5) Per serving: 342 Calories; 23.7g Fat; 4.3g Carbs; 31.7g Protein; 0.6g Fiber

Ingredients

1 pound ground beef 1 egg, beaten Salt and pepper, to taste 2 tablespoons olive oil 1 cup Swiss cheese, shredded 1 celery, grated 1 teaspoon garlic, minced 1 yellow onion, chopped 1 teaspoon Fajita seasoning mix

Directions

Mix all ingredients, except for cheese, until everything is well incorporated. Roll the mixture into small meatballs and bake at 365 degrees F for about 30 minutes.Bon appétit!

732.   Mexican-Style Avocado Fat Bombs

(Ready in about 20 minutes + chilling time | Servings 8) Per serving: 145 Calories; 12.6g Fat; 3.7g Carbs; 5.5g Protein; 1.7g Fiber

Ingredients

2 ounces bacon bits 1/2 teaspoon chili powder 1/4 teaspoon mustard powder 6 ounces avocado flash 6 ounces Cotija cheese 1 tablespoon cayenne pepper

Directions

Thoroughly combine all ingredients until everything is well incorporated. Roll the mixture into eight balls. Place in the refrigerator for about 1 hour. Bon appétit!

733.   Easy Peppery Ribs

(Ready in about 15 minutes | Servings 4) Per serving: 490 Calories; 44g Fat; 5.5g Carbs; 16.9g Protein; 0.6g Fiber

Ingredients

2 Italian peppers, deveined and thinly sliced 2 tablespoons scallions, chopped 1 pound ribs, cut into small chunks Salt and black pepper, to taste 1 tablespoon lard, at room temperature 1 teaspoon garlic, minced

 Directions

Melt the lard in a saucepan over medium-high heat. Cook the ribs for about 5 minutes or until the meat reaches an internal temperature of 160 degrees F. Add in the other ingredients and cook for 2 minutes more. Place under the preheated broiler until it is crispy in top.Bon appétit!

734.   Mini Meatloaves with Cheese and Pancetta

(Ready in about 30 minutes | Servings 6) Per serving: 276 Calories; 18.3g Fat; 1.2g Carbs; 29.2g Protein; 0.1g Fiber

Ingredients

2 ounces pancetta, chopped 4 ounces Teleme cheese, cubed 1/2 pound ground beef 1/2 ground pork 1 egg, beaten 1 teaspoon Dijon mustard 2 tablespoons scallions, chopped 2 garlic cloves, smashed Sea salt and pepper, to taste 1 teaspoon Italian herb mix

Directions

Begin by preheating your oven to 360 degrees F. In a mixing bowl, thoroughly combine the scallions, garlic, ground meat, pancetta, egg and mustard. Season with salt, black pepper, and Italian herb mix. Mix until well combined. Spoon the mixture into muffin cups. Insert one cube of cheese into each cup; seal the top to cover the cheese. Bake in the preheated oven for 18 to 20 minutes or until the internal temperature reaches 165 degrees F.Bon appétit!

735. Pillowy-Soft Chocolate Donuts

(Ready in about 25 minutes | Servings 6) Per serving: 218 Calories; 20g Fat; 6g Carbs; 4.8g Protein; 0.3g Fiber

Ingredients

1/4 cup coconut oil, room temperature 1/2 cup soft cheese 1/2 teaspoon cinnamon, ground 1/4 teaspoon grated nutmeg 1/3 cup coconut flour 1/3cup almond flour 1/4 cup Swerve 1 ½ teaspoons baking powder A pinch of coarse sea salt 1 egg 1 teaspoon vanilla extract For the Frosting: 1 cup whipping cream 1 cup bakers' chocolate chunks, unsweetened

Directions

Thoroughly combine the coconut flour, almond flour, Swerve, baking powder, cinnamon, nutmeg, and salt. In a separate bowl, thoroughly combine the coconut oil with cheese, egg, and vanilla. Beat until everything is well mixed. Add the cheese mixture to the dry flour mixture. Scrape the batter evenly into a lightly buttered donut pan. Bake in the preheated oven at 365 degrees F approximately 20 minutes. Meanwhile, warm the cream in a saucepan; then, fold in the chocolate chunks and whisk to combine well. Frost the prepared donuts.

736. Bacon and Turkey Roulade

(Ready in about 50 minutes | Servings 6) Per serving: 275 Calories; 9.5g Fat; 1.3g Carbs; 44.5g Protein; 0.5g Fiber

Ingredients

6 slices bacon 6 (4-ounce) turkey fillets 2 tablespoons fresh cilantro, roughly chopped 2 garlic cloves, chopped Salt and pepper, to taste 1/2 teaspoon chili pepper, chopped 1 tablespoon olive oil 3 tablespoons Dijon mustard

Directions

Rub the olive oil and Dijon mustard all over the turkey fillets. Place the fresh cilantro, garlic, chili pepper, salt, and pepper on each turkey fillet. Roll the fillets in the bacon and secure with a toothpick. Bake in the preheated oven at 395 degrees F for about 40 minutes.Bon appétit!

737. Vegetable Greek Mousaka

Ready in about: 50 minutes | Serves: 6 Per serving: Kcal 476, Fat 35g, Net Carbs 9.6g, Protein 33g

Ingredients

2 large eggplants, sliced 1 cup diced celery 1 cup diced carrots 1 small white onion, chopped 2 eggs 2 tbsp olive oil 3 cups Parmesan cheese, grated 1 cup ricotta cheese, crumbled 3 cloves garlic, minced 2 tsp Italian seasoning blend Salt to taste Sauce 1 ½ cups heavy cream ¼ cup butter, melted 1 cup mozzarella cheese, grated 2 tsp Italian seasoning ¾ cup almond flour Preheat the oven to 350°F.

Directions

Heat olive oil in a skillet over medium heat and sauté the onion, celery, and carrots for 5 minutes. Stir in the garlic and cook further for 30 seconds; set aside to cool. Mix the eggs, 1 cup of Parmesan cheese, ricotta cheese, and salt in a bowl. Pour the heavy cream into a pot and bring to heat over a medium fire while continually stirring. Stir in the remaining Parmesan cheese and 1 teaspoon of Italian seasoning. Turn the heat off and set aside. To lay the mousaka, spread a small amount of the sauce at the bottom of the baking dish. Make a single layer of eggplant slices on the sauce. Spread a layer of ricotta cheese on the eggplants, sprinkle some veggies over, and repeat the layering process until all the ingredients are exhausted. Evenly mix the melted butter, almond flour, and 1 teaspoon of Italian seasoning in a small bowl. Spread the top of the mousaka layers with it and sprinkle the top with mozzarella cheese. Cover the dish with foil and place it in the oven to bake for 25 minutes. Remove the foil and bake for 5 minutes until the cheese is slightly burned. Slice the mousaka and serve warm.

738.   Tofu Sesame Skewers with Warm Kale Salad

Ready in about: 30 minutes + marinating time | Serves: 4 Per serving: Kcal 263, Fat 12.9g, Net Carbs 6.1g, Protein 5.6g

Ingredients

14 oz firm tofu, cut into strips 4 tsp sesame oil 1 lemon, juiced 5 tbsp sugar-free soy sauce 4 tbsp coconut flour ½ cup sesame seeds Kale salad 4 cups kale, chopped 2 tbsp olive oil 1 white onion, thinly sliced 2 cloves garlic, minced 1 cup sliced white mushrooms 1 tsp fresh rosemary, chopped Salt and black pepper to taste 1 tbsp balsamic vinegar

DirectionsIn a bowl, mix sesame oil, lemon juice, soy sauce, and coconut flour. Stick the tofu on skewers, height-wise. Place onto a plate, pour the soy sauce mixture over, and turn in the sauce to coat. Cover the dish with cling film and marinate in the fridge for 2 hours. Heat a griddle pan over high heat. Roll the tofu skewers in the sesame seeds for a generous coat. Grill the tofu in the griddle pan until golden brown on both sides, about 12 minutes in total. Heat the olive oil in a skillet over medium heat and sauté onion to begin browning for 5 minutes with continuous stirring. Add in the mushrooms, garlic, rosemary, salt, pepper, and balsamic vinegar. Continue cooking for 5 minutes. Put the kale in a salad bowl. Pour the onion mixture over and toss well. Serve the tofu skewers with the warm kale salad and a peanut butter dipping sauce.

739.   Avocado & Tomato Burritos

Ready in about: 10 minutes | Serves: 4 Per serving: Kcal 303, Fat 25g, Net Carbs 6g, Protein 8g

Ingredients

2 cups cauli rice 6 low carb tortillas 2 cups sour cream sauce 1 ½ cups tomato herb salsa 2 avocados, peeled, pitted, sliced

DirectionsPour the cauli rice into a bowl, sprinkle with a bit of water, and soften in the microwave for 2 minutes. On the tortillas, spread the sour cream all over and distribute the salsa on top. Top with cauli rice and scatter the avocado evenly on top. Fold and tuck the burritos and cut them into two. Serve.

740.   Creamy Cucumber Avocado Soup

Ready in about: 15 minutes | Serves: 4 Per serving: Kcal 170, Fat 7.4g, Net Carbs 4.1g, Protein 3.7g

Ingredients

4 large cucumbers, seeded, chopped 1 large avocado, peeled and halved Salt and black pepper to taste 1 tbsp fresh cilantro, chopped 3 tbsp olive oil 2 limes, juiced 2 tsp minced garlic 2 tomatoes, chopped 1 avocado, chopped for garnish

DirectionsPour the cucumbers, avocado halves, salt, black pepper, olive oil, lime juice, cilantro, 2 cups water, and garlic in the food processor. Puree the ingredients for 2 minutes or until smooth. Pour the mixture into a bowl and top with chopped avocado and tomatoes. Serve chilled with zero-carb bread.

741.   Briam with Tomato Sauce

Ready in about: 40 minutes | Serves: 4 Per serving: Kcal 365, Fat 12g, Net Carbs 12.5g, Protein 11.3g

Ingredients

3 tbsp olive oil 1 large eggplant, halved and sliced 1 large onion, thinly sliced 3 cloves garlic, sliced 2 tomatoes, diced 1 rutabaga, diced 1 cup sugar-free tomato sauce 4 zucchinis, sliced ¼ cup water Salt and black pepper to taste ¼ tsp dried oregano 2 tbsp fresh parsley, chopped Preheat oven to 400°F.

Directions

Heat the olive oil in a skillet over medium heat and fry the eggplant and zucchini slices for 6 minutes until golden. Remove to a baking casserole and arrange them in a single layer. Sauté onion and garlic in the oil for 3 minutes. Remove to a bowl. Add in the tomatoes, rutabaga, tomato sauce, and water and mix well. Stir with salt, pepper, oregano, and parsley. Pour the mixture over the eggplant and zucchini. Place the dish in the oven and bake for 25-30 minutes. Serve the briam warm.

742. Vegetable Tempeh Kabobs

Ready in about: 30 minutes + chilling time | Serves: 4 Per serving: Kcal 228, Fat 15g, Net Carbs 3.6g, Protein 13.2g

Ingredients

1 yellow bell pepper, cut into chunks 10 oz tempeh, cut into chunks 1 red onion, cut into chunks 1 red bell pepper, cut chunks 2 tbsp olive oil 1 cup sugar-free barbecue sauce

Directions

Bring the 1 ½ cups water to boil in a pot over medium heat, and once it has cooked, turn the heat off, and add the tempeh. Cover the pot and let the tempeh steam for 5 minutes to remove its bitterness. Drain. Pour the barbecue sauce In a bowl, add in the tempeh, and coat with the sauce. Refrigerate for 2 hours. Preheat grill to 350°F. Thread the tempeh, yellow bell pepper, red bell pepper, and onion onto skewers. Brush the grate of the grill with olive oil, place the skewers on it, and brush with barbecue sauce. Cook the kabobs for 3 minutes on each side while rotating and brushing with more barbecue sauce. Serve.

743. Pumpkin Bake

Ready in about: 45 minutes | Serves: 6 Per serving: Kcal 125, Fat 4.8g, Net Carbs 5.7g, Protein 2.7g

Ingredients

3 large pumpkins, peeled and sliced 1 cup almond flour 1 cup grated mozzarella cheese 3 tbsp olive oil ½ cup fresh parsley, chopped Preheat oven to 350°F.

DirectionsArrange the pumpkin slices in a baking dish and drizzle with olive oil. Bake for 35 minutes. Mix almond flour, mozzarella cheese, and parsley and pour over the pumpkin. Place back in the oven and bake for another 5 minutes until the top is golden brown. Serve warm.

744. Jalapeño & Veggie Stew

Ready in about: 40 minutes | Serves: 4 Per serving: Kcal 65; Fat: 2.7g, Net Carbs: 9g, Protein: 2.7g

Ingredients

2 tbsp butter 1 cup leeks, chopped 1 garlic clove, minced ½ cup celery stalks, chopped ½ cup carrots, chopped 1 green bell pepper, chopped 1 jalapeño pepper, chopped 1 zucchini, chopped 1 cup mushrooms, sliced 1 ½ cups vegetable stock 2 tomatoes, chopped 2 tbsp fresh parsley, chopped 2 bay leaves Salt and black pepper to taste 1 tsp vinegar

DirectionsMelt the butter in a pot over medium heat. Add in garlic and leeks and sauté for 3 minutes until soft and translucent. Add in the celery, mushrooms, zucchini, and carrots and sauté for 5 more minutes. Stir in the rest of the ingredients. Season with salt and pepper. Bring to a boil and allow to simmer for 15-20 minutes or until cooked through. Divide between individual bowls and serve warm.

745. Baked Tomatoes with Pepita Seed Topping

Ready in about: 15 minutes | Serves: 6 Per serving: Kcal 161; Fat: 14g, Net Carbs: 7.2g, Protein: 4.6g

Ingredients

5 tomatoes, sliced ¼ cup olive oil 1 tbsp chili seasoning mix ½ cup pepitas seeds 1 tbsp nutritional yeast Salt and black pepper to taste ½ tsp nutmeg ½ tsp ginger powder 1 tsp garlic puree Preheat oven to 400°F.

Directions

Over the sliced tomatoes, drizzle olive oil. In a food processor, add pepita seeds, nutritional yeast, garlic puree, nutmeg, ginger powder, salt, and pepper and pulse until the desired consistency is attained. Transfer to a bowl and stir in the chili seasoning mix. Arrange the tomato slices on a baking pan and top them with the pepita seed mixture. Bake for 10 minutes. Remove and serve.

746.   Sautéed Celeriac with Tomato Sauce

Ready in about: 20 minutes | Serves: 4 Per serving: Kcal 135; Fat: 13.6g, Net Carbs: 3g, Protein: 0.9g

Ingredients

2 tbsp olive oil 1 garlic clove, crushed 1 celeriac, sliced ¼ cup vegetable stock Salt and black pepper to taste For the sauce 2 tomatoes, halved 2 tbsp olive oil ½ cup onions, chopped 2 cloves garlic, minced 1 chili, minced 1 bunch fresh basil, chopped 1 tbsp fresh cilantro, chopped Salt and black pepper to taste

Directions

Set a pan over medium heat and warm olive oil. Add in garlic and sauté for 1 minute. Stir in celeriac slices, stock and cook until softened. Sprinkle with pepper and salt. Brush the tomatoes with olive oil. Microwave for 5 minutes. Get rid of any excess liquid. Remove the tomatoes to a food processor. Add the rest of the ingredients for the sauce and puree to obtain the desired consistency. Serve the celeriac topped with tomato sauce.

747.   Pizza Bianca

Ready in about: 20 minutes | Serves: 1 Per serving: Kcal 591, Fat: 55g, Net Carbs: 2g, Protein: 22g 2

Ingredients

large eggs 1 tbsp water ½ jalapeño pepper, diced 1 oz Monterey Jack cheese, grated 1 chopped green onion 1 cup egg Alfredo sauce ¼ tsp cumin 2 tbsp olive oil Preheat the oven to 350°F.

DirectionsHeat the olive oil in a skillet over medium heat. Whisk the eggs along with water and cumin. Pour the eggs into the skillet. Cook until set. Top with the alfredo sauce and jalapeño pepper. Sprinkle the green onion and cheese over. Place in the oven and bake for 5 minutes. Serve.

748.   Parmesan Roasted Cabbage

Ready in about: 25 minutes | Serves: 4 Per serving: Kcal 268, Fat 19.3g, Net Carbs 4g, Protein 17.5g

Ingredients

1 large head green cabbage 4 tbsp melted butter 1 tsp garlic powder Salt and black pepper to taste 1 cup grated Parmesan cheese 1 tbsp fresh parsley, chopped Preheat oven to 400°F.

DirectionsLine a baking sheet with foil and grease with cooking spray. Stand the cabbage and run a knife from the top to bottom to cut the cabbage into wedges. Remove stems and wilted leaves. Place on the baking sheet. Mix the butter, garlic, salt, and black pepper until evenly combined. Brush the mixture on all sides of the cabbage wedges and sprinkle with some Parmesan cheese. Bake for 20 minutes to soften the cabbage and melt the cheese. Remove the cabbages when golden brown, plate, and sprinkle with remaining Parmesan cheese and parsley. Serve warm with pan-glazed tofu.

749.   Colorful Vegan Soup

Ready in about: 25 minutes | Serves: 6 Per serving: Kcal 142; Fat: 11.4g, Net Carbs: 9g, Protein: 2.9g

Ingredients

2 tsp olive oil 1 red onion, chopped 2 cloves garlic, minced 1 celery stalk, chopped 1 head broccoli, chopped 1 carrot, sliced 1 cup spinach, torn into pieces 1 cup collard greens, chopped Salt and black pepper to taste 2 thyme sprigs, chopped 1 rosemary sprig, chopped 2 bay leaves 6 cups vegetable stock 2 tomatoes, chopped 1 cup almond milk 1 tbsp white miso paste ½ cup arugula

Directions

Place a large pot over medium heat and warm oil. Add in carrot, celery, onion, broccoli, garlic, and sauté until soft, about 5 minutes. Place in spinach, salt, rosemary, tomatoes, bay leaves, black pepper, collard greens, thyme, and vegetable stock. Bring to a boil and simmer the mixture for 15 minutes while the lid is slightly open. Stir in white miso paste, arugula, and almond milk and cook for 5 more minutes.

750.   Cauliflower & Mushroom Stuffed Peppers

Ready in about: 40 minutes | Serves: 4 Per serving: Kcal: 77; Fat 4.8g, Net Carbs 8.4g, Protein 1.6g,

Ingredients

1 head cauliflower 4 bell peppers, cored and seeded 1 cup mushrooms, sliced 2 tbsp oil 1 onion, chopped 1 cup celery, chopped 1 garlic clove, minced 1 tsp chili powder 2 tomatoes, pureed Preheat oven to 360°F.

Directions

To prepare cauliflower rice, grate the cauliflower into rice-size. Set in a kitchen towel to attract and remove any excess moisture. Line a baking pan with a parchment paper. Warm the oil over medium heat. Add in garlic, celery, and onion and sauté until soft and translucent, about 3 minutes. Stir in chili powder, mushrooms, and cauliflower rice. Cook for 6 minutes until tender. Split the cauliflower mixture among the bell peppers. Place in the baking dish. Top with tomatoes. Bake for 20-25 minutes. Plate and serve warm.

751.Cheesy Cauliflower Falafel

Ready in about: 15 minutes | Serves: 4 Per serving: Kcal 315, Fat 26g, Net Carbs 2g, Protein 8g

Ingredients

1 head cauliflower, cut into florets ⅓ cup silvered ground almonds 2 tbsp cheddar cheese, shredded ½ tsp mixed spices Salt and chili pepper to taste 3 tbsp coconut flour 3 fresh eggs 4 tbsp ghee

Directions

Blend the cauli florets in a food processor until a grain meal consistency is formed. Pour the rice In a bowl, add the ground almonds, mixed spices, salt, cheddar, chili pepper, and coconut flour and mix well. Beat the eggs in a bowl until creamy in color and mix with the cauli mixture. Shape ¼ cup each into patties. Melt the ghee in a pan over medium heat and fry the patties for 5 minutes on each side until firm and browned. Remove onto a wire rack to cool, share into serving plates, and top with tahini sauce.

752.   Tomato Stuffed Avocado

Ready in about: 10 minutes | Serves: 4 Per serving: Kcal 263; Fat: 24.8g, Net Carbs: 5.5g, Protein: 3.5g

Ingredients

2 avocados 1 tomato, chopped ¼ cup walnuts, ground 2 carrots, chopped 1 garlic clove 1 tsp lemon juice 1 tbsp soy sauce Salt and black pepper to taste

DirectionsHalve and pit the avocados. Spoon out some of the pulp of each avocado. In a bowl, mix soy sauce, carrots, avocado pulp, tomato, lemon juice, and garlic. Add black pepper and salt. Fill the avocado halves with the mixture and scatter walnuts over to serve.

753.   Chili Stuffed Zucchini

Ready in about: 50 minutes | Serves: 4 Per serving: Kcal 148; Fat: 10g, Net Carbs: 9.8g, Protein: 7.5g

Ingredients

2 zucchinis, cut into halves, scoop out the insides 2 tbsp olive oil 12 oz firm tofu, crumbled 2 garlic cloves, pressed ½ cup onions, chopped 2 cups tomato sauce ¼ tsp turmeric Sea salt and chili pepper to taste 1 tbsp nutritional yeast ¼ cup almonds, chopped Set pan over medium heat and Warm the olive oil. Add in onion, garlic, and tofu and cook for 5 minutes. Place in scooped zucchini flesh, turmeric, and 1 cup of tomato sauce and cook for 6 more minutes. Preheat oven to 360°F.

Directions

Divide the tofu mixture among the zucchini shells. Arrange the stuffed zucchini shells in a greased baking dish. Pour in the remaining 1 cup of tomato sauce. Bake for about 30 minutes. Sprinkle with almonds and nutritional yeast and continue baking for 5 to 6 more minutes. Serve.

754.   Keto Flat Bread with Kulen

(Ready in about 30 minutes | Servings 6) Per serving: 464 Calories; 33.6g Fat; 5.1g Carbs; 31.1g Protein; 1.2g Fiber

Ingredients

10 ounces soft cheese, melted 3 tablespoons butter 1/2 cup tomato paste 12 large slices of kulen 4 large eggs, beaten 1/2 cup pork rinds, crushed 2 teaspoons baking powder 1/4 teaspoon sea salt 2 ½ cups Romano cheese, shredded

Directions

Thoroughly combine the cheese, eggs, butter, pork rinds, baking powder, and salt. Preheat a frying pan over a moderately-high flame. Cook your flatbread for about 5 minutes.Bon appétit!

755.   Basic Crustless Pizza

(Ready in about 15 minutes | Servings 4) Per serving: 266 Calories; 23.6g Fat; 6.6g Carbs; 9g Protein; 1g Fiber

Ingredients

2 bell peppers, chopped 1 cup tomatoes, chopped 1 teaspoon garlic, minced Salt and pepper, to season 2 tablespoons butter, melted 1/2 cup Colby cheese, shredded 1 3/4 cups soft cheese 2 tablespoons sour cream

Directions

In a large pan, melt the butter over medium heat. Spread the cheese on the bottom and cook for 4 to 5 minutes until it is crispy on top. Add the sour cream, garlic, bell peppers and tomatoes. Season with salt and pepper, and continue to cook for 2 to 3 minutes more.

756.   Autumn Pumpkin Pudding

(Ready in about 15 minutes + chilling time | Servings 6) Per serving: 368 Calories; 33.7g Fat; 5.6g Carbs; 13.8g Protein; 1.7g Fiber

Ingredients

1 cup double cream 1/2 teaspoon ground ginger 1/4 teaspoon ground cloves 1/2 teaspoon ground cinnamon 1/8 teaspoon grated nutmeg 1/8 teaspoon kosher salt 1 cup cream cheese 3 eggs 1 ¼ cups pumpkin puree 1/2 cup Swerve

Directions

Melt the cream, cheese, and Swerve in a sauté pan, whisking frequently. Whisk the eggs in a mixing bowl. Add in the eggs, whisking constantly and continue to cook for about 3 minutes, or until the mixture has reduced slightly. Remove from the heat and fold in the pumpkin puree and spices. Spoon the mixture into serving bowls and place in your refrigerator.Enjoy!

757.   Puffy Pancetta and Cheese Muffins

(Ready in about 25 minutes | Servings 5) Per serving: 240 Calories; 15.3g Fat; 7g Carbs; 16.1g Protein; 0.2g Fiber

Ingredients

4 slices pancetta 1/2 cup almond flour 1 teaspoon baking powder 1 cup goat cheese, diced Sea salt and black pepper, to taste 4 eggs, beaten

Directions Preheat a nonstick skillet over a moderately-high heat. Cook the pancetta for about 4 minutes until it is browned; place the pancetta on paper towels. Chop the pancetta and add in the remaining ingredients; stir to combine. Now, spoon the batter into paper-lined muffin cups (3/4 full). Bake in the preheated oven at 395 degrees F for 15 to 17 minutes.Bon appétit!

758.   Cauliflower Mac & Cheese

Ready in about: 20 minutes | Serves: 4 Per serving: Kcal 160, Fat: 12g, Net Carbs: 2g, Protein: 8.6g

Ingredients

1 cauliflower head, riced 1 ½ cups mozzarella cheese, grated 2 tsp paprika ¾ tsp rosemary 1 tsp turmeric Salt and black pepper to taste

DirectionsMicrowave the cauliflower for 5 minutes. Place it in cheesecloth and squeeze the extra juices out. Place the cauli in a pot over medium heat. Add paprika, turmeric, salt, pepper, and rosemary. Stir in mozzarella cheese and cook until the cheese is melted, about 10 minutes. Serve topped with rosemary.

759.   Chard Swiss Dip

Ready in about: 25 minutes | Serves: 6 Per serving: Kcal 105; Fat: 7.3g, Net Carbs: 7.9g, Protein: 2.9g

Ingredients

2 lb Swiss chard 1 cup tofu, pressed, crumbled ½ cup almond milk 2 tsp nutritional yeast 2 garlic cloves, minced 2 tbsp olive oil Salt and black pepper to taste ½ tsp paprika ½ tsp fresh mint leaves, chopped

DirectionsPlace a large pot of salted water over medium heat. Bring to a boil and add in the chard. Cook for 5 minutes until wilted. Drain and let cool. Transfer to a blender and add in the remaining ingredients. Puree until you get a homogeneous mixture. Serve alongside baked vegetables.

760.   Parsnip Chips with Avocado Dip

Ready in about: 20 minutes | Serves: 6 Per serving: Kcal 269; Fat: 26.7g, Net Carbs: 9.4g, Protein: 2.3g

Ingredients

2 avocados, mashed 2 tsp lime juice Salt and black pepper to taste 2 garlic cloves, minced 3 tbsp olive oil 3 cups parsnips, thinly sliced Preheat oven to 370ºF.

Directions

Set parsnip slices on a baking sheet. Season with salt and pepper and drizzle with some olive oil. Bake for 15 minutes until slices become dry. In a bowl, stir avocado with lime juice, remaining olive oil, garlic, salt, and pepper until combined. Serve the chips with the chilled avocado dip.

761. Morning Granola

Ready in about: 1 hour | Serves: 6 Per serving: Kcal 262; Fat: 24.3g, Net Carbs: 9.2g, Protein: 5.1g

Ingredients

1 tbsp coconut oil ⅓ cup almond flakes ½ cup almond milk ½ tbsp liquid stevia 1/8 tsp salt 1 tsp lime zest ½ tsp ground cinnamon ½ cup pecans, chopped ½ cup almonds, slivered 2 tbsp pepitas 3 tbsp sunflower seeds ¼ cup flax seeds Preheat the oven to 300°F.

Directions

Set a deep pan over medium heat and warm the coconut oil. Add almond flakes and toast for about 2 minutes. Stir in the remaining ingredients. Lay the mixture in an even layer onto a baking sheet lined with a parchment paper. Bake for 1 hour, making sure that you shake gently in intervals of 15 minutes. Serve alongside additional almond milk.

762. Morning Coconut Smoothie

Ready in about: 5 minutes | Serves: 4 Per serving: Kcal 247; Fat: 21.7g, Net Carbs: 6.9g, Protein: 2.6g

Ingredients

½ cup water 1 ½ cups coconut milk 1 cup frozen strawberries 2 cups fresh blueberries ¼ tsp vanilla extract 1 tbsp protein powder

Directions In a blender, Combine all the ingredients and pulse until you attain a uniform and creamy consistency. Divide between glasses and serve chilled.

763. Carrot Noodles with Cashew Sauce

Ready in about: 15 minutes | Serves: 4 Per serving: Kcal 145; Fat: 10.6g, Net Carbs: 7,9g, Protein: 5.5g

Ingredients

4 carrots, cut into long strips 2 tbsp olive oil Salt and black pepper to taste Cashew sauce ½ cup raw cashews 3 tbsp nutritional yeast Salt and black pepper to taste ¼ tsp onion powder ½ tsp garlic powder ¼ cup olive oil

DirectionsSet a pan over medium heat and warm the olive oil. Cook the carrots for 1 minute as you stir. Add in ½ cup water and cook for an additional 6 minutes. Sprinkle with salt and pepper. Place all the sauce ingredients in a food processor and pulse until you attain the required "cheese" consistency. Serve cooked noodles with a topping of cashew sauce.

764. Tofu Stir Fry with Asparagus

Ready in about: 30 minutes | Serves: 4 Per serving: Kcal 138; Fat: 8.9g, Net Carbs: 5.9g, Protein: 6.4g

Ingredients

1 lb asparagus, cut off stems 2 tbsp olive oil 2 blocks tofu, pressed and cubed 2 garlic cloves, minced 1 tsp cajun spice mix 1 tsp Dijon mustard 1 bell pepper, chopped ¼ cup vegetable broth Salt and black pepper to taste

Directions

In a large saucepan, warm the olive oil. Place in the asparagus and cook until tender for 10 minutes; set aside. Add the tofu cubes in the saucepan and cook for 6 minutes, stirring often. Place in garlic and cook for 30 seconds until soft. Stir in the rest of the ingredients, including reserved asparagus, and cook for an additional 4 minutes. Divide among plates and serve.

765. Artichoke & Cauliflower Bake

Ready in about: 30 minutes | Serves: 4 Per serving: Kcal 113; Fat: 6.7g, Net Carbs: 11.6g, Protein: 5g

Ingredients

1 head cauliflower, cut into florets 8 oz artichoke hearts, halved 2 garlic cloves, smashed 2 tomatoes, pureed ¼ cup coconut oil, melted 1 tsp chili paprika paste ¼ tsp marjoram ½ tsp curry powder Salt and black pepper to taste Preheat oven to 390°F.

DirectionsApply a cooking spray to a baking dish. Lay artichokes and cauliflower on the baking dish. Around the vegetables, scatter smashed garlic. Place in the pureed tomatoes. Sprinkle over melted coconut oil and stir in chili paprika paste, curry, black pepper, salt, and marjoram. Roast for 25 minutes, shaking often. Place on a serving plate and serve with green salad.

766. Coconut Cauliflower & Parsnip Soup

Ready in about: 25 minutes | Serves: 4 Per serving: Kcal 94; Fat: 7.2g, Net Carbs: 7g, Protein: 2.7g

Ingredients

4 cups vegetable broth 2 heads cauliflower, cut into florets 1 cup parsnips, chopped 1 onion, finely chopped 2 garlic cloves, finely chopped 2 tbsp coconut oil 2 tbsp lime juice 1 cup coconut milk ½ tsp red pepper flakes

DirectionsWarm the coconut oil in a pot over medium heat. Sauté the onion, parsnips, and garlic for 3 minutes. Add in the vegetable broth and cauliflower and bring to a boil. Cook for about 15 minutes. Puree the mixture with an immersion blender. After, stir in the coconut milk and red pepper flakes. Serve warm.

767. Fall Baked Vegetables

Ready in about: 45 minutes | Serves: 4 Per serving: Kcal 165; Fat: 14.3g, Net Carbs: 8.2g, Protein: 2.1g

Ingredients

3 mixed bell peppers, sliced ½ head broccoli, cut into florets 2 zucchinis, sliced 2 leeks, chopped 4 garlic cloves, halved 2 thyme sprigs, chopped 1 tsp dried sage, crushed 2 tbsp olive oil 2 tbsp vinegar Salt and black pepper to taste Salt to taste 1 tsp cayenne pepper Preheat oven to 425°F.

DirectionsApply nonstick cooking spray to a rimmed baking sheet. Mix in all the vegetables with olive oil, seasonings, and vinegar. Roast for 40 minutes, stirring every 10 minutes. Serve immediately.

768. Walnut-Crusted Tofu

Ready in about: 35 minutes | Serves: 4 Per serving: Kcal 232; Fat: 21.6g, Net Carbs: 5.3g, Protein: 8.3g

Ingredients

3 tsp olive oil 1 block extra-firm tofu, sliced 1 cup walnuts 2 tbsp tamari sauce 3 tbsp vegetable broth ½ tsp smashed garlic Salt and black pepper to taste 2 tsp sunflower seeds Preheat oven to 425°F.

Directions

Brush the tofu with tamari sauce. In a food processor, mix walnuts, vegetable broth, olive oil, garlic, sunflower seeds, salt, and pepper and blend until uniform. Coat the tofu with the walnut mixture and arrange on a lined baking dish. Bake for 25-30 minutes, flipping once until golden.

769.   Bell Pepper & Pumpkin with Avocado Sauce

Ready in about: 15 minutes | Serves: 4 Per serving: Kcal 233; Fat: 20.2g, Net Carbs: 11g, Protein: 1.9g

Ingredients

1 lb pumpkin, peeled ½ lb bell peppers 1 avocado, peeled and pitted 1 lemon, juiced and zested 2 tbsp sesame oil 2 tbsp fresh cilantro, chopped 1 onion, chopped 1 jalapeño pepper, minced 2 tbsp olive oil

Directions

Use a spiralizer to spiralize bell peppers and pumpkin. Warm the olive oil in a large skillet. Add in bell peppers and pumpkin and sauté for 8 minutes. In a blender, combine the remaining ingredients and pulse until you obtain a creamy mixture. Top the vegetable noodles with the avocado sauce and serve.

770.   Bell Pepper Stuffed Avocado

Ready in about: 10 minutes | Serves: 4 Per serving: Kcal 255; Fat: 23.2g, Net Carbs: 7.4g, Protein: 2.4g

Ingredients

2 avocados, pitted and halved 2 tbsp olive oil 3 cups green bell peppers, chopped 1 onion, chopped 1 tsp garlic puree Salt and black pepper to taste 1 tsp deli mustard 1 tomato, chopped

Directions

From each half of the avocados, scoop out 2 teaspoons of flesh; set aside. Warm the olive oil in a pan over medium heat. Cook the garlic, onion, and bell peppers until tender, about 5 minutes. Mix in the reserved avocado. Add in the tomato, salt, mustard, and black pepper. Separate the mixture and mix equally among the avocado halves. Serve.

771. Caprese Stuffed Tomatoes

Ready in about: 35 minutes | Serves: 4 Per serving: Kcal 306; Fat: 27.5g, Net Carbs: 4.4g, Protein: 11.3g

Ingredients

4 tomatoes 4 slices fresh mozzarella cheese ¼ cup sour cream 1 egg, whisked 1 clove garlic, minced 4 tbsp fresh scallions, chopped Salt and black pepper to taste 2 tbsp butter, softened Preheat oven to 360°F.

Directions

Lightly grease a rimmed baking sheet with cooking spray. Horizontally slice tomatoes into halves and get rid of the hard cores. Scoop out pulp and seeds. In a bowl, mix egg, salt, butter, black pepper, garlic, sour cream, and scallions. Split the filling between tomatoes, cover each one with a mozzarella slice and bake in the preheated oven for 30 minutes. Place on a wire rack and allow to cool for 5 minutes. Serve alongside fresh rocket leaves.

772. Homemade Pizza Crust

Ready in about: 8 minutes | Serves: 8 Per serving: Kcal: 234; Fat 16.7g, Net Carbs 7.9g, Protein 12.4g

Ingredients

3 cups almond flour 3 tbsp butter, then melted ⅓ tsp salt 3 large eggs Preheat oven to 350°F.

Directions

In a bowl, mix the almond flour, butter, salt, and eggs until a dough forms. Mold the dough into a ball and place it in between two wide parchment papers on a flat surface. Use a rolling pin to roll it out into a circle of a quarter-inch thickness. Slide the pizza dough into the pizza pan and remove the parchment papers. Bake the dough for 20 minutes.

773. Cheese Sticks with Mustard-Yogurt Dipping Sauce

Ready in about: 40 minutes | Serves: 6 Per serving: Kcal: 200; Fat 16.9g, Net Carbs 3.7g, Protein 9.4g

Ingredients

16 oz cheddar cheese with jalapeño peppers ¾ cup Grana Padano cheese, grated 2 tbsp almond flour 1 tbsp flax meal 1 tsp baking powder Salt to taste ¾ tsp red pepper flakes ⅓ tsp cumin powder ½ tsp dried oregano ⅓ tsp dried rosemary 2 eggs 2 tbsp olive oil Dipping sauce ¾ cup jarred fire-roasted red peppers, chopped 1 cup cream cheese ⅓ cup natural yogurt 1 tbsp mustard 1 chili pepper, deveined and minced 2 garlic cloves, chopped Salt and black pepper to taste

Directions

Chop cheddar cheese crosswise into sticks. In a bowl, mix the dry ingredients. In a separate bowl, whisk the eggs. Dip each cheese stick into the eggs and then roll in the dry mixture. Set cheese sticks on a wax paper-lined baking sheet. Freeze for 30 minutes. Mix all ingredients for the dipping sauce until smooth. In a skillet over medium heat, warm oil and fry cheese sticks for 5 minutes until the coating is golden brown and crisp. Set on paper towels to drain excess oil. Serve with the dipping sauce.

774. Broccoli Cheese Soup

Ready in about: 20 minutes | Serves: 4 Per serving: Kcal 296; Fat 14.1g, Net Carbs 7.4g, Protein 14.2g

Ingredients

2 tbsp butter ½ cup leeks, chopped 1 celery stalk, chopped 1 serrano pepper, finely chopped 1 tsp garlic puree ½ lb broccoli florets 3 cups chicken stock 1 cup coconut milk 1 tsp mustard powder 6 oz Monterey Jack cheese, grated Salt and black pepper to taste 2 tbsp fresh parsley, chopped

Directions

Set a pot over medium heat and melt butter. Add in serrano pepper, celery, and leeks and sauté for 5 minutes until soft. Stir in garlic puree and mustard powder for 1 minute. Pour in chicken stock and coconut milk. Bring to a Boil and reduce the heat. Allow simmering for 10 minutes. Add in the broccoli. Cook for another 5 minutes. Remove from the heat and fold in the cheese. Stir to ensure the cheese is melted, and you have a homogenous mixture. Adjust the seasoning, top with parsley, and serve warm.

775.   Chipotle Pizza with Cotija & Cilantro

Ready in about: 15 minutes | Serves: 2 Per serving: Kcal 397, Fat: 31g, Net Carbs: 8.1g, Protein: 22g

Ingredients

Pizza crust 4 eggs, beaten ¼ cup sour cream 2 tbsp flaxseed meal 1 tsp chipotle pepper ¼ tsp cumin ½ tsp dried ground coriander ¼ tsp salt 1 tbsp olive oil 2 tbsp tomato paste 2 oz Cotija cheese, shredded 1 tbsp fresh cilantro, chopped

Directions

Mix eggs, sour cream, flaxseed meal, chipotle pepper, cumin, coriander, and salt in a bowl. Set a pan over medium heat and warm ½ tablespoon oil. Ladle ½ of crust mixture into the pan and evenly spread out. Cook until the edges are set, flip, and cook on the second side. Repeat with the remaining crust mixture. Warm the remaining ½ tablespoon of oil in the pan. Spread each pizza crust with tomato paste, then scatter over the cotija cheese. In batches, bake in the oven for 8-10 minutes at 425°F until all the cheese melts. Garnish with cilantro and serve.

776.   Raspberry & Rum Omelet

Ready in about: 10 minutes | Serves: 1 Per serving: Kcal 488, Fat: 42g, Net Carbs: 8g, Protein: 15.3g

Ingredients

2 eggs 2 tbsp heavy cream ½ tsp ground cloves 1 tbsp coconut oil 2 tbsp mascarpone cheese 6 fresh raspberries, sliced ½ tsp powdered swerve sugar 1 tbsp rum

Directions

Beat the eggs with ground cloves and heavy cream. Set pan over medium heat and warm oil. Place in the egg mixture and cook for 3 minutes. Set the omelet onto a plate. Top with raspberries and mascarpone cheese. Roll it up and sprinkle with powdered swerve. Pour the warm rum over the omelet and ignite it. Let the flame die out and serve.

777.Cheesy Herb Omelet

Ready in about: 10 minutes | Serves: 2 Per serving: Kcal 431; Fat: 33.1g, Net Carbs: 2.7g, Protein: 30.3g

Ingredients

4 slices cooked bacon, crumbled 4 eggs, beaten 1 tsp basil, chopped 1 tsp parsley, chopped Salt and black pepper to taste ½ cup cheddar cheese, grated

Directions

In a frying pan, cook the bacon until sizzling, about 5 minutes. Add in eggs, parsley, black pepper, salt, and basil. Scatter the cheese over half of the omelet and, using a spatula, fold in half over the filling. Cook for 1 extra minute or until cooked through and serve immediately.

778.   Bacon Loaded Eggplants

Ready in about: 35 minutes | Serves: 4 Per serving: Kcal 245; Fat 12.8g, Net Carbs 9.5g, Protein 15.6g

Ingredients

2 eggplants, cut into halves 1 onion, chopped 4 bacon slices, chopped 4 eggs Salt and black pepper to taste ¼ tsp dried parsley Preheat oven at 380°F.

Directions

Scoop flesh from eggplant halves to make shells. Set the eggplant boats on a greased baking pan. Heat a skillet over medium heat and stir-fry the bacon for 5 minutes until crispy. Remove to a plate. Add the onion and eggplant flesh to the skillet and sauté for 5-7 minutes until tender. Season with salt, pepper, and parsley and stir in the bacon. Divide the mixture between the eggplant shells. Crack an egg in each half, sprinkle with salt and pepper, and bake for 30 minutes or until the boats become tender and the eggs are set. Serve with tomato salad.

779.   Vanilla-Coconut Cream Tart

Ready in about: 30 minutes + cooling time | Serves: 6 Per serving: Kcal 305, Fat: 30.6g, Net Carbs: 9.7g, Protein: 4.6g

Ingredients

½ cup butter ⅓ cup xylitol ¾ cup coconut flour ⅓ cup coconut shreds, unsweetened 2 ¼ cups heavy cream 3 egg yolks ⅓ cup almond flour ¾ cup water ½ tsp ground cinnamon ½ tsp star anise, ground ½ tsp vanilla extract 2 tbsp coconut flakes

Directions

Warm butter in a pan over medium heat. Stir in xylitol and cook until fully dissolved. Add in coconut shreds and coconut flour and cook for 2 minutes. Scrape the crust mixture into a baking dish. Refrigerate. In the same pan, warm 1 ¼ cups of heavy cream over medium heat. Fold in egg yolks and mix thoroughly. Mix in water and almond flour until thick. Place in cinnamon, vanilla, and anise star. Cook until thick. Let cool for 10 minutes; sprinkle over the crust. Place in the fridge for 2 hours. Beat the remaining heavy cream until stiff peaks start to form. Spread the cream all over the cake. Top with coconut flakes to serve.

780.   Egg & Cheese Stuffed Peppers

Ready in about: 35 minutes | Serves: 4 Per serving: Kcal 359; Fat: 29.7g, Net Carbs: 6.7g, Protein: 17.7g

Ingredients

4 bell peppers, tops sliced off and deseeded 6 oz cottage cheese, crumbled 6 oz blue cheese, crumbled ½ cup pork rinds, crushed 2 cloves garlic, smashed 1 ½ cups pureed tomatoes 1 tsp dried basil 1 tbsp olive oil ½ tsp chili pepper 2 eggs, beaten Preheat oven to 360°F.

Directions

 In a bowl, mix garlic, cottage cheese, pork rinds, blue cheese, eggs, tomatoes, chili pepper, and basil. Stuff the peppers and place them in a greased casserole dish. Pour in 1 cup of water. Drizzle with olive oil. Bake for 30 minutes until the peppers are tender. Serve with mixed salad.

781.   Carrot & Cheese Mousse

Ready in about: 15 minutes + cooling time | Serves: 6 Per serving: Kcal 368, Fat: 33.7g, Net Carbs: 5.6g, Protein: 13.8g

Ingredients

1 ½ cups half & half ½ cup cream cheese, softened ½ cup erythritol 3 eggs 1 ¼ cups canned carrots ½ tsp ground cloves ½ tsp ground cinnamon ¼ tsp grated nutmeg A pinch of salt

Directions

Heat a pan over medium heat, mix erythritol, cream cheese, and half & half and warm, stirring frequently. Remove from the heat. Beat the eggs; slowly place in ½ of the hot cream mixture to the beaten eggs. Pour the mixture back to the pan. Cook for 3 minutes, until thick. Kill the heat; add in carrots, cinnamon, salt, nutmeg, and cloves. Blend with a blender. Let cool before serving.

782.   Crabmeat & Cheese Stuffed Avocado

Ready in about: 25 minutes | Serves: 4 Per serving: Kcal 264, Fat: 24.4g, Net Carbs: 11g, Protein: 3.7g

Ingredients

1 tsp olive oil 1 cup crabmeat 2 avocados, halved and pitted 3 oz cream cheese ¼ cup almonds, chopped 1 tsp smoked paprika Preheat oven to 425°F.

Directions

In a bowl, mix crabmeat with cream cheese. Fill the avocado halves with crabmeat mixture and top with almonds. Bake for 18 minutes. Decorate with smoked paprika and serve.

783.   Cheese, Ham and Egg Muffins

Ready in about: 20 minutes | Serves: 6 Per serving: Kcal: 268; Fat 18.3g, Net Carbs 0.7g, Protein 26.2g

Ingredients

24 slices smoked ham 6 eggs, beaten Salt and black pepper to taste ¼ cup fresh parsley, chopped ¼ cup ricotta cheese ¼ cup Brie, chopped Preheat oven to 390°F.

DirectionsLine 2 slices of smoked ham into each greased muffin cup, to circle each mold. In a mixing bowl, mix the rest of the ingredients. Fill ¾ of the ham lined muffin cup with the egg/cheese mixture. Bake for 15 minutes. Serve warm!

784.   Prosciutto & Cheese Egg Cups

Ready in about: 30 minutes | Serves: 4 Per serving: Kcal 294, Fat: 21.4g, Net Carbs: 3.5g, Protein: 21g

Ingredients

4 slices prosciutto 4 eggs 2 green onions, chopped ½ cup cheddar cheese, shredded ¼ tsp garlic powder Salt and black pepper to taste Preheat oven to 390°F.

Directions

Line the prosciutto slices on greased ramekins. In a bowl, combine the remaining ingredients. Split the egg mixture among the cups. Bake for 20 minutes. Leave to cool before serving.

785. Chorizo Egg Balls

Ready in about: 10 minutes + cooling time | Serves: 6 Per serving: Kcal 174, Fat: 15.2g, Net Carbs: 4.3g, Protein: 5.9g

Ingredients

2 eggs ½ cup butter, softened 8 black olives, pitted and chopped 3 tbsp mayonnaise Salt to taste ½ tsp crushed red pepper flakes 1 lb cooked chorizo, chopped 2 tbsp chia seeds

Directions

In a food processor, place the eggs, olives, pepper flakes, mayo, butter, and salt and blitz until everything is incorporated. Stir in the chorizo. Refrigerate for 30 minutes. Form balls from the mixture. Roll the balls through the chia seeds to coat. Keep in the refrigerator until serving time.

786. Herbed Keto Bread

Ready in about: 40 minutes | Serves: 6 Per serving: Kcal 115, Fat: 10.2g, Net Carbs: 1g, Protein: 3.9g

Ingredients

5 eggs ½ tsp tartar cream 2 cups almond flour 3 tablespoons butter, melted 3 tsp baking powder 1 tsp salt ½ tsp dried oregano 1 tbsp sunflower seeds 2 tbsp sesame seeds Preheat oven to 360°F.

Directions

Combine the eggs with cream of tartar until the formation of stiff peaks happens. In a food processor, place in the baking powder, flour, salt, and butter and blitz to incorporate fully. Stir in the egg mixture. Scoop the batter into a greased loaf pan. Spread the loaf with sesame seeds, sunflower seeds, and oregano and bake for 35 minutes. Serve with butter.

787. Quatro Formaggio Pizza

Ready in about: 15 minutes | Serves: 4 Per serving: Kcal 266, Fat: 23.6g, Net Carbs: 6.6g, Protein: 9g

Ingredients

1 tbsp olive oil ½ cup cheddar cheese, shredded 1 ¼ cups mozzarella cheese, grated ½ cup mascarpone cheese ½ cup blue cheese 2 tbsp sour cream 2 garlic cloves, chopped 1 red bell pepper, sliced 1 green bell pepper, sliced 10 cherry tomatoes, halved 1 tsp oregano Salt and black pepper to taste

Directions

In a bowl, mix the cheeses. Set a pan over medium heat and warm olive oil. Spread the cheese mixture on the pan and cook for 5 minutes until cooked through. Scatter garlic and sour cream over the crust. Add in tomatoes and bell peppers; cook for 2 minutes. Sprinkle with pepper, salt, and oregano and serve.

788. Mini Egg Muffins

Ready in about: 40 minutes | Serves: 6 Per serving: Kcal 261; Fat: 16g, Net Carbs: 7.6g, Protein: 21.1g

Ingredients

2 tbsp olive oil 1 onion, chopped 1 bell pepper, chopped 6 slices bacon, chopped 6 eggs, whisked 1 cup gruyere cheese, shredded Salt and black pepper to taste ¼ tsp rosemary 1 tbsp fresh parsley, chopped Preheat oven to 390°F.

Directions

Place cupcake liners to your muffin pan. In a skillet over medium heat, warm the olive oil and sauté the onion and bell pepper for 4-5 minutes as you stir constantly until tender. Stir in bacon and cook for 3 more minutes. Add in the rest of the ingredients and mix well. Set the mixture to the lined muffin pan and bake for 23 minutes. Let muffins cool before serving.

789. Grilled Halloumi Cheese with Eggs

Ready in about: 20 minutes | Serves: 4 Per serving: Kcal 542; Fat: 46.4g, Net Carbs: 11.2g, Protein: 23.7g

Ingredients

4 slices halloumi cheese 2 tbsp olive oil 1 tsp dried Greek seasoning blend 6 eggs, beaten ½ tsp sea salt ¼ tsp crushed red pepper flakes 1 ½ cups avocado, pitted and sliced 1 cup grape tomatoes, halved 4 tbsp pecans, chopped

Directions

 Preheat your grill to medium. Set the halloumi in the center of a piece of heavy-duty foil. Sprinkle oil over the halloumi and apply Greek seasoning blend. Close the foil to create a packet. Grill for about 15 minutes. Then slice into four pieces. In a frying pan over medium heat, warm the olive oil and cook the eggs. Stir well to create large and soft curds. Season with salt and red pepper flakes. Put the eggs and grilled cheese on a serving bowl. Serve alongside tomatoes and avocado, decorated with chopped pecans.

790. Creamy Cheddar Deviled Eggs

Ready in about: 20 minutes | Serves: 4 Per serving: Kcal 177; Fat: 12.7g, Net Carbs: 4.6g, Protein: 11.4g

Ingredients

8 eggs ¼ cup mayonnaise 1 tbsp tomato paste 2 tbsp celery, chopped 2 tbsp carrot, chopped 2 tbsp chives, minced 2 tbsp cheddar cheese, grated Salt and black pepper to taste

Directions

Place the eggs in a pot and fill with water by about 1 inch. Bring the eggs to a boil over high heat, reduce the heat to medium; simmer for 10 minutes. Remove and rinse under running water until cooled. Peel and discard the shell. Slice each egg in half lengthwise and get rid of the yolks. Mix the yolks with the rest of the ingredients. Split the mixture amongst the egg whites and set deviled eggs on a plate to serve.

791.   Italian-Style Egg Muffins

(Ready in about 10 minutes | Servings 3) Per serving: 423 Calories; 34.1g Fat; 2.2g Carbs; 26.5g Protein; 0g Fiber

Ingredients

6 eggs 1 pound beef sausages, chopped 1 tablespoon olive oil 1 cup Romano cheese, freshly grated Sea salt and black pepper, to season 1/2 teaspoon cayenne pepper

Directions

Whisk the eggs until pale and frothy. Add in the remaining ingredients and stir to combine. Pour the mixture into a lightly greased muffin pan. Bake in the preheated oven at 400 degrees F for 5 to 6 minutes.Bon appétit!

792.   Classic Spicy Egg Salad

(Ready in about 15 minutes | Servings 8) Per serving: 174 Calories; 13g Fat; 5.7g Carbs; 7.4g Protein; 0.8g Fiber

Ingredients

10 eggs 1/2 cup onions, chopped 1/2 cup celery with leaves, chopped 2 cups butterhead lettuce, torn into pieces 3/4 cup mayonnaise 1 teaspoon hot sauce 1 tablespoon Dijon mustard 1/2 teaspoon fresh lemon juice Kosher salt and black pepper, to taste

Directions Place the eggs in a saucepan and cover them with water by 1 inch. Cover and bring the water to a boil over high heat. Boil for 6 to 7 minutes over medium-high heat. Peel the eggs and chop them coarsely. Add in the remaining ingredients and toss to combine.Bon appétit!

793.   Asiago, Pepperoni, and Pepper Casserole

(Ready in about 35 minutes | Servings 4) Per serving: 334 Calories; 23g Fat; 6.2g Carbs; 25.5g Protein; 4.9g Fiber

Ingredients

8 eggs Salt and pepper, to taste 1 cup Asiago cheese, grated 1/2 cup cream cheese 1 bell pepper, chopped 1 chili pepper, deveined and chopped 1 teaspoon yellow mustard 8 slices pepperoni, chopped

Directions In a mixing bowl, combine the eggs, salt, pepper, and cheese; spoon the mixture into a lightly greased baking dish. Add in the other ingredients. Bake in the preheated oven at 365 degrees F for about 30 minutes or until cooked through.Bon appétit!

794.   Festive Zucchini Boats

(Ready in about 35 minutes | Servings 3) Per serving: 506 Calories; 41g Fat; 4.5g Carbs; 27.5g Protein; 0.3g Fiber

Ingredients

3 medium-sized zucchinis, cut into halves and scoop out the pulp 6 eggs 1 tablespoon Dijon mustard 2 sausages, cooked and crumbled Salt and pepper, to taste 1/2 teaspoon dried basil

Directions

Place the zucchini boats on a lightly oiled baking sheet. Mix the Dijon mustard, sausages, salt, pepper, and basil. Spoon the sausage mixture into the zucchini shells. Crack an egg in each zucchini shell. Bake in the preheated oven at 390 degrees F for 30 to 35 minutes or until tender and cooked through.Enjoy!

795.   Nana's Pickled Eggs

(Ready in about 20 minutes | Servings 5) Per serving: 145 Calories; 9g Fat; 2.8g Carbs; 11.4g Protein; 0.9g Fiber

Ingredients

2 clove garlic, sliced 1 cup white vinegar 10 eggs 1 tablespoon yellow curry powder 1/2 cup onions, sliced 1 teaspoon fennel seeds 1 teaspoon mustard seeds 1 tablespoon sea salt 1 ¼ cups water

Directions

Place the eggs in a saucepan and cover them with water by 1 inch. Cover and bring the water to a boil over high heat. Boil for 6 to 7 minutes over medium-high heat. Peel the eggs and add them to a large-sized jar. Cook the other ingredients in a saucepan pan over moderately-high heat; bring to a boil. Immediately turn the heat to medium-low and continue to simmer for 5 to 6 minutes. Pour the mixture into the prepared jar.Bon appétit!

796.   Mushroom and Cheese Wraps

(Ready in about 20 minutes | Servings 4) Per serving: 172 Calories; 14g Fat; 3.4g Carbs; 9.5g Protein; 1g Fiber

Ingredients

For the Wraps:

2 tablespoons cream cheese 6 eggs, separated into yolks and whites 1 tablespoon butter, room temperature Sea salt, to taste

For the Filling:

1 cup Cremini mushrooms, chopped 4 slices of Swiss cheese Salt and pepper, to taste 6-8 fresh arugula 1 teaspoon olive oil 1 large vine-ripened tomatoes, chopped

Directions

Mix all ingredients for the wraps until well combined. Prepare four wraps in a frying pan and set them aside. Next, heat 1 teaspoon of olive oil over a moderate heat. Cook the mushrooms until they release the liquid; season with salt and pepper.

797.   Egg Drop Soup with Tofu

(Ready in about 15 minutes | Servings 3) Per serving: 153 Calories; 9.8g Fat; 2.7g Carbs; 15g Protein; 0.5g Fiber

Ingredients

2 eggs, beaten 1/2 teaspoon curry paste 1/2 pound extra-firm tofu, cubed 2 cups vegetable broth 1 tablespoon coconut aminos 1 teaspoon butter, softened 1/4 teaspoon cayenne pepper Salt and ground black ground, to taste

Directions

In a heavy-bottomed pot, cook the broth, coconut aminos and butter over high heat; bring to a boil. Immediately turn the heat to a simmer. Stir in the eggs and curry paste, whisking constantly, until well incorporated. Add in the salt, black pepper, cayenne pepper, and tofu. Partially cover and continue to simmer approximately 2 minutes.Enjoy!

798.   Cauliflower "Mac" and Cheese Casserole

(Ready in about 15 minutes | Servings 4) Per serving: 357 Calories; 32.5g Fat; 6.9g Carbs; 8.4g Protein; 1.3g Fiber

Ingredients

1 large-sized head cauliflower, broken into florets 1 cup Cottage cheese 1/2 cup milk 1/2 cup double cream 2 tablespoons olive oil 1 teaspoon garlic powder 1/2 teaspoon shallot powder 1 teaspoon dried parsley flakes Salt and pepper, to taste

Directions

Start by preheating your oven to 420 degrees F. In a lightly oiled baking dish, toss the cauliflower florets with the olive oil, salt, and pepper. Bake in the preheated oven for about 15 minutes. In a mixing dish, whisk the milk, cream, cheese, and spices. Pour the mixture over the cauliflower layer in the baking dish. Bake for another 10 minutes, until the top is hot and bubbly.Bon appétit!

799.   Baked Cheese-Stuffed Tomatoes

(Ready in about 45 minutes | Servings 5) Per serving: 306 Calories; 27.5g Fat; 4.4g Carbs; 11.3g Protein; 1.3g Fiber

Ingredients

2 teaspoons olive oil 1/4 cup Greek-style yogurt 1 egg, whisked 1 tablespoon fresh green garlic, minced 4 tablespoons fresh shallots, chopped 1 cup Ricotta cheese, at room temperature 1 ½ cups Swiss cheese, shredded 5 vine-ripened tomatoes, cut into halves and scoop out the pulp Salt and ground black pepper, to taste

Directions

Start by preheating your oven to 355 degrees F. Then, thoroughly combine the cheese, yogurt, egg, green garlic, shallots, salt, and pepper. Stuff the tomato halves with this filling. Brush the stuffed tomatoes with olive oil. Bake in the preheated oven for about 30 minutes.

800.   Spicy Cheese Omelet with Chervil

(Ready in about 15 minutes | Servings 2) Per serving: 490 Calories; 44.6g Fat; 4.5g Carbs; 22.7g Protein; 0.8g Fiber

Ingredients

4 eggs, beaten 1/2 cup Cheddar cheese, grated 2 tablespoons olive oil 1/2 teaspoon habanero pepper, minced 1/2 cup queso fresco cheese, crumbled 2 tablespoons fresh chervil, roughly chopped Salt and pepper, to taste

Directions

In a frying pan, heat the oil over a moderately high heat. Cook the eggs until the edges barely start setting. Add in the salt, pepper, habanero pepper, and cheese and cook an additional 4 minutes.Serve with fresh chervil. Bon appétit!

801. Scrambled Eggs with Crabmeat

(Ready in about 15 minutes | Servings 3) Per serving: 334 Calories; 26.2g Fat; 4.4g Carbs; 21.1g Protein; 0.4g Fiber

Ingredients

6 eggs, whisked 1 can crabmeat, flaked 1/2 teaspoon rosemary 1/2 teaspoon basil 1 tablespoon butter, room temperature For the Sauce: 1/2 teaspoon garlic, minced 3/4 cup cream cheese 1/2 cup onions, white and green parts, chopped 3 tablespoons mayonnaise Salt and black pepper, to taste

Directions

In a frying pan, melt the butter over a moderately high flame. Cook the eggs, gently stirring to create large soft curds. Cook until the eggs are barely set. Add in the crabmeat, rosemary and basil, and continue to cook, stirring frequently, until cooked through. Salt to taste. Make the sauce by whisking all ingredients.

802. Blue Cheese and Soppressata Balls

(Ready in about 15 minutes | Servings 8) Per serving: 168 Calories; 13g Fat; 2.5g Carbs; 10.3g Protein; 0.2g Fiber

Ingredients

6 slices Soppressata, chopped 6 ounces Parmigiano-Reggiano cheese, grated 1 teaspoon baking powder 1 teaspoon garlic, minced 1 egg, whisked 1/2 teaspoon dried basil 1/2 teaspoon dried oregano 6 ounces cream cheese Salt and pepper, to taste 1/4 cup almond meal

Directions

Thoroughly combine all ingredients until well combined. Roll the mixture into bite-sized balls and arrange them on a parchment-lined cookie sheet. Bake in the preheated oven at 400 degrees F approximately 15 minutes or until they are golden and crisp.

803. Alfredo Cheese Dip

(Ready in about 30 minutes | Servings 12) Per serving: 154 Calories; 13g Fat; 3.3g Carbs; 6.2g Protein; 0.1g Fiber

Ingredients

2 tablespoons butter 2 cloves garlic, chopped 1 ½ cups Swiss chard, chopped 1/2 cup Swiss cheese, grated 1 ½ cups Ricotta cheese, softened 1/2 cup Prosciutto, roughly chopped 6 ounces double cream 2 egg yolks Salt and pepper, to taste

Directions

Strat by preheating your oven to 355 degrees F. In a saucepan, melt the butter over medium-low heat. Cook the cream, salt and pepper for about 3 minutes. Add in the egg yolks and continue to cook for 4 to 5 minutes more, stirring continuously. Spoon the mixture into a baking dish. Add in the remaining ingredients and stir to combine. Bake in the preheated oven for 18 to 20 minutes.Enjoy!

804.   Genovese Salami and Egg Fat Bombs

(Ready in about 5 minutes | Servings 6) Per serving: 156 Calories; 12.2g Fat; 1.6g Carbs; 9.7g Protein; 0g Fiber

Ingredients

6 ounces Genovese salami, chopped 2 hard-boiled eggs, chopped 1 ½ tablespoons fresh cilantro, chopped 6 ounces cream cheese Salt and pepper, to taste

Directions

Thoroughly combine all ingredients until well incorporated. Shape into 12 balls.Enjoy!

805.   Asparagus & Tarragon Flan

Ready in about: 65 minutes | Serves: 4 Per serving: Kcal 264, Fat 11.6g, Net Carbs 2.5g, Protein 12.5g

Ingredients

16 asparagus, stems trimmed ½ cup whipping cream 1 cup almond milk 2 eggs + 2 egg yolks, beaten in a bowl 2 tbsp fresh tarragon, chopped Salt and black pepper to taste 2 tbsp Parmesan cheese, grated 2 tbsp butter, melted 1 tbsp butter, softened

Directions

Cover the asparagus with salted water and bring them to boil over medium heat for 6 minutes. Drain the asparagus, cut their tips, and reserve for garnishing. Chop the remaining asparagus into small pieces. In a blender, add chopped asparagus, whipping cream, almond milk, tarragon, salt, pepper, and Parmesan cheese. Process until smooth. Pour the mixture through a sieve into a bowl and whisk in the eggs. Preheat oven to 350°F. Grease 4 ramekins with softened butter and share the asparagus mixture among the ramekins. Pour the melted butter over each mixture and top with 2-3 asparagus tips. Pour 3 cups water into a baking dish, place in the ramekins, and insert in the oven. Bake for 45 minutes until their middle parts are no longer watery. Remove the ramekins and let cool. Garnish the flan with the asparagus tips and serve with chilled white wine.

806.   Tofu Sandwich with Cabbage Slaw

Ready in about: 10 minutes + marinating time | Serves: 4 Per serving: Kcal 386, Fat 33g, Net Carbs 7.8g, Protein 14g

Ingredients

½ lb firm tofu, sliced 4 zero carb buns 1 tbsp olive oil Marinade Salt and black pepper to taste 2 tsp allspice 1 tbsp erythritol 2 tsp chopped thyme 1 habanero pepper, minced 3 green onions, thinly sliced 2 cloves garlic ¼ cup olive oil Slaw ½ small cabbage, shredded 1 carrot, grated ½ red onion, grated ½ tsp swerve sugar 2 tbsp white vinegar 1 tsp Italian seasoning ¼ cup olive oil 1 tsp Dijon mustard Salt and black pepper to taste

DirectionsIn a food processor, make the marinade by blending the allspice, salt, black pepper, erythritol, thyme, habanero, green onions, garlic, and olive oil, for a minute. Pour the mixture into a bowl and put in the tofu. Toss to coat. Place in the fridge to marinate for 4 hours. In a large bowl, combine the white vinegar, swerve sugar, olive oil, mustard, Italian seasoning, salt, and pepper. Stir in the cabbage, carrot, and onion and place it in the refrigerator to chill. Heat 1 teaspoon of oil in a skillet over medium heat, remove the tofu from the marinade, and cook it in the oil to brown on both sides for 6 minutes in total. Remove onto a plate after and toast the buns in the skillet. In the buns, add the tofu and top with the slaw. Close the bread and serve with a sweet chili sauce.

807.   Lemon Cauliflower "Couscous" with Halloumi

Ready in about: 5 minutes | Serves: 4 Per serving: Kcal 185, Fat 15.6g, Net Carbs 2.1g, Protein 12g

Ingredients

4 oz halloumi, sliced 2 tbsp olive oil 1 cauliflower head, cut into florets ¼ cup chopped cilantro ¼ cup chopped parsley ¼ cup chopped mint ½ lemon juiced Salt and black pepper to taste 1 avocado, sliced to garnish

Directions

Warm the olive oil in a skillet over medium heat. Add the halloumi and fry for 2 minutes on each side until golden brown; set aside. Pour the cauli florets in a food processor and pulse until it crumbles and resembles couscous. Transfer to a bowl and steam in the microwave for 2 minutes. Remove the bowl from the microwave and let the cauli cool. Stir in cilantro, parsley, mint, lemon juice, salt, and pepper. Top couscous with avocado slices and serve with grilled halloumi and vegetable sauce.

808.   Zucchini Lasagna with Ricotta & Spinach

Ready in about: 50 minutes | Serves: 4 Per serving: Kcal 390, Fat 39g, Net Carbs 2g, Protein 7g

Ingredients

2 zucchinis, sliced Salt and black pepper to taste 2 cups ricotta cheese 2 cups shredded mozzarella cheese 3 cups tomato sauce 1 cup baby spinach Preheat oven to 370°F.

Directions

Put the zucchini slices in a colander and sprinkle with salt. Let sit and drain liquid for 5 minutes and pat dry with paper towels. Mix the ricotta cheese, mozzarella cheese, salt, and black pepper to evenly combine and spread ¼ cup of the mixture in the bottom of the baking dish. Layer ⅓ of the zucchini slices on top, spread 1 cup of tomato sauce over, and scatter a ⅓ cup of spinach on top. Repeat the layering process two more times to exhaust the ingredients while finally making sure to layer with the last ¼ cup of cheese mixture. Grease one end of foil with cooking spray and cover the baking dish with the foil. Bake for 35 minutes, remove foil, and bake further for 5 to 10 minutes or until the cheese has a nice golden brown color. Remove the dish, sit for 5 minutes, make slices of the lasagna, and serve warm.

809.   Creamy Vegetable Stew

Ready in about: 25 minutes | Serves: 4 Per serving: Kcal 310, Fat 26.4g, Net Carbs 6g, Protein 8g

Ingredients

2 tbsp ghee 1 tbsp onion-garlic puree 2 medium carrots, chopped 1 head cauliflower, cut into florets 2 cups green beans, halved Salt and black pepper to taste 1 cup water 1 ½ cups heavy cream

Directions

Melt the ghee in a saucepan over medium heat and sauté onion-garlic puree to be fragrant, 2 minutes. Stir in carrots, cauliflower, and green beans for 5 minutes. Season with salt and black pepper. Pour in the water, stir again, and cook on low heat for 15 minutes. Mix in the heavy cream to be incorporated and turn the heat off. Serve the stew with almond flour bread

810.   Salami & Prawn Pizza

Ready in about: 35 minutes | Serves: 6 Per serving: Kcal 267, Fat 13.3g, Net Carbs 4.3g, Protein 9.5g

Ingredients

1 low carb pizza crust (see "Homemade Pizza Crust") 1 cup sugar-free pizza sauce 2 ¼ cups mozzarella cheese, grated 4 oz Hot Salami, thinly sliced 3 tomatoes, thinly sliced 16 prawns, deveined and halved 2 cloves garlic, finely sliced 2 cups baby arugula 2 tbsp toasted pine nuts 1 tbsp olive oil Salt and black pepper to taste 10 basil leaves Preheat oven to 450ºF.

Directions

With the pizza bread on the pizza pan, spread the pizza sauce on it and sprinkle with half of the mozzarella cheese. Top with the salami, tomatoes, prawns, and garlic, then sprinkle the remaining cheese over it. Place the pizza in the oven to bake for 15 minutes. Once the cheese has melted, top with the basil leaves. In a bowl, toss the arugula and pine nuts with olive oil and adjust its seasoning to taste. Section the pizza with a slicer and serve with the arugula mixture.

811. Pork & Vegetable Tart

Ready in about: 45 minutes | Serves: 6 Per serving: Kcal 415; Fat: 26.3g, Net Carbs: 4.2g, Protein: 35g

Ingredients

2 lb ground pork 1 onion, chopped 1 bell pepper, chopped Salt and black pepper to taste 2 zucchinis, sliced 2 tomatoes, sliced ¼ cup whipping cream 8 eggs ½ cup Monterey Jack cheese, grated Preheat oven to 360ºF.

Directions

In a bowl, mix onion, bell pepper, ground pork, pepper, and salt. Layer the mixture on a greased baking dish. Spread zucchini slices on top, followed by tomato slices. Bake for 30 minutes. In a separate bowl, combine cheese, eggs, and whipping cream. Top the tart with the creamy mixture and bake for 10 minutes until the edges and top become brown. Let cool slightly, slice, and serve.

812.   Ham & Egg Salad

Ready in about: 20 minutes | Serves: 4 Per serving: Kcal: 284; Fat 21.3g, Net Carbs 6.8g, Protein 16.7g

Ingredients

4 eggs 1 cup mayonnaise 1 green onion, sliced diagonally ½ tsp mustard 1 tsp lime juice Salt and black pepper to taste 1 small lettuce, torn ½ cup ham, chopped

Directions

Boil the eggs in salted water for 10 minutes. Remove and run under cold water. Peel and chop them. Remove to a mixing bowl together with the mayonnaise, mustard, black pepper, ham, lime juice, and salt. Lay on a bed of lettuce. Scatter the green onion over and serve.

813.   Greek Yogurt & Cheese Alfredo Sauce

Ready in about: 10 minutes | Serves: 12 Per serving: Kcal 154; Fat: 13g, Net Carbs: 3.3g, Protein: 6.2g

Ingredients

2 tbsp butter 6 oz heavy cream Salt and black pepper to taste 2 cloves garlic, chopped ¾ cup sour cream ½ cup Gruyere cheese, grated 1 cup goat cheese ½ cup cooked bacon, chopped 1 cup Greek yogurt

Directions

Set a pan over medium heat and warm butter. Stir in heavy cream and cook for 2-3 minutes. Sprinkle with black pepper and salt; mix in the Greek yogurt and cook for 2 minutes. Stir in the remaining ingredients to mix well until smooth. Serve.

814.   Broccoli Rabe Pizza with Parmesan

Ready in about: 40 minutes | Serves: 2 Per serving: Kcal 673, Fat 47g, Net Carbs 10.7g, Protein 32.6g

Ingredients

1 cauliflower pizza crust 2 tbsp olive oil 2 parsnips, chopped Salt and black pepper to taste 2 cups broccoli rabe 2 hard-boiled eggs, chopped ½ cup largely diced bacon 1 cup grated Parmesan cheese 2 tbsp chopped basil leaves Preheat oven to 400°F.

Directions

 Drizzle the parsnips with some olive oil and sprinkle with salt and pepper. Place on a baking sheet. Bake for 20 minutes; set aside. Toss the broccoli rabe with 2 tablespoons of olive oil in a bowl, season with salt and pepper, and drain any liquid from the bowl. Bake the crust for 7 minutes. Let cool for a few minutes and brush with the remaining olive oil. Scatter the parsnips all over, top with the broccoli rabe, bacon, and eggs, and sprinkle with Parmesan cheese. Bake for 6-8 minutes until the cheese is melted. Garnish with basil and section with a pizza cutter. Serve with sundried tomato salad.

815.   Chorizo Scotch Eggs

Ready in about: 35 minutes | Serves: 4 Per serving: Kcal 247; Fat 11.4g, Net Carbs 0.6g, Protein 33.7g

Ingredients

4 whole eggs 1 egg, beaten ½ cup pork rinds, crushed 1 lb chorizo sausages, skinless ¼ cup Grana Padano cheese, grated 1 garlic clove, minced ¼ tsp onion powder ¼ tsp chili pepper Salt and black pepper to taste

Directions

Cook the eggs in boiling salted water over medium heat for 10 minutes. Rinse under running water and remove the shell; reserve. Preheat oven to 370°F. In a mixing dish, mix the other ingredients, except for the beaten egg and pork rinds. Take a handful of the mixture and wrap around each of the boiled eggs. With fingers, mold the mixture until sealed to form balls. Dip the balls in the beaten eggs, coat with rinds, and place in a greased baking dish. Bake for 25 minutes, until golden brown and crisp. Serve chilled.

816.   Mediterranean Cheese Balls

Ready in about: 5 minutes | Serves: 6 Per serving: Kcal 217; Fat: 18.7g, Net Carbs: 2.1g, Protein: 10g

Ingredients

4 oz prosciutto, chopped 4 oz goat cheese, crumbled ½ cup aioli ½ cup black olives, chopped ½ tsp red pepper flakes 2 tbsp fresh basil, finely chopped

DirectionsIn a bowl, mix aioli, prosciutto, goat cheese, red pepper flakes, and black olives. Form 10 balls from the mixture. Roll them in the basil. Arrange on a serving platter and serve immediately.

817.   Ham & Egg Mug Cups

Ready in about: 5 minutes | Serves: 2 Per serving: Kcal: 244; Fat 17.5g, Net Carbs 2.9g, Protein 19.2

Ingredients

4 eggs 4 tbsp coconut milk ¼ cup ham, cubed ½ tsp chili pepper Salt and black pepper to taste 2 tbsp chives, chopped

DirectionsMix all ingredients, excluding chives. Divide the egg mixture into 2 greased microwave-safe cups. Microwave for 1 minute. Decorate with chives before serving.

818.   Cauliflower & Gouda Cheese Casserole

Ready in about: 25 minutes | Serves: 4 Per serving: Kcal 215, Fat 15g, Net Carbs 4g, Protein 12g

Ingredients

2 heads cauliflower, cut into florets 2 tbsp olive oil 2 tbsp butter, melted 1 white onion, chopped Salt and black pepper to taste ¼ almond milk ½ cup almond flour 1 ½ cups gouda cheese, grated Preheat oven to 350°F.

DirectionsPut the cauli florets in a large microwave-safe bowl. Sprinkle with a bit of water, and steam in the microwave for 4 to 5 minutes. Warm the olive oil in a saucepan over medium heat and sauté the onion for 3 minutes. Add the cauliflower, season with salt and pepper, and mix in almond milk. Simmer for 3 minutes. Mix the melted butter with almond flour. Stir into the cauliflower as well as half of the cheese. Sprinkle the top with the remaining cheese and bake for 10 minutes until the cheese has melted and golden brown on the top. Plate the bake and serve with salad.

819.   Cremini Mushroom Stroganoff

Ready in about: 25 minutes | Serves: 4 Per serving: Kcal 284, Fat 28g, Net Carbs 1,5g, Protein 8g

Ingredients

3 tbsp butter 1 white onion, chopped 4 cups cremini mushrooms, cubed ½ cup heavy cream ½ cup Parmesan cheese, grated 1 ½ tbsp dried mixed herbs

Directions

Melt the butter in a saucepan over medium heat and sauté the onion for 3 minutes until soft. Stir in the mushrooms and cook until tender, about 5 minutes. Add 2 cups water and bring to boil. Cook for 10-15 minutes until the water reduces slightly. Pour in the heavy cream and Parmesan cheese. Stir to melt the cheese. Mix in the dried herbs and season. Simmer for 5 minutes. Serve warm.

820.   Sriracha Tofu with Yogurt Sauce

Ready in about: 40 minutes | Serves: 4 Per serving: Kcal 351; Fat: 25.9g, Net Carbs: 8.1g, Protein: 17.5g

Ingredients

12 oz tofu, pressed and sliced 1 cup green onions, chopped 1 garlic clove, minced 2 tbsp vinegar 1 tbsp sriracha sauce 2 tbsp olive oil Yogurt sauce 2 cloves garlic, pressed 2 tbsp fresh lemon juice Salt and black pepper to taste 1 tsp fresh dill weed 1 cup Greek yogurt 1 cucumber, shredded

Directions

Put tofu slices, garlic, sriracha sauce, vinegar, and green onions in a bowl. Allow to settle for 30 minutes. Set a nonstick skillet to medium heat and add oil to warm. Cook tofu for 5 minutes until golden brown. For the preparation of the sauce: In a bowl, mix garlic, salt, yogurt, black pepper, lemon juice, and dill. Add in shredded cucumber as you stir to combine. Serve the tofu with a dollop of yogurt sauce.

821.   Wild Mushroom & Asparagus Stew

Ready in about: 25 minutes | Serves: 4 Per serving: Kcal 114; Fat: 7.3g, Net Carbs: 9.5g, Protein: 2.1g

Ingredients

2 tbsp olive oil 1 onion, chopped 2 garlic cloves, pressed 1 celery stalk, chopped 2 carrots, chopped 1 cup wild mushrooms, sliced 2 tbsp dry white wine 2 rosemary sprigs, chopped 1 thyme sprig, chopped 2 cups vegetable stock ½ tsp chili pepper 1 tsp smoked paprika 2 tomatoes, chopped 1 tbsp flaxseed meal

Directions

Warm the olive oil in a pot over medium heat. Add in onions and cook until tender, about 3 minutes. Place in carrots, celery, and garlic and cook until soft for 4 more minutes. Add in mushrooms and cook until the liquid evaporates; set aside. Stir in wine to deglaze the pot's bottom. Place in thyme and rosemary. Pour in tomatoes, vegetable stock, paprika, and chili pepper, add in reserved vegetables, and bring to a boil. Reduce the heat to low and let the mixture to simmer for 15 minutes. Stir in flaxseed meal to thicken the stew, about 2-3 minutes. Spoon into individual bowls and serve warm.

822.   Keto Pizza Margherita

Ready in about: 25 minutes | Serves: 2 Per serving: Kcal 510, Fat: 39g, Net Carbs: 3.7g, Protein: 31g

Ingredients

Crust 6 oz mozzarella cheese, grated 2 tbsp cream cheese, softened 2 tbsp Parmesan cheese, grated 1 tsp dried oregano ½ cup almond flour 2 tbsp psyllium husk Topping 4 oz cheddar cheese, grated ¼ cup marinara sauce 1 bell pepper, sliced 1 tomato, sliced 2 tbsp fresh basil, chopped Preheat oven to 400°F.

Directions

Melt the mozzarella cheese in a microwave. Combine the remaining crust ingredients in a large bowl and add the mozzarella cheese. Mix with your hands to combine. Divide the dough in two. Roll out the two crusts in circles and place on a lined baking sheet. Bake for 10 minutes. Remove and spread the marinara sauce evenly. Top with cheddar cheese, bell pepper, and tomato slices. Return to the oven and bake for 10 more minutes. Serve sliced sprinkled with basil.

823.   Cauliflower Risotto with Mushrooms

Ready in about: 15 minutes | Serves: 4 Per serving: Kcal 264, Fat: 18g, Net Carbs: 8.4g, Protein: 11g

Ingredients

2 shallots, diced 2 tbsp olive oil ¼ cup veggie broth ⅓ cup Parmesan cheese, shredded 2 tbsp butter 3 tbsp chives, chopped 1 lb mushrooms, sliced 4 cups cauliflower rice Salt and black pepper to taste

DirectionsHeat olive oil in a saucepan over medium heat. Add the mushrooms and shallots and cook for 5 minutes until tender. Set aside. Add in the cauliflower, broth, salt, and pepper and cook until the liquid is absorbed, about 4-5 minutes. Stir in butter and Parmesan cheese until the cheese is melted. Serve warm.

824.   Walnut Tofu Sauté

Ready in about: 15 minutes | Serves: 4 Per serving: Kcal 320, Fat 24g, Net Carbs 4g, Protein 18g

Ingredients

1 tbsp olive oil 1 (8 oz) block firm tofu, cubed 1 tbsp tomato paste 1 garlic clove, minced 1 onion, chopped 1 tbsp balsamic vinegar Salt and black pepper to taste ½ tsp mixed dried herbs 1 cup chopped raw walnuts

DirectionsHeat the oil in a skillet over medium heat and cook the tofu for 3 minutes until brown. Stir in the garlic, onion, tomato paste, and vinegar and cook for 4 minutes. Season with salt and pepper. Add in the herbs and walnuts. Stir and cook on low heat for 3 minutes. Spoon on plates and serve warm.

825.   Spaghetti Squash with Eggplant & Parmesan

Ready in about: 15 minutes | Serves: 4 Per serving: Kcal 139, Fat: 8.2g, Net Carbs: 6.8g, Protein: 6.9g

Ingredients

2 tbsp butter 1 cup cherry tomatoes 1 eggplant, cubed ¼ cup Parmesan cheese, shredded 3 tbsp scallions, chopped 1 cup snap peas 1 tsp lemon zest 2 cups spaghetti squash, cooked Salt and black pepper to taste

DirectionsMelt butter in a saucepan and cook eggplant for 5 minutes until tender. Add in the tomatoes and peas and cook for 5 minutes. Stir in the zest, scallions, salt, and pepper. Remove the pan from heat. Stir in spaghetti squash and Parmesan cheese and serve.

826.   Fried Tofu with Mushrooms

Ready in about: 40 minutes | Serves: 2 Per serving: Kcal 223; Fat: 15.9g, Net Carbs: 8.1g, Protein: 15.6g

Ingredients

12 oz extra-firm tofu, cubed 1 ½ tbsp flaxseed meal Salt and black pepper to taste 1 tsp garlic clove, minced ½ tsp paprika 1 tsp onion powder 2 tbsp olive oil 1 cup mushrooms, sliced 1 jalapeño pepper, deveined, sliced

Directions

In a bowl, add onion powder, tofu, salt, paprika, black pepper, jalapeño pepper, flaxseed, and garlic. Toss the mixture to coat and allow to marinate for 30 minutes. Warm the olive oil in a pan over medium heat. Cook mushrooms for 5 minutes until tender, stirring continuously. Add in the tofu mixture and stir. Cook for 4-5 more minutes. Divide between plates and serve warm.

827.   Vegetable Tempura

Ready in about: 20 minutes | Serves: 4 Per serving: Kcal 218, Fat 17g, Net Carbs 0.9g, Protein 3g

Ingredients

½ cup coconut flour + extra for dredging Salt and black pepper to taste 3 egg yolks 2 red bell peppers, cut into strips 1 squash, peeled and cut into strips 1 broccoli, cut into florets 1 cup chilled water 4 tbsp olive oil 4 lemon wedges ½ cup sugar-free soy sauce

Directions

In a deep frying pan, heat the olive oil over medium heat. Beat the eggs lightly with ½ cup of coconut flour and water. The mixture should be lumpy. Dredge the vegetables lightly in some flour, shake off the excess flour, dip it in the batter, and then into the hot oil. Fry in batches for 1 minute each, not more, and remove with a perforated spoon onto a wire rack. Sprinkle with salt and pepper and serve with the lemon wedges and soy sauce.

828.   Spanish-Style Sausage and Eggs

(Ready in about 20 minutes | Servings 2) Per serving: 462 Calories; 40.6g Fat; 7.1g Carbs; 16.9g Protein; 2.1g Fiber

Ingredients

6 ounces Chorizo sausage, crumbled 4 eggs, whisked 1/2 cup Hojiblanca olives, pitted and sliced 1 teaspoon garlic paste 1 teaspoon ancho chili pepper, deveined and minced 2 tablespoons canola oil 1/2 cup red onions, chopped 2 rosemary sprigs, leaves picked and chopped Salt and black pepper to the taste

Directions

In a frying pan, heat the oil over a moderate flame; cook red onions until just tender and fragrant, about 4 to 5 minutes. Add in the garlic, pepper, salt, black pepper, sausage, and olives; continue to cook, stirring constantly, for 7 to 8 minutes. Stir in the eggs and rosemary leaves; cook for 4 to 5 minutes, lifting and folding the eggs until thickened.Enjoy!

829.   Keto Belgian Waffles

(Ready in about 30 minutes | Servings 6) Per serving: 316 Calories; 25g Fat; 1.5g Carbs; 20.2g Protein; 0.1g Fiber

Ingredients

3 smoked Belgian sausages, crumbled 1 cup Limburger cheese, shredded 1/2 teaspoon ground cloves 6 eggs 6 tablespoons milk Sea salt and pepper, to taste

Directions

Whisk the eggs with the milk and spices until pale and frothy. Add in the crumbled Belgian sausage and Limburger cheese. Mix until everything is well combined. Brush a waffle iron with a nonstick cooking spray. Pour the batter into waffle iron and cook until golden and cooked through. Repeat until all the batter is used.Enjoy!

830. Scotch Eggs with Ground Pork

(Ready in about 20 minutes | Servings 8) Per serving: 247 Calories; 11.4g Fat; 0.6g Carbs; 33.7g Protein; 0.1g Fiber

Ingredients

8 eggs 1 ½ pounds ground pork 1/2 cup Romano cheese, freshly grated 1 teaspoon garlic, smashed 1/2 teaspoon onion powder 1/2 teaspoon red pepper flakes, crushed 1 teaspoon Italian seasoning mix

Directions

Place the eggs in a saucepan and cover them with water by 1 inch. Cover and bring water to a boil over high heat. Boil for 6 to 7 minutes over medium-high heat; peel the eggs and rinse them under running water. Thoroughly combine the remaining ingredients. Divide the mixture into 8 pieces; now, using your fingers, shape the meat mixture around the eggs. Bake in the preheated oven at 365 degrees F for 20minutes until golden brown.

831. Chipotle Cheese Frittata

(Ready in about 25 minutes | Servings 6) Per serving: 225 Calories; 17g Fat; 5.1g Carbs; 13.2g Protein; 0.9g Fiber

Ingredients

1/3 cup Crema Mexicana 1 Spanish pepper, chopped 1 teaspoon chipotle paste 1 ½ cups spinach 1 tablespoon butter, room temperature 1 large onion, chopped 2 garlic cloves, minced 10 eggs Salt and black pepper, to taste 1/2 cup Mexican cheese blend, shredded

Directions

Preheat your oven to 365 degrees F. In an oven-proof skillet, melt the butter over a moderately high flame. Sauté the onion until caramelized and fragrant. Add in the garlic, Spanish peppers, and chipotle paste, and continue to cook for about 4 minutes more. Add in the spinach and continue to cook for 2 minutes or until it wilts. Whisk the eggs, salt, pepper and Crema Mexicana. Spoon the egg/cheese mixture into the skillet. Bake in the preheated oven for 8 to 10 minutes or until your frittata is golden on top. Top with the Mexican cheese blend and bake an additional 5 minutes or until the cheese is hot and bubbly.

832. Nutty Cheese Logs

(Ready in about 10 minutes + chilling time | Servings 15) Per serving: 209 Calories; 18.9g Fat; 3.7g Carbs; 6.6g Protein; 0.3g Fiber

Ingredients

1 tablespoon Mediterranean spice mix 1 teaspoon lemon juice 14 ounces Ricotta cheese, at room temperature 14 ounces Swiss cheese, grated 1/2 cup mayonnaise 1/2 cup pine nuts, finely chopped

Directions

Combine all ingredients, except for the pine nut, in a mixing bowl. Place the mixture in your refrigerator for about 4 hours or until firm. Shape the mixture into two logs and roll them over chopped pine nuts.Enjoy!

833. Vegetarian Tacos with Guacamole

(Ready in about 10 minutes | Servings 6) Per serving: 370 Calories; 30g Fat; 4.9g Carbs; 19.5g Protein; 4g Fiber

Ingredients

1 pound Monterey-Jack cheese, grated 1 teaspoon taco seasoning mix 1 ½ cups guacamole 1 cup cream cheese 2 cups arugula

Directions

Thoroughly combine the cheese and taco seasoning mix. On a parchment-lined baking sheet, place 1/4 cup piles of cheese 2 inches apart. Press the cheese down lightly. Bake at 350 degrees F for about 7 minutes or until the edges of your tacos are brown.Enjoy!

834. Dad's Cheeseburger Quiche

(Ready in about 45 minutes | Servings 6) Per serving: 310 Calories; 18.3g Fat; 3.8g Carbs; 30.7g Protein; 0.6g Fiber

Ingredients

1 Italian pepper, chopped 1/2 pound ground beef 1/2 ground pork 1 medium leek, chopped 1 garlic clove, chopped 2 zucchinis, thinly sliced 2 tomatoes, thinly sliced 1/4 cup double cream 8 eggs 1/2 cup Colby cheese, grated Salt and pepper, to taste

Directions

Preheat a lightly greased nonstick skillet over medium-high heat. Now, brown the ground meat, leek, garlic and Italian pepper for about 5 minutes, stirring periodically. Season with salt and pepper to taste. Spoon the meat layer on the bottom of a lightly greased baking pan. Place the zucchini slices on top. Top with tomato slices. Beat the cream, eggs and cheese in a mixing dish. Spread this mixture on the top of the vegetables. Bake in the preheated oven at 360 degrees F for about 45 minutes or until cooked through.Enjoy!

835. Italian Burgers with Mushrooms

(Ready in about 20 minutes | Servings 4) Per serving: 370 Calories; 30g Fat; 4.7g Carbs; 16.8g Protein; 2.2g Fiber

Ingredients

1/2 stick butter, softened 1 teaspoon garlic, minced 2 cups Cremini mushrooms, chopped 6 tablespoons blanched almond flour 6 tablespoons ground flax seeds 1 tablespoon Italian seasoning mix 1 teaspoon Dijon mustard 2 eggs, whisked ½ cup Romano cheese, grated

Directions

In a frying pan, melt 1 tablespoon of butter over medium-high heat. Sauté the garlic and mushrooms until just tender and fragrant; drain excess water. Add in the remaining ingredients and mix to combine well. Shape the mixture into 4 patties. In the same frying pan, melt the remaining butter; once hot, fry the patties for 6 to 7 minutes per side. Bon appétit!

836.   Rich Chia Pudding

(Ready in about 35 minutes | Servings 4) Per serving: 93 Calories; 5.1g Fat; 7.2g Carbs; 4.4g Protein; 0.7g Fiber

Ingredients

3/4 cup coconut milk, preferably homemade 1/4 cup water 3 tablespoons orange flower water 2 tablespoons chocolate chunks, unsweetened 2 tablespoons peanut butter 1/2 cup chia seeds 1 teaspoon liquid Monk fruit

Directions

Thoroughly combine the coconut milk, water, peanut butter, chia seeds, Monk fruit, and orange flower water. Let the mixture stand for 30 minutes in your refrigerator. Scatter the chopped chocolate over the top of each serving.

837.   Bacon and Mascarpone Fat Bombs

(Ready in about 15 minutes | Servings 4) Per serving: 88 Calories; 6.5g Fat; 0.7g Carbs; 6.5g Protein; 0.3g Fiber

Ingredients

4 bacon slices, chopped 1 teaspoon paprika 1 teaspoon onion powder 1/2 teaspoon garlic powder 1/2 cup mascarpone cheese 1/2 teaspoon smoke flavor 1/4 teaspoon apple cider vinegar

Directions

Thoroughly combine all ingredients until well combined. Roll the mixture into bite-sized balls.

838.   Prosciutto and Cheddar Muffins

(Ready in about 30 minutes | Servings 9) Per serving: 294 Calories; 21.4g Fat; 3.5g Carbs; 21g Protein; 0.2g Fiber

Ingredients

9 slices prosciutto, chopped 1/2 cup cheddar cheese, shredded 1/4 teaspoon garlic powder 1/2 teaspoon cayenne pepper Sea salt and pepper, to taste 9 eggs 1/2 cup green onions, chopped

Directions

Thoroughly combine all ingredients in a mixing bowl. Spoon the batter into a lightly oiled muffin pan. Bake in the preheated oven at 395 degrees F for about 25 minutes.Bon appétit!

839.   Avocado Stuffed with Tomato and Cheese

(Ready in about 25 minutes | Servings 4) Per serving: 264 Calories; 24.4g Fat; 6g Carbs; 3.7g Protein; 5g Fiber

Ingredients

2 avocados, halved and pitted 1/2 cup tomatoes, chopped 3 ounces mascarpone cheese 1 teaspoon olive oil 8 black olives, pitted and sliced

Directions

Mix the olive oil, tomatoes, cheese and black olives in a bowl. Spoon the mixture into the avocado halves. Bake in the preheated oven at 365 degrees F for about 20 minutes or until everything is cooked through.Bon appétit!

840.   Mom's Homemade Bread

(Ready in about 40 minutes | Servings 6) Per serving: 109 Calories; 10.2g Fat; 1g Carbs; 3.9g Protein; 0.8g Fiber

Ingredients

5 eggs whites 1/2 teaspoon sea salt 1 tablespoon poppy seeds 1 tablespoon flax seeds 1 tablespoon sesame seeds 1/2 teaspoon cream of tartar 1/4 cup butter, softened 1 teaspoon baking powder 1 teaspoon baking soda 1 3/4 cups almond flour 1/4 cup psyllium husk flour

Directions

Start by preheating your oven to 365 degrees F. Beat the eggs with the cream of tartar using your electric mixer until stiff peaks form. Add in the flour, butter, baking powder, baking soda, and salt; blend until everything is well combined. Add the egg mixture to the flour mixture; add in seeds and stir again. Spoon the batter into a lightly buttered loaf pan. Bake in the preheated oven for about 30 minutes.

841.   Cheesy Mashed Cauliflower

(Ready in about 15 minutes | Servings 4) Per serving: 230 Calories; 17.7g Fat; 7.2g Carbs; 11.9g Protein; 3.5g Fiber

Ingredients

1 ½ pounds cauliflower florets 1/2 teaspoon dried oregano 2 cups goat cheese, crumbled Salt and pepper, to taste 2 tablespoons butter, softened 1 thyme sprig, chopped 1 teaspoon dried basil 1 teaspoon garlic, minced

Directions

Steam the cauliflower florets for about 10 minutes or until they are crisp-tender. Puree the cauliflower in your blender or food processor, adding the cooking liquid periodically. Add in the remaining ingredients and pulse until everything is well combined.

842.   Italian Savory Panna Cotta

(Ready in about 15 minutes + chilling time | Servings 6) Per serving: 489 Calories; 47.4g Fat; 6.9g Carbs; 12.7g Protein; 1.6g Fiber

Ingredients

2 ounces button mushrooms, chopped 8 ounces goat cheese 1 cup Greek-style yogurt 1 tablespoon canola oil 1 teaspoon Italian herb mix 1/4 cup almonds, slivered 2 teaspoons powdered gelatin 1 1/3 cups double cream

Directions

Heat the oil in a saucepan over medium-high heat; once hot, sauté the mushrooms for 4 to 5 minutes until they release the liquid. Add in the gelatin and cream and continue to cook for 3 to 4 minutes more. Remove from the heat. Add in the remaining ingredients and transfer to your refrigerator until set.Enjoy!

843.   French-Style Bacon Fat Bombs

(Ready in about 15 minutes + chilling time | Servings 5) Per serving: 206 Calories; 16.5g Fat; 0.6g Carbs; 13.4g Protein; 0.1g Fiber

Ingredients

1/2 teaspoon red pepper flakes, crushed 6 ounces Camembert 3 ounces bacon 1 chili pepper, seeded and minced

Directions

Cook the bacon over a moderately high flame until it is browned on all sides; chop the bacon and set aside. Mix the remaining ingredients until well blended. Place the mixture in your refrigerator for 1 hour. Roll the mixture into bite-sized balls; roll the balls over chopped bacon.Serve well chilled!

844.   Festive Triple Cheese Fondue

(Ready in about 15 minutes | Servings 10) Per serving: 148 Calories; 10.2g Fat; 1.5g Carbs; 9.3g Protein; 0.2g Fiber

Ingredients

1 tomato, pureed 1 tablespoon xanthan gum 1/2 teaspoon garlic, minced 1 teaspoon onion powder 3/4 cup dry white wine 1/2 tablespoon lime juice Cayenne pepper, to taste 1/3 pound soft cheese, chopped 1/3 pound goat cheese, shredded 1/2 cup Parmesan, freshly grated

Directions

Melt the cheese in a double boiler; add in the remaining ingredients and stir to combine. Then, place the cheese mixture under the preheated broiler for about 7 minutes, until the cheese is hot and bubbly.Enjoy!

845.   Chicken Skin Chips

(Ready in about 15 minutes | Servings 4) Per serving: 119 Calories; 10.5g Fat; 1.1g Carbs; 5.1g Protein; 0.3g Fiber

Ingredients

Skin from 4 chicken wings 1/4 cup soft cheese 2 tablespoons Greek-style yogurt 1 tablespoon butter 1/2 teaspoon mustard seeds 2 tablespoons scallions, chopped Salt and pepper, to season

Directions

Bake the chicken skins in the preheated oven at 365 degrees F for about 10 minutes; cut the skin into small pieces. Meanwhile, mix the remaining ingredients to make the sauce.Enjoy!

846.   Spicy Chorizo with Vegetables

(Ready in about 25 minutes | Servings 4) Per serving: 227 Calories; 18g Fat; 7g Carbs; 7.1g Protein; 0.7g Fiber

Ingredients

2 chorizo sausages, sliced 1 tablespoon olive oil 1 teaspoon Taco seasoning mix 1 poblano pepper, minced 2 Spanish peppers, sliced 2 cloves garlic, minced 2 zucchinis, sliced 1 celery, sliced

Directions

In a large skillet, heat the olive oil over a moderately-high heat. Sear the sausage for 7 to 8 minutes. Add in the other ingredients and continue to cook, partially covered, for about 15 minutes.Enjoy!

847.   Cheese Bites with Celery Chips

(Ready in about 25 minutes | Servings 8) Per serving: 177 Calories; 12.9g Fat; 6.8g Carbs; 8.8g Protein; 1.3g Fiber

Ingredients

1 cup Swiss cheese, shredded 1 teaspoon Italian herb mix 2 tablespoons chili pepper, minced Salt and pepper, to taste 1 cup Parmesan cheese, freshly grated 1/2 cup Greek-style yogurt 2 tablespoons tomato paste For Celery Chips: 2 tablespoons avocado oil 1 pound celery, cut into sticks Salt and pepper, to taste

Directions

Mix the Swiss cheese, Parmesan cheese, Greek-style yogurt, tomato paste, Italian herb mix, chili pepper, salt, and pepper in a bowl. Roll the mixture into balls and place in your refrigerator. Toss the celery with avocado oil, salt, and pepper. Roast in the preheated oven at 420 degrees F for about 20 minutes.

848.   Italian Bacon and Gorgonzola Waffles

(Ready in about 20 minutes | Servings 3) Per serving: 453 Calories; 37g Fat; 4.5g Carbs; 25.6g Protein; 1.8g Fiber

Ingredients

6 large-sized eggs, separated 3 tablespoons tomato paste 3 ounces bacon, chopped 3 ounces Gorgonzola cheese, shredded 1 teaspoon baking powder 4 tablespoons butter 1 teaspoon Italian seasoning mix Salt and pepper, to taste

Directions

Combine the egg yolks, baking powder, butter, salt, pepper, and Italian seasoning mix. Beat the egg whites with an electric mixer until pale and frothy. Fold in the egg whites into the egg yolk mixture. Heat you waffle iron. Cook 1/4 cup of the batter until golden. Repeat with the remaining ingredients; you will have six waffles. Spread your toppings onto three waffle; top with remaining waffles and cook until the cheese is melted. Enjoy!

849. Greek-Style Loaded Cheeseburgers

(Ready in about 20 minutes | Servings 6) Per serving: 252 Calories; 15.5g Fat; 1.2g Carbs; 26g Protein; 0.3g Fiber

Ingredients

3 ounces Cheddar cheese, grated 1/2 pound ground beef 1/2 pound ground lamb 1/2 cup onions, chopped 1 teaspoon garlic, chopped 2 ounces soft cheese 2 tablespoons olive oil Se salt and black pepper, to taste 1/2 teaspoon red pepper flakes

Directions

Thoroughly combine the ground meat, onions, garlic, salt, black pepper, and red pepper. Roll the mixture into six balls; flatten them using your hands to make 6 burgers. In a separate bowl, combine soft cheese with Cheddar cheese. Place the cheese into the center of each ball, and enclose inside the meat mixture. Heat the olive oil in a frying pan over a moderately-high flame. Cook your burgers approximately 5 minutes per side.Bon appétit!

850. Mushroom & Bell PepperPizza

Ready in about: 35 minutes | Serves: 4 Per serving: Kcal 295, Fat 20g, Net Carbs 8g, Protein 15g

Ingredients

2 tsp olive oil 1 cup button mushrooms, chopped ½ cup mixed bell peppers, sliced Salt and black pepper to taste 2 cauliflower pizza crusts 1 cup tomato sauce ½ cup Parmesan cheese, grated 2 tbsp sugar-free berry juice

Directions

Warm the olive oil in a skillet over medium heat. Sauté the mushrooms and bell peppers for 10 minutes until softened. Season with salt and black pepper. Put the pizza crusts on a large pan and bake in the oven at 400°F for 10 minutes. Remove and let sit for 5 minutes. Spread the tomato sauce all over the top. Scatter vegetables evenly on top. Season with a little more salt and sprinkle with some Parmesan cheese. Return to the oven and bake for 5-10 minutes until the vegetables are soft and the cheese has melted and is bubbly. Garnish with extra Parmesan cheese. Serve with chilled berry juice.

851. Zesty Frittata with Roasted Chilies

Ready in about: 20 minutes | Serves: 4 Per serving: Kcal 153, Fat 10.3g, Net Carbs 2.3g, Protein 6.4g

Ingredients

2 large green bell peppers, chopped 4 red and yellow chilies, roasted 2 tbsp red wine vinegar 1 knob butter, melted 2 tbsp fresh parsley, chopped 8 eggs, beaten 4 tbsp olive oil ½ cup Parmesan cheese, grated ¼ cup goat cheese, crumbled 2 cloves garlic, minced 1 cup arugula Preheat oven to 400°F.

Directions

With a knife, seed the chilies, cut into long strips, and pour into a bowl. Mix in the vinegar, butter, parsley, half of the olive oil, and garlic; set aside. In another bowl, whisk the eggs with salt, pepper, bell peppers, and Parmesan cheese. Heat the remaining oil in a pan over medium heat and pour the egg mixture along with the goat cheese. Let cook for 3 minutes. Transfer the pan to the oven. Bake the frittata for 4 more minutes, remove, and top with the chili mixture. Garnish the frittata with arugula and serve for lunch.

852.   Cajun Stuffed Cremini Mushrooms

Ready in about: 35 minutes | Serves: 4 Per serving: Kcal 206; Fat: 13.4g, Net Carbs: 10g, Protein: 12.7g

Ingredients

1 lb cremini mushrooms, stems removed ½ head broccoli, cut into florets 2 tbsp coconut oil 1 onion, chopped 1 garlic clove, minced 1 bell pepper, chopped 1 tsp cajun seasoning Salt and black pepper to taste 1 cup cheddar cheese, shredded Preheat oven to 360°F.

Directions

Bake mushroom caps until tender for 8 to 12 minutes. In a food processor, pulse broccoli florets until they become like small rice-like granules. Warm the coconut oil in a skillet over medium heat. Stir in bell pepper, garlic, and onion and sauté until fragrant, about 5 minutes. Sprinkle with black pepper, salt, and cajun seasoning. Fold in broccoli rice. Equally, separate the filling mixture among mushroom caps. Cover with cheddar cheese and bake for 15 more minutes. Serve warm.

853.   Buffalo Salad with Baked Cauliflower

Ready in about: 50 minutes | Serves: 4 Per serving: Kcal 255; Fat: 23.2g, Net Carbs: 5.5g, Protein: 4.1g

Ingredients

1 Iceberg lettuce, chopped ½ cup Tabasco hot sauce 1 tbsp avocado oil 1 head cauliflower, cut into florets ½ cup almond milk 3/4 cup almond flour 2 tsp garlic powder 2 tsp onion powder 1 tsp paprika Salt and black pepper to taste ¼ fennel bulb, sliced 1 cup cherry tomatoes, halved 1 large avocado, sliced 1 carrot, shredded ½ cup Ranch dressing Preheat the oven to 425°F.

Directions

In a bowl, combine the almond flour, almond milk, garlic powder, onion powder, paprika, ½ cup water, salt, and pepper. Add in the cauliflower and toss to coat. Spread the cauliflower on a baking sheet in a single layer and bake for 20 minutes. In a bowl, whisk the Tabasco sauce with avocado oil. Shake and sprinkle the cauliflower with the hot sauce. Return in the oven and bake for 20 more minutes. In a salad bowl, combine the lettuce, fennel, cherry tomatoes, and carrot and drizzle with the Ranch dressing. Top with roasted cauliflower

854.   Garlicky Bok Choy Stir-Fry

Ready in about: 20 minutes | Serves: 4 Per serving: Kcal 118; Fat: 7g, Net Carbs: 13.4g, Protein: 2.9g

Ingredients

2 pounds bok choy, chopped 2 tbsp avocado oil 2 garlic cloves, sliced 2 tbsp pine nuts ½ tsp red pepper flakes Salt and black pepper, to the taste

Directions

Toast the pine nuts in a dry pan over medium heat for 2 minutes, shaking often; set aside. Warm the avocado oil in the pan and sauté the garlic for 30 seconds until soft. Stir in the bok choy for 4-5 minutes. Season with salt, black pepper, and red pepper flakes. Top with the pine nuts and serve.

855.   Cauliflower & Hazelnut Salad

Ready in about: 15 minutes + chilling time | Serves: 4 Per serving: Kcal 221; Fat: 18g, Net Carbs: 6.6g, Protein: 4.2g

Ingredients

1 head cauliflower, cut into florets 1 cup green onions, chopped 4 oz roasted peppers, chopped ¼ cup extra-virgin olive oil 1 tbsp red wine vinegar 1 tsp yellow mustard Salt and black pepper to taste ½ cup black olives, chopped ½ cup hazelnuts, chopped

Directions

Place the cauliflower florets in a steamer basket over boiling water. Cover and steam for 5 minutes. Remove to a bowl and let cool. Add in the roasted peppers and green onions and stir. In a small dish, Combine salt, olive oil, mustard, pepper, and vinegar. Sprinkle the mixture over the veggies. Top with hazelnuts and black olives and serve.

856.   Zoodles with Avocado & Olives

Ready in about: 15 minutes | Serves: 4 Per serving: Kcal 449, Fat: 42g, Net Carbs: 8.4g, Protein: 6.3g

Ingredients

4 zucchinis, spiralized ½ cup pesto 2 avocados, sliced 1 cup Kalamata olives, chopped ¼ cup fresh basil, chopped 2 tbsp olive oil ¼ cup sun-dried tomatoes, chopped Salt and black pepper to taste

Directions

Heat olive oil in a pan over medium heat. Cook the zoodles for 4 minutes. Transfer to a plate. In a bowl, stir pesto, basil, salt, pepper, tomatoes, and olives. Pour over the zoodles and top with avocado slices.

857.   Autumn Cheese and Pepper Dip

(Ready in about 35 minutes | Servings 10) Per serving: 228 Calories; 17.2g Fat; 5.7g Carbs; 10.2g Protein; 0.5g Fiber

Ingredients

1 jar (17-ounce) roasted red peppers, drained and chopped 1 teaspoon deli mustard 1 ¼ cups Colby cheese, grated 10 ounces cream cheese, room temperature 1 cup mayonnaise Salt and black pepper, to taste

Directions

In a mixing bowl, combine the ingredients until everything is well combined. Spoon the mixture into a lightly greased baking pan. Bake in the preheated oven at 355 degrees F for about 30 minutes, rotating the baking pan halfway through the cook time.Enjoy!

858.   Cheese and Sardine Stuffed Avocado

(Ready in about 25 minutes | Servings 4) Per serving: 286 Calories; 23.9g Fat; 6g Carbs; 11.2g Protein; 6g Fiber

Ingredients

2 ounces canned sardines, flaked 2 tablespoons chives, chopped Salt and pepper, to taste 2 tablespoons fresh parsley, chopped 1/2 cup cucumbers, diced 2 large-sized avocados, halved and pitted 4 ounces Asiago cheese, grated

Directions

In a mixing bowl, combine the sardines, chives, salt, pepper, parsley, and cucumber. Stuff your avocado halves. Place the stuffed avocado in a parchment-lined baking pan. Bake in the preheated oven at 355 degrees F for about 20 minutes.Bon appétit!

859.   Breakfast Eggs in a Mug

(Ready in about 5 minutes | Servings 2) Per serving: 197 Calories; 13.8g Fat; 2.7g Carbs; 15.7g Protein; 0.1g Fiber

Ingredients

4 eggs 1 garlic clove, minced 1/4 teaspoon turmeric powder 1/4 cup milk 1/4 cup Swiss cheese, freshly grated Salt and pepper, to taste

Directions

Combine the ingredients until well incorporated. Brush 2 microwave-safe mugs with a nonstick cooking spray (butter-flavored). Spoon the egg mixture into the mugs. Microwave for about 40 seconds. Stir and microwave for 1 minute more or until they're done.Enjoy!

860.   Cheese and Prosciutto Stuffed Avocado

(Ready in about 15 minutes | Servings 6) Per serving: 308 Calories; 27g Fat; 6.4g Carbs; 8.8g Protein; 4.9g Fiber

Ingredients

2/3 cup Ricotta cheese 1 teaspoon stone-ground mustard Salt and pepper, to taste 1 teaspoon hot paprika 1/3 cup Queso Fresco, crumbled 1 cup prosciutto, chopped 3 avocados, cut into halves and pitted

Directions Scoop out the avocados; combine avocado flesh with the remaining ingredients; stir until everything is well incorporated. Spoon the mixture into the avocado halves.Bon appétit!

861.   Simple and Quick Egg Muffins

(Ready in about 5 minutes | Servings 2) Per serving: 244 Calories; 17.5g Fat; 2.9g Carbs; 19.2g Protein; 0.9g Fiber

Ingredients

2 tablespoons onions, chopped 4 tablespoons Greek-style yogurt 1/4 cup Feta cheese, crumbled 4 eggs Salt and pepper, to taste

Directions

Mix all of the above ingredients in a bowl. Spoon the mixture into lightly greased mugs. Microwave for about 70 seconds.Bon appétit!

862. Cheese Sticks with Peppery Dipping Sauce

(Ready in about 40 minutes | Servings 8) Per serving: 200 Calories; 16.9g Fat; 3.7g Carbs; 9.4g Protein; 1.1g Fiber

Ingredients

2 eggs 3 tablespoons almond meal 1 teaspoon baking powder Salt and red pepper flakes, to serve 1/3 teaspoon cumin powder 1/3 teaspoon dried rosemary 2 (8-ounce) packages Colby cheese, cut into sticks 3/4 cup Romano cheese, grated For Roasted Red Pepper Dip: 3/4 cup roasted red peppers, drained and chopped 1 tablespoon yellow mustard 1 cup Ricotta cheese 1/3 cup sour cream 1 teaspoon fresh garlic, minced Black pepper to taste

Directions

In a shallow bowl, whisk the eggs until pale and frothy. In a separate shallow bowl, mix the Romano cheese, almond meal, baking powder, and spices. Dip the cheese stick into the eggs, and then dredge them into dry mixture. Place in your freezer for about 30 minutes. Deep fry the cheese sticks for 5 to 6 minutes. Prepare the sauce by whisking the ingredients.Enjoy!

863. Mediterranean-Style Fat Bombs

(Ready in about 5 minutes | Servings 6) Per serving: 217 Calories; 18.7g Fat; 2.1g Carbs; 9.9g Protein; 0.4g Fiber

Ingredients

4 ounces salami, chopped 2 tablespoons cilantro, finely chopped 1/2 cup black olives, pitted and chopped 1/2 teaspoon paprika 4 ounces Feta cheese, crumbled 1/4 cup mayonnaise

Directions

In a mixing bowl, thoroughly combine all of the above ingredients. Roll the mixture into 10 to 12 balls.Enjoy!

864. Movie Night Cheese Crisps

(Ready in about 10 minutes | Servings 4) Per serving: 205 Calories; 15g Fat; 2.9g Carbs; 14.5g Protein; 0g Fiber

Ingredients

1 thyme sprig, minced 2 cups Monterey-Jack cheese, shredded 1/2 teaspoon garlic powder 1/4 teaspoon onion powder 1/2 teaspoon ancho chili powder

Directions

Begin by preheating your oven to 390 degrees F. Line baking sheets with Silpat mat. Place small piles of the cheese mixture on the prepared baking sheets. Bake for 6 to 7 minutes; then, let them cool at room temperature.Enjoy!

865.   Pickle, Cheese, and Broccoli Bites

(Ready in about 15 minutes | Servings 6) Per serving: 407 Calories; 26.8g Fat; 5.8g Carbs; 33.4g Protein; 1.1g Fiber

Ingredients

1/4 teaspoon dried dill weed 1/2 teaspoon onion powder 4 cups broccoli, grated 1/2 pound salami, chopped 12 ounces Cottage cheese curds 1 cup Swiss cheese, freshly grated 1 teaspoon garlic, minced 1/2 teaspoon mustard seeds 1/2 cup dill pickles, chopped and thoroughly squeezed Salt and black pepper, to taste 1 cup crushed pork rinds 1 teaspoon smoked paprika

Directions

Thoroughly combine all ingredients, except for the pork rinds and paprika. Roll the mixture into 18 balls. In a shallow dish, mix the pork rinds with the smoked paprika. Roll each ball over the paprika mixture until completely coated. Fry these balls in a preheated skillet for 5 to 6 minutes.Enjoy!

866.   Cheese and Basil Keto Balls

(Ready in about 10 minutes | Servings 10) Per serving: 105 Calories; 7.2g Fat; 2.8g Carbs; 7.5g Protein; 0.2g Fiber

Ingredients

1/3 cup black olives, pitted and chopped 1 ½ cups Cottage cheese, at room temperature 18 fresh basil leaves, snipped 1 ½ cups Colby cheese, shredded 1 ½ tablespoons tomato ketchup, no sugar added 1 teaspoon red pepper flakes Salt and freshly ground black pepper

Directions

Mix all of the above ingredients until well combined. Roll the mixture into 18 to 20 balls.Enjoy!

867.   Mediterranean Eggs with Aioli

(Ready in about 20 minutes | Servings 8) Per serving: 285 Calories; 22.5g Fat; 1.8g Carbs; 19.5g Protein; 0.3g Fiber

Ingredients

1/2 Feta cheese, crumbled 1/3 cup Greek-style yogurt 1/2 cup scallions, finely chopped 8 eggs 2 cans anchovies, drained 1 cup butterhead lettuces, torn into pieces 1/2 tablespoon deli mustard For Aioli: 1 egg 1/2 cup olive oil 2 medium cloves garlic, minced 1 tablespoon fresh lime juice Salt, to taste

Directions

Place the eggs in a saucepan and cover them with water by 1 inch. Cover and bring the water to a boil over high heat. Boil for 6 to 7 minutes over medium-high heat. Peel and chop the eggs. Add in the anchovies, lettuce, scallions, Feta cheese, Greek-style yogurt, mustard. To make the aioli, blend the egg, garlic, and lemon juice until well combined. Gradually pour in the oil and continue to blend until everything is well incorporated. Salt to taste. Toss the salad with the prepared aioli.Enjoy!

868.   Old-Fashioned Stuffed Peppers

(Ready in about 45 minutes | Servings 4) Per serving: 359 Calories; 29.7g Fat; 6.7g Carbs; 17.7g Protein; 2.5g Fiber

Ingredients

4 bell peppers 12 ounces Cottage cheese, room temperature 1/2 cup pork rinds, crushed 1 teaspoon garlic, smashed 1 ½ cups pureed tomatoes 1 teaspoon Italian herb mix

Directions

Parboil the peppers in salted water for about 5 minutes. In a mixing bowl, combine the cheese, pork rinds, and garlic until everything is well incorporated. Divide the filling among bell peppers. Whisk the pureed tomatoes with the Italian herb mix until well combined. Pour the tomato mixture over the stuffed pepper. Bake in the preheated oven at 350 degrees F for 35 to 40 minutes.

869.   Egg and Bacon Salad

(Ready in about 20 minutes | Servings 4) Per serving: 284 Calories; 21.3g Fat; 6.8g Carbs; 16.7g Protein; 0.7g Fiber

Ingredients

8 eggs 1/2 cup bacon bits 1 ½ teaspoons fresh lemon juice Salt and pepper, to taste 1/3 cup mayonnaise 1 tablespoon scallions, chopped 1/2 teaspoon deli mustard 2 cups Iceberg lettuce leaves

Directions

Place the eggs in a saucepan and cover them with water by 1 inch. Cover and bring the water to a boil over high heat. Boil for 6 to 7 minutes over medium-high heat. Peel and chop the eggs. Add in the remaining ingredients; gently stir to combine.Bon appétit!

870.   Pepperoni and Vegetable Frittata

(Ready in about 25 minutes | Servings 4) Per serving: 310 Calories; 26.2g Fat; 3.9g Carbs; 15.4g Protein; 0.8g Fiber

Ingredients

8 pepperoni slices 8 eggs, whisked 1 habanero pepper, chopped 1 celery rib, chopped 1/2 stick butter, at room temperature 1/2 cup onions, chopped 2 garlic cloves, minced Salt and pepper, to season

Directions

In a skillet, melt the butter over a moderately high flame. Sauté the onions and garlic for about 3 minutes, stirring continuously to ensure even cooking. Add in the habanero pepper and celery, and continue to cook for 4 to 5 minutes longer or until just tender and fragrant. Spoon the mixture into a lightly greased baking dish. Top with the pepperoni slices. Pour the whisked eggs over the pepperoni layer; season with salt and pepper to taste. Bake for 15 to 18 minutes.Enjoy!

871.   Baked Avocado Boats

(Ready in about 20 minutes | Servings 4) Per serving: 342 Calories; 30.4g Fat; 6.5g Carbs; 11.1g Protein; 4.8g Fiber

Ingredients

2 avocados, halved and pitted, skin on 2 eggs, beaten Salt and pepper, to taste 1/2 teaspoon garlic powder 1 tablespoon fresh parsley, coarsely chopped 2 ounces goat cheese, crumbled 2 ounces Swiss cheese, grated

Directions

Start by preheating your oven to 355 degrees F. Place the avocado halves in a baking dish. In a mixing dish, thoroughly combine the eggs with cheese, salt, pepper, garlic powder, and parsley. Spoon the mixture into the avocado halves. Bake for about 18 minutes or until everything is cooked through.Bon appétit!

872.   Keto Salad with Cheese Balls

(Ready in about 20 minutes | Servings 6) Per serving: 234 Calories; 16.7g Fat; 5.9g Carbs; 12.4g Protein; 4.3g Fiber

Ingredients

For the Cheese Balls:

3 eggs 1 cup almond meal 1 teaspoon baking powder Salt and pepper, to taste 1 cup blue cheese, crumbled 1/2 cup Romano cheese, shredded

For the Salad:

1 cup grape tomatoes, halved 1/3 cup mayonnaise 1 teaspoon Mediterranean seasoning blend 1/2 cup scallions, thinly sliced 1/2 cup radishes, thinly sliced 1 head Iceberg lettuce

Directions

Thoroughly combine all ingredients for the cheese balls. Roll the mixture into bite-sized balls. Bake the cheese balls in the preheated oven at 380 degrees F for 8 to 10 minutes. Toss all the salad ingredients in a large bowl. Serve on your salad and enjoy!

873.   Decadent Scrambled Eggs

(Ready in about 15 minutes | Servings 4) Per serving: 495 Calories; 45g Fat; 6.3g Carbs; 19.5g Protein; 0.3g Fiber

Ingredients

8 eggs, well beaten 1/4 cup milk 2 tablespoons butter Salt, to taste For the Swiss Chard Pesto: 1/2 cup olive oil 1 cup Pecorino Romano cheese, grated 2 tablespoons fresh lime juice 1 teaspoon garlic, minced 2 cups Swiss chard A pinch of ground cloves

Directions

Melt the butter in a cast-iron skillet over moderately-high flame. Beat the eggs with the milk; salt to taste. When the butter is just hot, cook the egg mixture, gently stirring to create large soft curds. Cook until the eggs are barely set. Add all the ingredients for the pesto, except the olive oil, to your blender. Pulse until your ingredients are coarsely chopped. With the machine running, gradually pour in the olive oil and blend until creamy and uniform.

874.   Gorgonzola and Pancetta Cups

(Ready in about 20 minutes | Servings 6) Per serving: 268 Calories; 18.3g Fat; 0.7g Carbs; 26.2g Protein; 0.3g Fiber

Ingredients

2 ounces Gorgonzola cheese, diced 12 small thin slices of pancetta 1/4 cup scallions, chopped 2 ounces soft cheese 6 eggs, whisked Salt and pepper, to season

Directions

Line 6 ramekins with 2 slices of pancetta each. Mix the remaining ingredients until everything is well incorporated. Divide the egg mixture between ramekins. Cover with a double layer of foil. Bake in the preheated oven at 395 degrees F for 15 to 18 minutes or until the top is golden brown. Enjoy!

875.   Old Bay Crabmeat Frittata

(Ready in about 25 minutes | Servings 3) Per serving: 265 Calories; 15.8g Fat; 7.1g Carbs; 22.9g Protein; 0.6g Fiber

Ingredients

4 ounces crabmeat, flaked 1 tablespoon butter, melted 1 teaspoon Old Bay seasoning mix 6 eggs, slightly beaten 1/2 cup sour cream 1 yellow onion, chopped 1 teaspoon garlic, minced

Directions

Begin by preheating your oven to 360 degrees F. Heat the oil in an oven-proof skillet over moderately-high heat. Sauté the onions until they are tender and translucent; add the crabmeat and garlic and continue to cook for 2 minutes or until fragrant. Mix the eggs and sour cream until well combined; pour the egg mixture into the skillet. Bake for 18 to 20 minutes or until the eggs are puffed and opaque.

876.   Easy Mexican Quesadilla

(Ready in about 15 minutes | Servings 4) Per serving: 323 Calories; 24g Fat; 7.4g Carbs; 18.8g Protein; 2.3g Fiber

Ingredients

1 pound cauliflower florets 1/2 cup Muenster cheese, shredded 1/2 pound bacon, cut into strips 1 cup whipping cream 1 tablespoon butter 2 garlic cloves, minced 2 tablespoons white vinegar

Directions

In a preheated sauté pan, cook the bacon for 2 to 3 minutes and reserve. Melt the butter in the same pan. Sauté the cauliflower florets in the pan drippings until they are crisp-tender. Pour the whipping cream into the pan. Add in the garlic and vinegar and continue to cook for 3 minutes longer, stirring frequently. Add in the reserved bacon along with cheese; continue to cook for 2 to 3 minutes, or until the cheese has melted.

877. Caramel Cheese Balls

(Ready in about 5 minutes | Servings 4) Per serving: 180 Calories; 17.3g Fat; 3.4g Carbs; 5.3g Protein; 1.1g Fiber

Ingredients

3 ounces walnuts, chopped 1/2 teaspoon caramel flavoring 3 ounces soft cheese 1/4 teaspoon ground cinnamon

Directions

Pulse all ingredients in your blender until well combined. Roll the mixture into 8 balls.

878. Egg, Olive and Pancetta Balls

(Ready in about 35 minutes | Servings 6) Per serving: 174 Calories; 15.2g Fat; 4.3g Carbs; 5.9g Protein; 0.6g Fiber

Ingredients

3 eggs 3 tablespoons aioli Salt and pepper, to taste 3 slices pancetta, chopped 1/4 cup butter, softened 8 Kalamata olives, pitted and coarsely chopped 2 tablespoons sesame seeds, toasted

Directions

Thoroughly combine the eggs, butter, Kalamata olives, aioli, salt and pepper. Fold in the chopped pancetta. Roll the mixture into balls. Place the sesame seeds in a shallow dish; roll your balls over the seeds to coat on all sides.Bon appétit!

879. French-Style Cheese Sauce

(Ready in about 15 minutes | Servings 6) Per serving: 110 Calories; 10.5g Fat; 0.7g Carbs; 3.4g Protein; 0.2g Fiber

Ingredients

1/3 cup double cream 1/2 teaspoon dried dill 1/2 teaspoon garlic powder 1 teaspoon onion powder 1/3 teaspoon cayenne pepper 1 ½ tablespoons butter 3 tablespoons coconut milk 1/2 cup Roquefort cheese 1/3 cup Brie, grated

Directions

Melt the double cream and butter in a sauté pan over a moderate heat. Once hot, add in the cheese along with the other ingredients. Cook for 4 to 5 minutes, stirring continuously.Enjoy!

880. Butter Rum Pancakes

(Ready in about 25 minutes | Servings 6) Per serving: 243 Calories; 19.6g Fat; 5.5g Carbs; 11g Protein; 0.1g Fiber

Ingredients

6 ounces soft cheese 1/4 cup almond meal 1 ½ teaspoons baking powder 1/2 teaspoon ground cinnamon 6 eggs 4 tablespoons Erythritol For the Syrup: 1 tablespoon ghee 3/4 cup Erythritol 1 tablespoon rum extract 3/4 cup water

Directions Thoroughly combine the soft cheese, eggs, Erythritol, almond meal, baking powder, and cinnamon. Brush a frying pan with nonstick cooking oil and cook your pancakes over a moderate flame until the edges begin to brown. Flip and cook your pancake on the other side for about 3 minutes more. Whisk the water, ghee, Erythritol, and rum extract in a saucepan over medium heat; let it simmer for 5 to 6 minutes or until thickened and reduced.Bon appétit!

881. Iced Bulletproof Coffee

(Ready in about 10 minutes | Servings 4) Per serving: 161 Calories; 13.7g Fat; 4.4g Carbs; 0.7g Protein; 0.4g Fiber

Ingredients

4 cups coffee, chilled 4 teaspoons MCT oil 1/4 cup almond milk 1 teaspoon vanilla liquid stevia 1/4 teaspoon ground cinnamon 4 tablespoons coconut whipped cream

Directions

Blend the coffee with the remaining ingredients, except for the heavy cream. Spoon your coffee along with ice cubes into four chilled glasses. Enjoy!

882. Roasted Asparagus with Spicy Eggplant Dip

Ready in about: 35 minutes | Serves: 6 Per serving: Kcal 149; Fat: 12.1g, Net Carbs: 9g, Protein: 3.6g

Ingredients

1 ½ lb asparagus spears, trimmed ¼ cup + 2 tbsp olive oil ½ tsp paprika Eggplant dip 1 lb eggplants ½ cup scallions, chopped 2 cloves garlic, minced 1 tbsp fresh lemon juice ½ tsp chili pepper Salt and black pepper to taste ¼ cup fresh cilantro, chopped Preheat oven to 390°F.

Directions

Line a parchment paper to a baking sheet. Add in the asparagus. Toss with 2 tbsp of the olive oil, paprika, black pepper, and salt. Roast until cooked through for 9 minutes. Remove. Place the eggplants on a lined cookie sheet. Bake in the oven for about 20 minutes. Let the eggplants cool. Peel them and discard the stems. Warm the remaining olive oil in a frying pan over medium heat and add in the garlic and scallions. Sauté for 3 minutes until tender. In a food processor, pulse together black pepper, roasted eggplants, salt, lemon juice, scallion mixture, and chili pepper. Add in cilantro and serve alongside roasted asparagus spears.

883. Portobello Mushroom Burgers

Ready in about: 15 minutes | Serves: 4 | Per serving: Kcal 339, Fat 29.4g, Net Carbs 3.5g, Protein 10g

Ingredients

8 large portobello mushroom caps 1 clove garlic, minced ½ cup mayonnaise ½ tsp salt 4 tbsp olive oil ½ cup roasted red peppers, sliced 2 medium tomatoes, chopped 4 halloumi slices, ½-inch thick 1 tbsp red wine vinegar 2 tbsp Kalamata olives, chopped ½ tsp dried oregano 2 cups baby spinach

Directions

Preheat a grill pan over medium-high heat. In a bowl, crush the garlic with salt using the back of a spoon. Stir in half of the oil and brush the mushroom caps and halloumi cheese with the mixture. Place the "buns" on the pan and grill them on both sides for 8 minutes until tender. Add the halloumi cheese slices to the grill. Cook for 2 minutes per side or until golden brown grill marks appear. In a bowl, mix the red peppers, tomatoes, olives, vinegar, oregano, baby spinach, and the remaining olive oil; toss to coat. Spread the mayonnaise on 4 mushroom "buns", add a halloumi slice, a scoop of vegetables, and cover with the remaining mushroom caps. Serve and enjoy!

884.   Grilled Cheese the Keto Way

Ready in about: 15 minutes | Serves: 1 Per serving: Kcal 623, Fat: 51g, Net Carbs: 6.1g, Protein: 25g

Ingredients

2 eggs ½ tsp baking powder 2 tbsp butter 2 tbsp almond flour 1 ½ tbsp psyllium husk powder 2 oz cheddar cheese, shredded

Directions

Whisk together all ingredients, except 1 tbsp butter and cheddar cheese. Place in a square oven-proof bowl and microwave for 90 seconds. Flip the bun over and cut in half. Place the cheddar cheese on one half of the bun and top with the other. Melt the remaining butter in a skillet. Add the sandwich and grill until the cheese is melted and the bun is crispy.

885.   Vegetarian Burgers

Ready in about: 20 minutes | Serves: 2 Per serving: Kcal 637, Fat: 55g, Net Carbs: 8.5g, Protein: 23g

Ingredients

1 garlic clove, minced 2 portobello mushrooms, sliced 1 tbsp coconut oil, melted 1 tbsp fresh basil, chopped 2 eggs, fried 2 low carb buns 2 tbsp mayonnaise 2 lettuce leaves Salt to taste

Directions

Combine the melted coconut oil, garlic, basil, and salt in a bowl. Add in the mushrooms and toss to coat. Form into burger patties. Preheat the grill to medium heat. Grill the patties for 2 minutes per side. Cut the buns in half. Add the lettuce, mushrooms, eggs, and mayonnaise. Top with the other bun half. Serve.

886.   Classic Tangy Ratatouille

Ready in about: 47 minutes | Serves: 6 Per serving: Kcal 154, Fat 12.1g, Net Carbs 5.6g, Protein 1.7g

Ingredients

2 eggplants, chopped 3 zucchinis, chopped 2 red onions, diced 1 (28 oz) can tomatoes, diced 2 red bell peppers, cut into chunks 1 yellow bell pepper, cut into chunks 3 garlic cloves, sliced ½ cup fresh basil leaves, chopped 4 sprigs thyme 1 tbsp balsamic vinegar 2 tbsp olive oil ½ lemon, zested

Directions

In a casserole pot, heat the olive oil over medium heat and sauté the eggplants, zucchinis, and bell peppers for 5 minutes. Spoon the veggies into a large bowl. In the same pan, sauté garlic, onions, and thyme leaves for 5 minutes. Add in the canned tomatoes, balsamic vinegar, basil, salt, and black pepper. Return the cooked veggies to the pan. Stir and cover the pot. Cook the ingredients on low heat for 30 minutes. Open the lid and stir in the remaining basil leaves, lemon zest, and adjust the seasoning. Turn the heat off. Plate the ratatouille and serve with some low carb crusted bread.

887.   Smoked Tofu with Rosemary Sauce

Ready in about: 20 minutes | Serves: 4 Per serving: Kcal 336; Fat: 22.2g, Net Carbs: 9.3g, Protein: 27.6g

Ingredients

10 oz smoked tofu, cubed 2 tbsp sesame oil 1 onion, chopped 1 tsp garlic, minced ½ cup vegetable broth ½ tsp turmeric powder Salt and black pepper to taste 2 tbsp olive oil 1 cup tomato sauce 2 tbsp white wine 1 tsp fresh rosemary, chopped 1 tsp chili garlic sauce

Directions

Warm the sesame oil in a pan over medium heat. Brown the tofu for about 5 minutes. Stir in turmeric powder, onion, garlic, salt, pepper for 3 minutes Pour in broth and cook until all liquid evaporates. Warn the olive oil in another pan over medium heat. Place in tomato sauce and heat until cooked through. Place in the rest of the ingredients and simmer for 10 minutes. Pour over the tofu and serve

888.   Mushroom & Bell PepperPizza

Ready in about: 35 minutes | Serves: 4 Per serving: Kcal 295, Fat 20g, Net Carbs 8g, Protein 15g

Ingredients

2 tsp olive oil 1 cup button mushrooms, chopped ½ cup mixed bell peppers, sliced Salt and black pepper to taste 2 cauliflower pizza crusts 1 cup tomato sauce ½ cup Parmesan cheese, grated 2 tbsp sugar-free berry juice

Directions

Warm the olive oil in a skillet over medium heat. Sauté the mushrooms and bell peppers for 10 minutes until softened. Season with salt and black pepper. Put the pizza crusts on a large pan and bake in the oven at 400°F for 10 minutes. Remove and let sit for 5 minutes. Spread the tomato sauce all over the top. Scatter vegetables evenly on top. Season with a little more salt and sprinkle with some Parmesan cheese. Return to the oven and bake for 5-10 minutes until the vegetables are soft and the cheese has melted and is bubbly. Garnish with extra Parmesan cheese. Serve with chilled berry juice.

889.   Spicy Cauliflower Steaks with Steamed Green Beans

Ready in about: 20 minutes | Serves: 4 Per serving: Kcal 118, Fat 9g, Net Carbs 4g, Protein 2g

Ingredients

2 heads cauliflower, sliced lengthwise into 'steaks' ¼ cup olive oil ¼ cup chili sauce 1 tsp erythritol Salt and black pepper to taste 2 shallots, diced 1 bunch green beans, trimmed 2 tbsp fresh lemon juice 2 tbsp fresh parsley, chopped

Directions

In a bowl, mix the olive oil, chili sauce, and erythritol. Brush the cauliflower with the mixture. Place them on the preheated grill. Close the lid and grill for 12 minutes, flipping once. Remove the grilled steaks to a plate and sprinkle with salt, black pepper, shallots, and parsley. Bring salted water to boil over high heat, place the green beans in a sieve, and set over the steam from the boiling water. Cover with a clean napkin to keep the steam trapped in the sieve. Cook for 6 minutes. Remove to a bowl and toss with lemon juice. Add them to the cauliflower steaks and serve.

890.   Vegetable Burritos

Ready in about: 10 minutes | Serves: 4 Per serving: Kcal 373, Fat 23.2g, Net Carbs 5.4g, Protein 17.9g

Ingredients

2 large low carb tortillas 2 tsp olive oil 1 small onion, sliced 1 bell pepper, seeded and sliced 1 ripe avocado, pitted and sliced 1 cup lemon cauli couscous Salt and black pepper to taste ⅓ cup sour cream 3 tbsp Mexican salsa

Directions

Heat the olive oil in a skillet over medium heat. Sauté the onion and bell pepper until they start to brown on the edges, about 4 minutes. Lay the tortillas on a flat surface and top each one with the bell pepper mixture, avocado, and cauli couscous. Season with salt and black pepper Top with sour cream and Mexican salsa. Fold in each tortilla's sides and roll them in and over the filling to be completely enclosed. Wrap with foil, cut in halves, and serve.

891.   Zesty Frittata with Roasted Chilies

Ready in about: 20 minutes | Serves: 4 Per serving: Kcal 153, Fat 10.3g, Net Carbs 2.3g, Protein 6.4g

Ingredients

2 large green bell peppers, chopped 4 red and yellow chilies, roasted 2 tbsp red wine vinegar 1 knob butter, melted 2 tbsp fresh parsley, chopped 8 eggs, beaten 4 tbsp olive oil ½ cup Parmesan cheese, grated ¼ cup goat cheese, crumbled 2 cloves garlic, minced 1 cup arugula Preheat oven to 400°F.

Directions

With a knife, seed the chilies, cut into long strips, and pour into a bowl. Mix in the vinegar, butter, parsley, half of the olive oil, and garlic; set aside. In another bowl, whisk the eggs with salt, pepper, bell peppers, and Parmesan cheese. Heat the remaining oil in a pan over medium heat and pour the egg mixture along with the goat cheese. Let cook for 3 minutes. Transfer the pan to the oven. Bake the frittata for 4 more minutes, remove, and top with the chili mixture. Garnish the frittata with arugula and serve for lunch

892.   Onion & Nut Stuffed Mushrooms

Ready in about: 30 minutes | Serves: 4 Per serving: Kcal 139; Fat: 11.2g, Net Carbs: 7.4g, Protein: 4.8g

Ingredients

2 tbsp sesame oil 1 onion, chopped 1 garlic clove, minced 1 lb mushrooms, stems removed Salt and black pepper to taste ¼ cup raw pine nuts Preheat oven to 360°F.

Directions

Warm the sesame oil in a frying pan over medium heat. Place in garlic and onion and cook for 3 minutes. Chop mushroom stems and add to the pan. Cook for 3-4 minutes until tender. Sprinkle with pepper and salt and add in pine nuts. Stuff the mushroom caps with the mixture. Set on a greased baking sheet. Bake the stuffed mushrooms for 30 minutes. Let cool slightly and serve.

893.   Greek-Style Zucchini Pasta

Ready in about: 15 minutes | Serves: 4 Per serving: Kcal 231, Fat: 19.5g, Net Carbs: 6.5g, Protein: 6.5g

Ingredients

¼ cup sun-dried tomatoes 2 garlic cloves, minced 1 cup spinach, chopped 2 large zucchinis, spiralized ¼ cup feta cheese, crumbled ¼ cup halloumi cheese, shredded 10 kalamata olives, halved 2 tbsp olive oil 2 tbsp fresh parsley, chopped

Directions

Heat the olive oil in a pan over medium heat. Add in zoodles, garlic, and spinach and cook for 5 minutes. Stir in the olives, tomatoes, feta, and parsley for 2 more minutes. Top with halloumi cheese and serve.

894.   Cajun Stuffed Cremini Mushrooms

Ready in about: 35 minutes | Serves: 4 Per serving: Kcal 206; Fat: 13.4g, Net Carbs: 10g, Protein: 12.7g

Ingredients

1 lb cremini mushrooms, stems removed ½ head broccoli, cut into florets 2 tbsp coconut oil 1 onion, chopped 1 garlic clove, minced 1 bell pepper, chopped 1 tsp cajun seasoning Salt and black pepper to taste 1 cup cheddar cheese, shredded Preheat oven to 360°F.

Directions

 Bake mushroom caps until tender for 8 to 12 minutes. In a food processor, pulse broccoli florets until they become like small rice-like granules. Warm the coconut oil in a skillet over medium heat. Stir in bell pepper, garlic, and onion and sauté until fragrant, about 5 minutes. Sprinkle with black pepper, salt, and cajun seasoning. Fold in broccoli rice. Equally, separate the filling mixture among mushroom caps. Cover with cheddar cheese and bake for 15 more minutes. Serve warm.

895.   Greek Salad with Poppy Seed Dressing

Ready in about: 3 hours 15 minutes | Serves: 4 Per serving: Kcal 208; Fat: 15.6g, Net Carbs: 6.7g, Protein: 7.6g

Ingredients

Dressing 1 cup poppy seeds 2 cups water 2 tbsp green onions, chopped 1 garlic clove, minced 1 lime, freshly squeezed Salt and black pepper to taste ¼ tsp dill, minced 2 tbsp almond milk Salad 1 head lettuce, separated into leaves 3 tomatoes, diced 3 cucumbers, sliced 2 tbsp kalamata olives, pitted

Directions

Put all dressing ingredients, except for the poppy seeds, in a food processor and pulse until well incorporated. Add in poppy seeds and mix well with a fork. Mix and divide the salad ingredients between 4 plates. Add the dressing to each and shake to coat. Serve.

896.   Brussels Sprouts with Tofu

Ready in about: 20 minutes | Serves: 4 Per serving: Kcal 179; Fat: 11.7g, Net Carbs: 9.1g, Protein: 10.5g

Ingredients

2 tbsp olive oil 2 garlic cloves, minced ½ cup onions, chopped 10 oz tofu, crumbled 2 tbsp water 2 tbsp soy sauce 1 tbsp tomato puree ½ lb Brussels sprouts, quartered Salt and black pepper to taste

Directions

Set a saucepan over medium heat and Warm the olive oil. Add onion and garlic and cook until tender, 3 minutes. Place in the soy sauce, water, and tofu. Cook for 5 minutes until the tofu starts to brown. Add in Brussels sprouts; adjust the seasonings. Cook for 13 minutes while stirring frequently. Serve warm.

897.   Spicy Green Cabbage with Tofu

Ready in about: 25 minutes | Serves: 4 Per serving: Kcal 182; Fat: 10.3g, Net Carbs: 8.3g, Protein: 8.1g

Ingredients

2 tbsp olive oil 14 oz block tofu, pressed and cubed 1 celery stalk, chopped 1 bunch of scallions, chopped 1 tsp cayenne pepper 1 tsp garlic powder 2 tbsp Worcestershire sauce Salt and black pepper to taste 1 lb green cabbage, shredded ½ tsp turmeric ¼ tsp dried basil

Directions

Warm the olive oil a large skillet over medium heat. Stir in tofu cubes and cook for 8 minutes. Set aside. Add scallions, celery, and garlic in the same pan and sauté for 5 minutes until soft. Stir in cayenne pepper, Worcestershire sauce, garlic powder, turmeric, basil, salt, and pepper for 2 more minutes. Add in the green cabbage and cook for 8-10 minutes, stirring often. Serve topped with the tofu.

898.   Easy Cauliflower & Kale

Soup Ready in about: 35 minutes | Serves: 4 Per serving: Kcal 172; Fat: 10.3g, Net Carbs: 11.8g, Protein: 8.1g

Ingredients

2 tbsp olive oil 1 onion, finely chopped 2 garlic cloves, minced 1 head cauliflower, cut into florets 1 cup kale, chopped 4 cups vegetable broth ½ cup almond milk ½ tsp salt ½ tsp red pepper flakes 1 tbsp fresh parsley, chopped ½ cup cheddar cheese, grated

Directions

Set a pot over medium heat and warm the oil. Add garlic and onion and sauté until softened. Place in vegetable broth, kale, and cauliflower and cook for 10 minutes until the mixture boils. Stir in the pepper flakes, salt, and almond milk; reduce the heat and simmer the soup for 10-15 minutes. Remove from the heat and stir in the cheddar cheese. Blitz the soup with an immersion blender to achieve the desired consistency. Top with parsley and serve immediately.

899. Crispy-Topped Baked Vegetables

Ready in about: 40 minutes | Serves: 4 Per serving: Kcal 242; Fat: 16.3g, Net Carbs: 8.6g, Protein: 16.3g

Ingredients

2 tbsp olive oil 1 onion, chopped 1 celery stalk, chopped 2 carrots, grated ½ lb turnips, sliced 1 cup vegetable broth 1 tsp turmeric Salt and black pepper to taste ½ tsp liquid smoke 1 cup Parmesan cheese, shredded 2 tbsp fresh chives, chopped Preheat oven to 360°F.

Directions

Set a skillet over medium heat and warm olive oil. Sweat the onion until soft. Place in the turnips, carrots, and celery and cook for 4 minutes. Remove to a greased baking dish. Combine vegetable broth with turmeric, pepper, liquid smoke, and salt. Spread this mixture over the vegetables. Sprinkle with Parmesan cheese and bake for about 30 minutes. Garnish with chives to serve.

900. Butternut Squash Risotto with Almonds

Ready in about: 25 minutes | Serves: 4 Per serving: Kcal 492; Fat: 39g, Net Carbs: 9.4g, Protein: 7.2g

Ingredients

1 leek, chopped 2 lb butternut squash, peeled, cubed ¼ cup almonds, chopped 2 tbsp olive oil 2 garlic cloves, minced Salt and black pepper to taste 2 cups almond milk 1 lime, juiced 1 celery stalk, chopped 2 cups baby spinach 2 tbsp fresh cilantro, chopped

Directions

In a food processor, pulse butternut squash until it becomes like small rice-like granules. Place in a bowl. Warm the olive oil in a large saucepan over medium heat. Add the leek, garlic, and celery and cook for 3 minutes until tender. Stir in the butternut rice for 2-3 minutes. Sprinkle with salt and pepper. Pour in the almond milk and cook for 5-7 minutes. Stir in the spinach for 2-3 more minutes until it is wilted. Drizzle with the lime juice, scatter almonds all over, and top with cilantro. Serve warm.

901. Easy Vanilla Granola

Ready in about: 1 hour | Serves: 6 Per serving: Kcal 449; Fat: 44.9g, Net Carbs: 5.1g, Protein: 9.3g

Ingredients

½ cup hazelnuts, chopped 1 cup walnuts, chopped ⅓ cup flax meal ⅓ cup coconut milk ⅓ cup poppy seeds ⅓ cup pumpkin seeds 8 drops stevia ⅓ cup coconut oil, melted 1 ½ tsp vanilla paste 1 tsp ground cloves 1 tsp grated nutmeg 1 tsp lemon zest Preheat oven to 300°F.

Directions

Line a parchment paper to a baking sheet. In a bowl, combine all ingredients and mix well. Stir in ⅓ cup water. Spread the mixture onto the baking sheet in an even layer. Bake for 55 minutes as you stir at intervals of 15 minutes. Let cool at room temperature. Serve.

902.   Tasty Cauliflower Dip

Ready in about: 10 minutes | Serves: 4 Per serving: Kcal 100; Fat: 8.2g, Net Carbs: 4.7g, Protein: 3.7g

Ingredients

1 head cauliflower, cut into florets ¼ cup olive oil Salt and black pepper to taste 1 garlic clove, smashed 1 tbsp sesame paste ½ tsp garam masala

Directions

Boil cauliflower until tender for 7 minutes in salted water in a large pot. Transfer to a blender and pulse until you attain a rice-like consistency. Place in garam masala, olive oil, black paper, garlic, salt, and sesame paste. Blend the mixture until well combined. Drizzle with some olive oil and serve.

903.   Creamy Almond & Turnip Soup

Ready in about: 25 minutes | Serves: 4 Per serving: Kcal 114; Fat: 6.5g, Net Carbs: 9.2g, Protein: 3.8g

Ingredients

2 tbsp olive oil 1 onion, chopped 1 celery stalk, chopped 2 turnips, peeled and chopped 4 cups vegetable broth Salt and white pepper to taste ¼ cup ground almonds 1 cup almond milk 1 tbsp fresh cilantro, chopped

Directions

Set a pot over medium heat and warm the olive oil. Add in celery and onion and sauté for 6 minutes. Stir in white pepper, vegetable broth, salt, and almonds. Boil the mixture. Simmer for 17 minutes. Blend the soup with an immersion blender. Stir in the almond milk and decorate with cilantro before serving.

904.   Spiced Cauliflower with Garlic & Peppers

Ready in about: 35 minutes | Serves: 4 Per serving: Kcal 166; Fat: 13.9g, Net Carbs: 7.4g, Protein: 3g

Ingredients

1 head cauliflower, cut into florets 2 red bell peppers, cut into squares ¼ cup olive oil Salt and black pepper to taste ½ tsp cayenne pepper 2 garlic cloves, sliced Preheat oven to 425°F.

Directions

Line a parchment paper to a baking sheet. Set the cauliflower, bell peppers, and garlic on the sheet. Sprinkle with cayenne pepper, salt, and black pepper and drizzle with olive oil; stir. Roast for 30 minutes as you toss in intervals until they start to brown. Serve with tomato dip.

905. Curried Asparagus Frittata

(Ready in about 20 minutes | Servings 4) Per serving: 248 Calories; 17.1g Fat; 6.2g Carbs; 17.6g Protein; 1.6g Fiber

Ingredients

8 eggs, beaten 1 cup asparagus spears, chopped 1/2 teaspoon Fresno pepper, minced 1 teaspoon curry paste Salt and pepper, to your liking 3/4 cup Cheddar cheese, grated 1/4 cup fresh parsley, to serve 2 tablespoons olive oil 1/2 cup onions, chopped

Directions

Begin by preheating your oven to 370 degrees F. In an oven-proof skillet, heat the oil over a medium heat. Sauté the onions until they are tender and caramelized. Add in the asparagus and cook until they've softened. Stir in the eggs, Fresno pepper, curry paste, salt, and pepper. Cook the eggs until the edges barely start setting. Scatter the cheese over the top of your frittata. Bake your frittata in the preheated oven for about 15 minutes. Serve with fresh parsley and enjoy!

906. Black Pepper, Tomato and Cheese Omelet

(Ready in about 15 minutes | Servings 2) Per serving: 307 Calories; 25g Fat; 2.5g Carbs; 18.5g Protein; 1g Fiber

Ingredients

4 eggs 1/4 cup goat cheese, crumbled 1/4 cup Appenzeller cheese, shredded 1 tablespoon olive oil 1/4 teaspoon black peppercorns, crushed 1 cup cherry tomatoes, halved Salt, to taste

Directions

In a frying pan, heat the olive oil over a moderate heat. Pour in the eggs; swirl the eggs around using a spatula. Season the eggs with salt and black pepper. When the eggs are just set and no visible liquid egg remains, top them with the cheese. Fold gently in half with the spatula.Bon appétit!

907. Eggs with Prosciutto di Parma and Cheese

(Ready in about 10 minutes | Servings 2) Per serving: 431 Calories; 33.1g Fat; 2.7g Carbs; 30.3g Protein; 0.3g Fiber

Ingredients

4 slices Prosciutto di Parma, chopped 4 eggs, beaten 1 teaspoon Italian herb mix Sea salt and black pepper, to season 4 ounces Asiago cheese, grated

Directions

Preheat a slightly greased frying pan over medium-high heat. Add in the eggs, Italian herb mix, salt, and black pepper. When the eggs are just set and no visible liquid egg remains, top with Asiago cheese. Fold gently in half with the spatula. Cook an additional 1 to 2 minutes or until cooked through.Bon appétit!

908. Goat Cheese Deviled Eggs

(Ready in about 20 minutes | Servings 5) Per serving: 177 Calories; 12.7g Fat; 4.6g Carbs; 11.4g Protein; 0.4g Fiber

Ingredients

10 eggs 2 tablespoons bell peppers, minced 2 tablespoons goat cheese, crumbled 1/4 cup mayonnaise 2 tablespoons shallot, finely chopped 2 tablespoons celery, finely chopped 1/2 teaspoon red pepper flakes   Salt and black pepper, to taste

Directions

Place the eggs in a saucepan and cover them with water by 1 inch. Cover and bring the water to a boil over high heat. Boil for 6 to 7 minutes over medium-high heat. Peel the eggs and slice them in half lengthwise; mix the yolks with the remaining ingredients. Divide the mixture between the egg whites and arrange the deviled eggs on a nice serving platter.

909. Greek-Style Egg and Apple Muffins

(Ready in about 20 minutes | Servings 6) Per serving: 81 Calories; 3.5g Fat; 6.7g Carbs; 5.5g Protein; 2.1g Fiber

Ingredients

1/4 cup Greek-style yogurt 3 eggs, beaten 1 apple, sliced 3/4 Feta cheese 2 tablespoons ground almonds 4 tablespoons Swerve 1/2 teaspoon vanilla paste

Directions

Begin by preheating an oven to 365 degrees F. Thoroughly combine all ingredients until well mixed. Spoon the batter into lightly buttered muffin cups. Bake in the preheated oven for about 15 minutes. Place on a wire rack before unmolding.Enjoy!

910. The Best Cauliflower Fritters Ever

(Ready in about 35 minutes | Servings 6) Per serving: 199 Calories; 13.8g Fat; 6.8g Carbs; 13g Protein; 2.8g Fiber

Ingredients

1 ½ tablespoons butter, room temperature 1 small onion, chopped 1 garlic clove, minced 1 pound cauliflower, grated 4 tablespoons almond meal 2 tablespoons ground flaxseed ½ cup Colby cheese, shredded 1 cup Romano cheese 2 eggs, beaten Sea salt and pepper, to taste

Directions

Begin by preheating your oven to 390 degrees F. Melt the butter in a nonstick skillet over medium heat. Cook the onion and garlic until they are tender and fragrant. Add in the remaining ingredients and stir until well combined. Form the mixture into patties. Bake in the preheated for about 30 minutes, flipping them halfway through the cook time.Bon appétit!

911. Mediterranean-Style Panna Cotta

(Ready in about 40 minutes | Servings 8) Per serving: 155 Calories; 12.7g Fat; 6.2g Carbs; 4.6g Protein; 0.4g Fiber

Ingredients

1 ½ cups double cream 1 cup chive cream cheese 2 teaspoons powdered gelatin 4 bell peppers, sliced 1 tablespoon olive oil, room temperature 1/4 cup fresh parsley, chopped Salt and pepper, to taste 1/2 teaspoon mustard seeds 1/2 teaspoon paprika

Directions

Strat by preheating your oven to 450 degrees F. Brush the bell peppers with olive oil and roast them for about 30 minutes, until the skin is charred in spots. Peel the peppers and chop them. In the meantime, cook the remaining ingredients for about 10 minutes until thoroughly warmed. Fold in the chopped peppers and stir to combine. Divide the mixture between eight lightly oiled ramekins. Place in your refrigerator overnight.Enjoy!

912.   Easy Mini Frittatas

(Ready in about 40 minutes | Servings 5) Per serving: 261 Calories; 16g Fat; 6.6g Carbs; 21.1g Protein; 0.9g Fiber

Ingredients

8 eggs, whisked 1 cup Asiago cheese, shredded 1/2 teaspoon chipotle powder 1 tablespoon olive oil 1 onion, chopped 1 Italian pepper, chopped 1 cup spinach, torn into pieces 3 slices bacon, chopped Salt and pepper, to taste 1 tablespoon fresh coriander, chopped

Directions

Begin by preheating your oven to 380 degrees F. Heat the oil in frying pan over medium-high heat; cook the onion for about 6 minutes or until caramelized. Add in the pepper and spinach, and continue to sauté for 4 to 5 minutes. Add in the bacon and continue to cook for 3 to 4 minutes. Stir in the remaining ingredients. Spoon the mixture into a lightly oiled muffin pan. Bake in the preheated oven for about 22 minutes.Bon appétit!

913.   Spanish-Style Cheese Crisps

(Ready in about 18 minutes | Servings 2) Per serving: 100 Calories; 8g Fat; 0g Carbs; 7g Protein; 0.4g Fiber

Ingredients

3 cups Manchego cheese, grated 1 teaspoon dried Perejil 1/2 teaspoon Spanish pimentón Sea salt and black pepper, to taste 1/2 teaspoon granulated garlic

Directions

Start by preheating your oven to 410 degrees F. Mix all of the above ingredients. Place about 2 tablespoons of the mixture into small mounds on a parchment-lined baking sheet. Bake for 13 to 15 minutes or until golden and crisp.Enjoy!

914.   Baked Eggs Provencal

(Ready in about 20 minutes | Servings 5) Per serving: 444 Calories; 35.3g Fat; 2.7g Carbs; 29.8g Protein; 1g Fiber

Ingredients

1 teaspoon Herbes de Provence 1/4 cup chicken broth 5 eggs 1 ½ cups Comté cheese, shredded 4 slices Bayonne ham, chopped 1/2 cup onions, chopped 1/2 cup fire-roasted tomatoes, diced 1 clove garlic, minced 1 tablespoon butter

Directions

In an oven-proof pan, melt the butter over medium-high heat. Now, cook the Bayonne ham for about 5 minutes until crisp; reserve. Then, sauté the onions in the pan drippings. Add in the tomatoes, garlic, Herbes de Provence, and broth; continue to cook for 5 to 6 minutes more. Now, create 5 holes in the vegetable mixture. Crack an egg into each hole. Bake in the preheated oven at 350 degrees F for about 18 minutes until the egg whites are completely cooked through. Top with reserved Bayonne ham.Enjoy!

915.   French-Style Gorgonzola Cheese Soup

(Ready in about 20 minutes | Servings 4) Per serving: 296 Calories; 14.1g Fat; 6.4g Carbs; 14.2g Protein; 1.5g Fiber

Ingredients

6 ounces Gorgonzola cheese, shredded 1 ½ cups milk 1 celery stalk, chopped 1 chili pepper, finely chopped 1 teaspoon ginger-garlic paste 1 ½ tablespoons flaxseed meal 2 cups water 2 tablespoons butter 1/2 cup white onions, chopped Salt and pepper, to taste

Directions

Melt the butter in a heavy-bottomed pot over a moderately high heat. Sauté the onions, celery and pepper until tender and fragrant. Add in the garlic paste, flaxseed meal, water, and milk and bring to a boil; immediately, turn the heat to medium-low. Partially cover, and continue to simmer for 8 to 10 minutes. Fold in the Gorgonzola cheese and remove from the heat. Season with salt and pepper.

916.   Cheese Stuffed Mushrooms

Ready in about: 30 minutes | Serves: 2 Per serving: Kcal 334, Fat: 29g, Net Carbs: 5.5g, Protein: 14g

Ingredients

4 portobello mushrooms, stems removed 2 tbsp olive oil 2 cups lettuce 1 cup blue cheese, crumbled Preheat oven to 350°F.

Directions

Fill the mushrooms with blue cheese and place on a lined baking sheet. Bake for 20 minutes. Serve with lettuce drizzled with olive oil.

917. Cream of Zucchini with Avocado

Ready in about: 35 minutes | Serves: 4 Per serving: Kcal 165 Fat: 13.4g, Net Carbs: 9g, Protein: 2.2g

Ingredients

3 tsp vegetable oil 1 onion, chopped 1 carrot, sliced 1 turnip, sliced 3 cups zucchinis, chopped 1 avocado, peeled and diced Salt and black pepper to taste 4 cups vegetable broth 1 tomato, pureed

Directions

In a pot, warm the oil and sauté onion until translucent, about 3 minutes. Add in turnip, zucchini, and carrot and cook for 7 minutes until tender. Season with salt and black pepper. Mix in pureed tomato and vegetable broth. Bring to a boil. Simmer for 20 minutes. Lift from the heat. Add the soup and avocado to a blender. Puree until creamy and smooth. Serve warm.

918. Buffalo Salad with Baked Cauliflower

Ready in about: 50 minutes | Serves: 4 Per serving: Kcal 255; Fat: 23.2g, Net Carbs: 5.5g, Protein: 4.1g

Ingredients

1 Iceberg lettuce, chopped ½ cup Tabasco hot sauce 1 tbsp avocado oil 1 head cauliflower, cut into florets ½ cup almond milk 3/4 cup almond flour 2 tsp garlic powder 2 tsp onion powder 1 tsp paprika Salt and black pepper to taste ¼ fennel bulb, sliced 1 cup cherry tomatoes, halved 1 large avocado, sliced 1 carrot, shredded ½ cup Ranch dressing Preheat the oven to 425°F.

Directions

In a bowl, combine the almond flour, almond milk, garlic powder, onion powder, paprika, ½ cup water, salt, and pepper. Add in the cauliflower and toss to coat. Spread the cauliflower on a baking sheet in a single layer and bake for 20 minutes.

In a bowl, whisk the Tabasco sauce with avocado oil. Shake and sprinkle the cauliflower with the hot sauce. Return in the oven and bake for 20 more minutes. In a salad bowl, combine the lettuce, fennel, cherry tomatoes, and carrot and drizzle with the Ranch dressing. Top with roasted cauliflower and serve.

919. Vegetable Burritos

Ready in about: 10 minutes | Serves: 4 Per serving: Kcal 373, Fat 23.2g, Net Carbs 5.4g, Protein 17.9g

Ingredients

2 large low carb tortillas 2 tsp olive oil 1 small onion, sliced 1 bell pepper, seeded and sliced 1 ripe avocado, pitted and sliced 1 cup lemon cauli couscous Salt and black pepper to taste ⅓ cup sour cream 3 tbsp Mexican salsa

Directions

Heat the olive oil in a skillet over medium heat. Sauté the onion and bell pepper until they start to brown on the edges, about 4 minutes. Lay the tortillas on a flat surface and top each one with the bell pepper mixture, avocado, and cauli couscous. Season with salt and black pepper Top with sour cream and Mexican salsa. Fold in each tortilla's sides and roll them in and over the filling to be completely enclosed. Wrap with foil, cut in halves, and serve.

920.   Greek-Style Zucchini Pasta

Ready in about: 15 minutes | Serves: 4 Per serving: Kcal 231, Fat: 19.5g, Net Carbs: 6.5g, Protein: 6.5g

Ingredients

¼ cup sun-dried tomatoes 2 garlic cloves, minced 1 cup spinach, chopped 2 large zucchinis, spiralized ¼ cup feta cheese, crumbled ¼ cup halloumi cheese, shredded 10 kalamata olives, halved 2 tbsp olive oil 2 tbsp fresh parsley, chopped

DirectionsHeat the olive oil in a pan over medium heat. Add in zoodles, garlic, and spinach and cook for 5 minutes. Stir in the olives, tomatoes, feta, and parsley for 2 more minutes. Top with halloumi cheese and serve. Blue

921.   Cream of Zucchini with Avocado

Ready in about: 35 minutes | Serves: 4 Per serving: Kcal 165 Fat: 13.4g, Net Carbs: 9g, Protein: 2.2g

Ingredients

3 tsp vegetable oil 1 onion, chopped 1 carrot, sliced 1 turnip, sliced 3 cups zucchinis, chopped 1 avocado, peeled and diced Salt and black pepper to taste 4 cups vegetable broth 1 tomato, pureed

DirectionsIn a pot, warm the oil and sauté onion until translucent, about 3 minutes. Add in turnip, zucchini, and carrot and cook for 7 minutes until tender. Season with salt and black pepper. Mix in pureed tomato and vegetable broth. Bring to a boil. Simmer for 20 minutes. Lift from the heat. Add the soup and avocado to a blender. Puree until creamy and smooth. Serve warm.

922.   Roasted Brussels Sprouts with Sunflower Seeds

Ready in about: 45 minutes | Serves: 6 Per serving: Kcal: 186; Fat 17g, Net Carbs 8g, Protein 2.1g

Ingredients

¼ cup olive oil 3 lb brussels sprouts, halved Salt and black pepper to taste 1 tsp sunflower seeds 2 tbsp fresh chives, chopped Preheat oven to 390ºF.

DirectionsArrange sprout halves on a greased baking sheet. Shake in pepper, salt, sunflower seeds, and olive oil. Roast for 40 minutes until the cabbage becomes soft. Top with chives and serve.

923.   Mexican-Style Frittata

Ready in about: 25 minutes | Serves: 6 Per serving: Kcal: 225; Fat 17g, Net Carbs 5.1g, Protein 13.2g

Ingredients

10 eggs Salt and black pepper to taste ⅓ cup chive and onion cream cheese 3 tbsp butter 1 onion, chopped 1 tsp garlic paste 2 red bell peppers, chopped ½ green bell pepper, chopped 1 tsp chipotle paste 2 cups kale ½ cup cotija cheese, shredded Preheat oven to 370ºF.

DirectionsMix the eggs with onion-cream cheese, black pepper, and salt. Warm butter in a skillet over medium heat. Sauté the onion for 3 minutes until soft. Add in chipotle paste, bell peppers, and garlic paste and cook for 4 minutes. Place in kale and cook for 2 minutes. Add in the egg/cheese mixture. Spread the mixture evenly over the skillet and insert it in the oven. Bake for 8 minutes or until the frittata's top becomes golden brown but still slightly wobbly in the middle. Sprinkle with cotija cheese and bake for 3 minutes or until the cheese melts completely. Slice and serve.

924.   Roasted Vegetable & Goat Cheese Pizza

Ready in about: 45 minutes | Serves: 4 Per serving: Kcal 315, Fat 16g, Net Carbs 7.3g, Protein 12g

Ingredients

1 cauliflower pizza crust 1 sweet onion, cut into chunks 1 eggplant, cut into chunks 1 red bell pepper, cut into pieces 1 medium zucchini, cut into pieces 2 tbsp olive oil Salt and black pepper to taste ½ cup pesto sauce ½ cup goat cheese, crumbled Preheat oven to 425°F.

Directions

Bake the pizza crust in a greased baking sheet for 7 minutes. Let cool. In a bowl, mix the onion, eggplant, red bell pepper, and zucchinis with olive oil, salt, and pepper. Pour the mixture into a baking sheet and spread it well around. Bake for 30 minutes, stirring at 10 minutes intervals. Remove the veggies and set aside. Spread the pesto on the pizza crust. Arrange the roasted veggies on top and sprinkle with goat cheese. Bake the pizza for 5-6 minutes until the cheese is melted. Serve.

925.   Tuna & Monterey Jack Stuffed Avocado

Ready in about: 20 minutes | Serves: 4 Per serving: Kcal: 286; Fat 23.9g, Net Carbs 9g, Protein 11.2g

Ingredients

2 avocados, halved and pitted 4 oz Monterey Jack cheese, grated 2 oz canned tuna, flaked 2 tbsp chives, chopped Salt and black pepper to taste ½ cup curly endive, chopped Preheat oven to 360°F.

Directions

Set avocado halves in an ovenproof dish. In a mixing bowl, mix Monterey Jack cheese, chives, black pepper, salt, and tuna. Stuff the cheese/tuna mixture in avocado halves. Bake for 15 minutes or until the top is golden brown. Serve with curly endive for garnish.

926.   Italian-Style Roasted Butternut Squash Cups

Ready in about: 40 minutes | Serves: 4 Per serving: Kcal 155; Fat: 12.7g, Carbs 6.2g, Protein: 4.6g

Ingredients

2 lb butternut squash, sliced 2 tbsp coconut oil, melted ¼ cup fresh basil, chopped 1 cup heavy cream ½ cup buttermilk 1 cup ricotta cheese, crumbled 2 tsp powdered unflavored gelatin 1 tbsp fresh rosemary, chopped Celery salt to taste ¼ tsp onion flakes ½ tsp fennel seeds ½ tsp cayenne pepper Preheat oven to 360°F.

Directions

Place the squash slices in a baking dish and sprinkle with coconut oil and celery salt. Toss to coat. Roast for 30 minutes. Het a pan on low heat, add in the rest of the ingredients. Cook until heated through, about 3-4 minutes. Transfer to a food processor, add in the roasted squash, and pulse to obtain a smooth and creamy mixture. Fold in pureed squash and stir to mix well. Ladle the mixture into ramekins. Refrigerate overnight. Flip the ramekin onto serving plates.

927.   Sopressata & Cheese Bake

Ready in about: 1 hour | Serves: 4 Per serving: Kcal 334; Fat: 23g, Net Carbs: 6.2g, Protein: 25.5g

Ingredients

8 eggs Salt to taste 1 cup cheddar cheese, grated ½ cup goat cheese 1 bell pepper, chopped 1 poblano pepper, chopped ½ tsp dried dill weed 1 tsp mustard 4 slices soppressata, chopped 4 slices pancetta, chopped 6 cups hot water Preheat oven to 360°F.

Directions

Beat the eggs in a bowl, add cheddar, mustard, and salt and mix to incorporate everything. Place the mixture in a greased casserole. Stir in the remaining ingredients. Set a roasting pan with hot water in the middle of the oven. Insert the casserole dish into the roasting pan. Bake for around 1 hour. Let cool for some minutes before cutting into squares. Serve while warm!

928.   Chorizo & Emmental Baked Eggs

Ready in about: 20 minutes | Serves: 4 Per serving: Kcal 444; Fat: 35.3g, Net Carbs: 2.7g, Protein: 29.8g

Ingredients

2 tbsp olive oil 4 slices chorizo, chopped ½ cup chives, chopped 10 broccoli florets, chopped 1 clove garlic, minced 1 tsp fines herbes ¼ cup vegetable broth 4 eggs 1 ½ cups Emmental cheese, grated

Directions

Warm the oil in a pan over medium heat. Add the chorizo and cook for 4 minutes until brown; set aside. In the same pan, add the chives, garlic, and broccoli and sauté for 3 minutes until soft as you stir occasionally. Stir in broth and fines herbes and cook for 6 more minutes. Make 4 holes in the mixture until you are able to see the bottom of your pan. Crack an egg into each hole. Spread cheese over the top and cook for 6 more minutes. Scatter the reserved chorizo over and serve.

929.   Cauli Mac & Cheese

Ready in about: 15 minutes | Serves: 4 Per serving: Kcal 357; Fat: 32.5g, Net Carbs: 10.9g, Protein: 8.4g

Ingredients

1 head cauliflower, cut into florets 2 tbsp ghee, melted Salt and black pepper to taste ½ cup crème fraiche ½ cup half-and-half 1 cup cream cheese ½ tsp turmeric powder 1 tsp garlic paste ½ tsp onion flakes Preheat oven to 450°F.

Directions

 Shake cauliflower florets with melted ghee, salt, and black pepper. Arrange on a greased baking sheet and roast for 15 minutes. In a saucepan over medium heat, pour the remaining ingredients and heat through, stirring frequently. Reduce heat to low and simmer for 2-3 minutes until thickened. Coat the cauliflower florets in the cheese sauce and serve immediately in serving bowls.

930. Chicken Meatloaf Cups with Pancetta

Ready in about: 30 minutes | Serves: 6 Per serving: Kcal 276, Fat: 18.3g, Net Carbs: 1.2g, Protein: 29.2g

Ingredients

2 tbsp onion, chopped 1 tsp garlic, minced 1 lb ground chicken 2 oz cooked pancetta, chopped 1 egg, beaten 1 tsp mustard Salt and black pepper to taste ½ tsp crushed red pepper flakes 1 tsp dried basil ½ tsp dried oregano 4 oz cheddar cheese, cubed

Directions

In a bowl, mix mustard, onion, ground chicken, egg, pancetta, and garlic. Season with oregano, red pepper, black pepper, basil, and salt. Split the mixture into greased muffin cups. Lower one cube of cheddar cheese into each meatloaf cup. Close the top to cover the cheese. Bake in the oven at 345°F for 20 minutes, or until the meatloaf cups become golden brown. Let cool for 10 minutes before transferring from the muffin pan. Serve. Spicy Cheese Chips Ready in about: 18 minutes | Serves: 2 Per serving: Kcal: 100; Fat 8g, Net Carbs 0g, Protein 7g 3 cups cheddar cheese, grated ⅓ tsp salt ½ tsp garlic powder ½ tsp cayenne pepper ½ tsp dried rosemary ⅓ tsp chili powder Preheat oven to 420°F. Line a parchment paper on a baking sheet. Mix the grated cheddar cheese with spices in a bowl. Create 2 tablespoons of cheese mixture into small mounds on the baking sheet. Bake for about 15 minutes; allow to cool to harden the chips.

931. Gingery Tuna Mousse

Ready in about: 20 minutes + chilling time | Serves: 4 Per serving: Kcal 100; Fat: 5.8g, Net Carbs: 4.1g, Protein: 8g

Ingredients

1 ½ tsp gelatin, powdered 2 oz ricotta cheese 3 tbsp mayonnaise 1 tsp mustard 3 oz canned tuna, flaked ¼ cup onions, chopped 1 garlic clove, minced Salt and black pepper to taste ⅓ tsp ginger, grated

Directions

Cover the gelatin with cold water in a small bowl. Let dissolve for 5 minutes. Set a pan over medium heat and warm ricotta cheese. Place in gelatin and mix to blend well; let the mixture cool. Place in the other ingredients and stir. Split the mixture among 4 mousse molds and refrigerate overnight. Invert the molds over a platter to serve.

932. Italian Cakes with Gorgonzola & Salami

Ready in about: 25 minutes | Serves: 4 Per serving: Kcal 240, Fat: 15.3g, Net Carbs: 10g, Protein: 16.1g

Ingredients

3 slices salami 4 eggs, beaten ½ cup coconut flour 1 cup gorgonzola cheese, crumbled A pinch of salt ½ tsp grated nutmeg

Directions

Place a frying pan over medium heat. Add in salami and cook as you turn with tongs until browned. Place on paper towels to absorb the excess fat. Chop the salami and stir with the other ingredients to mix. Grease cake molds. Fill them with batter (¾ full). Set oven to 390°F and bake for 15 minutes. Serve.

933. Crêpes with Lemon-Buttery Syrup

Ready in about: 25 minutes | Serves: 6 Per serving: Kcal 243, Fat: 19.6g, Net Carbs: 5.5g, Protein: 11g

Ingredients

Crêpes 6 oz mascarpone cheese, softened 6 eggs 1 ½ tbsp granulated swerve sugar ¼ cup almond flour 1 tsp baking soda 1 tsp baking powder Syrup ¾ cup water 2 tbsp lemon juice 1 tbsp butter ¾ cup swerve, powdered 1 tbsp vanilla extract ½ tsp xanthan gum

Directions

In a bowl, beat the mascarpone cheese, eggs, swerve sugar, almond flour, baking soda, and baking powder with an electric mixer until well incorporated. Let sit for 5-10 minutes. Heat pan over medium heat and grease it with butter. Pour in a ladleful of the batter. Swirl the pan quickly to spread the dough around the skillet and cook the crepe until the edges start to brown, about 2 minutes. Flip over and cook the other side for 2 minutes. Repeat with the remaining batter. In the same pan, mix swerve sugar, butter, and water. Simmer for 6 minutes as you stir. Transfer the mixture to a blender with a ¼ teaspoon of xanthan gum and vanilla and mix well. Place in the remaining xanthan gum, lemon juice, and allow to sit until the syrup is thick. Pour over the crepes and serve.

934. Chili Egg Pickles

Ready in about: 20 minutes | Serves: 4 Per serving: Kcal: 145; Fat 9g, Net Carbs 2.8g, Protein 11.4g

Ingredients

8 eggs ½ cup onions, sliced 2 cardamom pods ½ tsp chili powder 1 tsp fennel seeds 2 clove garlic, sliced 1 cup vinegar 1 ¼ cups water 1 tbsp salt

Directions

Boil eggs in salted water until hard-cooked, about 10 minutes. Rinse them under running water, peel, and discard the shells. Place the peeled eggs onto a large jar. Set a pan over medium heat. Stir in all remaining ingredients and bring to a boil. Reduce heat to low and allow to simmer for 6 minutes. Spoon the mixture into the jar. Store in the refrigerator for up to 2 to 3 weeks.

935. Cheese & Pumpkin Chicken Meatballs

Ready in about: 35 minutes | Serves: 4 Per serving: Kcal 378; Fat: 24.5g, Net Carbs: 4.7g, Protein: 36g

Ingredients

1 egg, beaten 1 ½ lb ground chicken ½ cup pumpkin, grated 2 garlic cloves, minced 1 onion, chopped 1 tbsp Italian mixed herbs Salt and black pepper to taste 2 tbsp olive oil 1 cup cheddar cheese, shredded Preheat oven to 360°F.

Directions

Combine all the ingredients, excluding the cheddar cheese. Form meatballs from the mixture and set them on a parchment-lined baking sheet. Bake for 25 minutes, flipping once. Spread cheese over the balls and bake for 7 more minutes or until all cheese melts. Serve.

936. Baked Chicken Legs with Cheesy Spread

Ready in about: 45 minutes | Serves: 4 Per serving: Kcal 119; Fat: 10.5g, Net Carbs: 1.1g, Protein: 5.1g

Ingredients

4 chicken legs ¼ cup goat cheese 2 tbsp sour cream 1 tbsp butter, softened 1 onion, chopped Sea Salt and black pepper to taste Preheat oven to 360°F and season the legs with salt and black pepper.

DirectionsRoast in a greased baking dish for 25-30 minutes until crispy and browned. In a mixing bowl, mix the rest of the ingredients to form the spread. Scatter the spread over the chicken and serve with green salad.

937. One-Pot Cheesy Cauliflower & Bacon

Ready in about: 15 minutes | Serves: 4 Per serving: Kcal 323, Fat: 24g, Net Carbs: 7.4g, Protein: 18.8g

Ingredients

2 tbsp butter ½ lb bacon, cut into strips 1 head cauliflower, cut into florets ¼ cup sour cream ¾ cup heavy whipping cream 1 tsp garlic puree 2 tbsp apple cider vinegar ½ cup queso fresco, crumbled

DirectionsSet a frying pan over medium heat and melt the butter; brown the bacon for 3 minutes. Set aside. Add in cauliflower and cook until tender, about 4-5 minutes. Add in the whipping and sour cream, then the vinegar and garlic, and cook until warmed fully. Take the reserved bacon back to the pan. Fold in queso fresco and cook for 2 minutes, or until cheese melts.

938. Cilantro & Chili Omelet

Ready in about: 15 minutes | Serves: 2 Per serving: Kcal 319; Fat: 25g, Net Carbs: 10g, Protein: 14.9g

Ingredients

1 tsp butter 1 spring onion, chopped 1 spring garlic, chopped 4 eggs ¼ cup sour cream 1 tomato, sliced ½ green chili pepper, minced 1 tbsp fresh cilantro, chopped Salt and black pepper to taste

DirectionsSet a pan over high heat and warm the butter. Sauté garlic and onion until tender, about 3 minutes. Whisk the eggs with sour cream. Pour into the pan and use a spatula to smooth the surface. Cook until eggs become puffy and brown to bottom. Add cilantro, chili pepper, and tomato to one side of the omelet. Season with black pepper and salt. Fold the omelet in half and slice into wedges.

939. Cajun Crabmeat Frittata

Ready in about: 25 minutes | Serves: 4 Per serving: Kcal 265; Fat: 15.8g, Net Carbs: 7.1g, Protein: 22.9g

Ingredients

2 tbsp olive oil 1 shallot, chopped 4 oz crabmeat, chopped 1 tsp cajun seasoning 6 large eggs, slightly beaten ½ cup Greek yogurt Preheat oven to 350°F.

Directions

Set a large skillet over medium heat and warm the oil. Add in shallot and sauté until soft, about 3 minutes. Stir in crabmeat and cook for 2 more minutes. Season with cajun seasoning. Whisk the eggs with yogurt. Transfer to the skillet. Set the skillet in the oven and bake for about 18 minutes or until eggs are cooked through. Slice into wedges and serve warm.

940. Zucchini with Blue Cheese & Walnuts

Ready in about: 15 minutes | Serves: 4 Per serving: Kcal 489; Fat: 47.4g, Net Carbs: 6.9g, Protein: 12.7g

Ingredients

2 tbsp olive oil 2 lb zucchinis, sliced 1 ⅓ cups heavy cream 1 cup sour cream 4 oz blue cheese, crumbled 1 tsp Italian seasoning ¼ cup walnut halves Salt and black pepper to taste

Directions

Set a grill pan over medium heat. Season zucchinis with Italian seasoning, salt, and black pepper and drizzle with olive oil. Grill the zucchini until lightly charred. Remove to a serving platter. In a dry pan over medium heat, toast the walnuts for 2-3 minutes and set aside. Add the heavy cream, blue cheese, and sour cream to the pan and mix until everything is well combined. Let cool for a few minutes and scatter over the grilled zucchini. Top with walnuts and serve.

941. Three-Cheese Fondue with Walnuts & Parsley

Ready in about: 15 minutes | Serves: 10 Per serving: Kcal 148; Fat: 10.2g, Net Carbs: 1.5g, Protein: 9.3g

Ingredients

½ lb brie cheese, chopped ⅓ lb Swiss cheese, shredded ½ cup Emmental cheese, grated 1 tbsp xanthan gum ½ tsp onion powder ¾ cup white wine ½ tbsp lemon juice Black pepper to taste 1 cup walnuts, chopped

Directions

In a skillet, thoroughly mix onion powder, brie, Emmental, Swiss cheese, and xanthan gum. Pour in lemon juice and wine and sprinkle with black pepper. Set the skillet under the broiler for 6-7 minutes until the cheese browns. Garnish with walnuts. Serve.

942. Pureed Broccoli with Roquefort Cheese

Ready in about: 15 minutes | Serves: 4 Per serving: Kcal 294, Fat: 24.7g, Net Carbs: 4.3g, Protein: 9.2g

Ingredients

1 ½ lb broccoli, broken into florets 2 tbsp butter 1 garlic clove, minced 1 cup almond milk ½ cup Roquefort cheese, crumbled 2 tbsp almond flour

Directions

Warm the butter in a saucepan over low heat and stir in the almond flour for 2 minutes. Remove from the heat. Using a whisk, slowly stir in the almond milk. Return to the heat and bring to a simmer. Add in the cheese and cook for 1-2 minutes until the cheese melts. Set aside covered. Place salted water in a deep pan over medium heat. Add in broccoli and Boil for 8 minutes. Drain and remove to a food processor. Add in the cheese mixture and blend until smooth and creamy. Serve.

943. Juicy Beef Cheeseburgers

Ready in about: 20 minutes | Serves: 6 Per serving: Kcal 252; Fat: 15.5g, Net Carbs: 1.2g, Protein: 26g

Ingredients

1 lb ground beef ½ cup green onions, chopped 2 garlic cloves, finely chopped Salt and black pepper to taste ¼ tsp cayenne pepper, 2 oz mascarpone cheese 3 oz Pecorino Romano cheese, grated 2 tbsp olive oil

Directions

In a mixing bowl, mix ground beef, garlic, cayenne pepper, black pepper, green onions, and salt. Shape into 6 balls; then flatten to make burgers. In a separate bowl, mix mascarpone cheese with grated Pecorino Romano cheeses. Split the cheese mixture among prepared patties. Wrap the meat mixture around the cheese mixture to ensure that the filling is sealed inside. Warm oil in a skillet over medium heat. Cook the burgers for 5 minutes each side. Serve.

944. Goat Cheese Muffins with Ajillo Mushrooms

Ready in about: 45 minutes | Serves: 6 Per serving: Kcal 263, Fat: 22.4g, Net Carbs: 6.1g, Protein: 10g

Ingredients

1 ½ cups heavy cream 5 oz goat cheese, crumbled 3 eggs Salt and black pepper to taste 1 tbsp butter, softened 2 cups mushrooms, chopped 2 garlic cloves, minced 1 tbsp fresh parsley, chopped Preheat oven to 320°F.

Directions

Insert 6 ramekins into a large pan. Add in boiling water up to 1-inch depth. In a pan over medium heat, warm heavy cream. Reduce the heat and stir in goat cheese and cook until melted. Remove from the heat. Beat the eggs in a bowl and gradually add the cream mixture. Sprinkle with pepper and salt. Spoon the mixture into ramekins. Bake for 40 minutes. Melt butter in a pan over medium heat. Add garlic and mushrooms, season with salt and pepper, and sauté for 5 minutes until tender. Spread the ajillo mushrooms on top of each cooled muffin to serve.

945. Chili Chicken Breasts Wrapped in Bacon

Ready in about: 35 minutes | Serves: 6 Per serving: Kcal 275, Fat: 9.5g, Net Carbs: 1.3g, Protein: 44.5g

Ingredients

6 chicken breasts, flatten 2 tbsp fresh parsley, chopped 3 garlic cloves, chopped 1 chili pepper, chopped 1 tsp tarragon Salt and black pepper to taste 1 tsp hot paprika 6 slices bacon Preheat oven to 390°F.

Directions

Mix garlic, tarragon, hot paprika, salt, chili pepper, and black pepper in a bowl and rub onto the chicken. Roll the fillets in the bacon slices. Arrange on a greased and bake for 30 minutes. Plate the chicken and serve sprinkled with fresh parsley.

946. Jamon & Queso Balls

Ready in about: 15 minutes | Serves: 8 Per serving: Kcal: 168; Fat 13g, Net Carbs 2.5g, Protein 10.3g

Ingredients

1 egg 6 slices Jamon serrano, chopped 6 oz cotija cheese 6 oz Manchego cheese, grated Salt and black pepper to taste ¼ cup almond flour 1 tsp baking powder 1 tsp garlic powder Preheat oven to 420 °F.

Directions

Whisk the egg in a bowl. Place in the remaining ingredients and mix well. Split the mixture into 16 balls. Set them on a baking sheet lined with parchment paper. Bake for 13 minutes or until they turn golden brown and become crispy. Serve.

947. Fried Brie Cheese Bites

Ready in about: 15 minutes + chilling time | Serves: 4 Per serving: Kcal 625; Fat: 53.9g, Net Carbs: 0.7g, Protein: 28.7g

Ingredients

1 celery stalk, cut into julienne strips 1 cup almond flour 2 eggs, beaten ½ cup vegetable oil 1 cup pork rinds, crushed 12 oz brie cheese, cubed ½ tsp chili pepper ¼ tsp parsley flakes 1 cup hot pepper sauce

Directions

In a bowl, mix the almond flour with parsley and chili pepper. Pour the pork rinds in another one. Dip the brie cubes into the eggs first and then roll them in the almond flour mixture. Dip again in the eggs and coat with the pork rinds. Put on a plate. Warm the vegetable oil in a pan over medium heat. Fry the brie cubes in batches until golden brown on all sides, about 5 minutes. Remove to kitchen paper to soak up excess fat. Serve with hot pepper sauce and celery sticks. Serve garnished with parsley, with cranberry sauce on the side for dipping.

948. Eggs in a Mug

Ready in about: 5 minutes | Serves: 2 Per serving: Kcal 197; Fat: 13.8g, Net Carbs: 2.7g, Protein: 15.7g

Ingredients

4 eggs ¼ cup coconut milk ¼ cup cheddar cheese, grated 1 garlic clove, minced ¼ tsp dried dill ¼ tsp turmeric powder Salt to taste ¼ tsp red pepper flakes

Directions

In a mixing bowl, mix the eggs, cheddar cheese, red pepper, garlic, coconut milk, turmeric powder, and salt. Divide the mixture between 2 microwave-safe mugs. Place in the microwave for 40 seconds. Stir well and continue microwaving for 70 seconds. Sprinkle with dried dill and serve.

949.   Chorizo & Cheese Gofre

Ready in about: 20 minutes | Serves: 3 Per serving: Kcal 453, Fat: 37g, Net Carbs: 4.5g, Protein: 25.6g

Ingredients

6 eggs, separate egg whites, and egg yolks ½ tsp baking powder 6 tbsp almond flour 4 tbsp butter, melted ¼ tsp salt ½ tsp dried rosemary 3 tbsp tomato puree 3 oz smoked chorizo, chopped 3 oz cheddar cheese, shredded

Directions

In a mixing bowl, mix egg yolks, almond flour, rosemary, butter, baking powder, and salt. Beat the egg whites until pale and combine with the egg yolk mixture. Grease waffle iron and set over medium heat, add in ¼ cup of the batter and cook for 3 minutes until golden. Repeat with the remaining batter. Place one waffle back to the waffle iron. Sprinkle 1 tbsp of tomato puree to the waffle. Apply a topping of 1 ounce of cheese and 1 ounce of chorizo. Cover with another waffle and cook until all the cheese melts. Do the same with all remaining ingredients. Serve.

950.   Cheesy Bites with Turnip Chips

Ready in about: 25 minutes | Serves: 4 Per serving: Kcal 177; Fat: 12.9g, Net Carbs: 6.8g, Protein: 8.8g,

Ingredients

1 cup Monterey Jack cheese, grated ½ cup natural yogurt 1 cup Pecorino cheese, grated 2 tbsp tomato puree ½ tsp dried rosemary ½ tsp dried thyme Salt and black pepper to taste 1 lb turnips, sliced 2 tbsp olive oil

Directions

In a mixing bowl, mix cheese, tomato puree, black pepper, salt, rosemary, yogurt, and thyme. Place in foil liners-candy cups and refrigerate until ready to serve. Preheat oven to 430°F. Coat turnips with salt, black pepper, and oil. Arrange in a single layer on a cookie sheet. Bake for 20 minutes, shaking once or twice. Dip turnip chips in cheese cups.

951.   Homemade Spanish Salsa Aioli

Ready in about: 10 minutes | Serves: 6 Per serving: Kcal 116; Fat: 13.2g, Net Carbs: 0.2g, Protein: 0.4g

Ingredients

1 tbsp lemon juice 1 egg yolk, at room temperature 2 garlic cloves, crushed Salt and black pepper to taste ½ cup olive oil ¼ cup fresh parsley, chopped

Directions

In a blender, place the egg yolk, salt, lemon juice, and garlic and pulse to get a smooth and creamy mixture. Set blender to slow speed. Slowly sprinkle in olive oil and combine to ensure the oil incorporates well. Stir in parsley and black pepper. Refrigerate the mixture until ready.

952. Tuna Caprese Salad

Ready in about: 10 minutes | Serves: 4 Per serving: Kcal 360, Fat 31g, Net Carbs 1g, Protein 21g

Ingredients

2 (10 oz) cans tuna in water, drained 2 tomatoes, sliced 8 oz fresh mozzarella cheese, sliced 6 basil leaves 2 tbsp extra virgin olive oil ½ lemon, juiced Place the tuna in the center of a serving platter.

Directions

Arrange the cheese and tomato slices around the tuna. Alternate a slice of tomato, cheese, and a basil leaf. Drizzle with olive oil and lemon juice and serve.

953. Genoa Salami and Goat Cheese Waffles

(Ready in about 20 minutes | Servings 2) Per serving: 470 Calories; 40.3g Fat; 2.9g Carbs; 24.4g Protein; 0.6g Fiber

Ingredients

2 tablespoons olive oil Salt and black pepper, to your liking 1/2 teaspoon chili pepper flakes 4 eggs 1/2 cup goat cheese, crumbled 4 slices Genoa

salami, chopped

Directions

Strat by preheating your waffle iron and brush it with a nonstick cooking oil. Mix all ingredients until everything is well combined. Pour the batter into waffle iron and cook until golden and cooked through. Repeat until all the batter is used.Enjoy!

954. Mediterranean Mezze Platter

(Ready in about 20 minutes | Servings 4) Per serving: 542 Calories; 46.4g Fat; 6.2g Carbs; 23.7g Protein; 4g Fiber

Ingredients

12 ounces Halloumi cheese, cut into 1/4-1/3-inch slices 3 teaspoons olive oil 1 teaspoon Greek seasoning blend 1 tablespoon olive oil 6 eggs Sea salt and ground black pepper, to taste 1 ½ cups avocado, pitted and sliced 1 cup grape tomatoes, halved 4 tablespoons Kalamata olives

Directions

Preheat a grill pan over medium-high heat, about 395 degrees F. Grill your halloumi for about 3 minutes or until golden brown grill marks appear. Heat the oil in a nonstick skillet over moderately-high plate; scramble the eggs with a wide spatula.

955.   Anchovy and Cheese Mousse

(Ready in about 20 minutes + chilling time | Servings 5) Per serving: 100 Calories; 5.8g Fat; 4.1g Carbs; 8g Protein; 0.5g Fiber

Ingredients

3 ounces anchovies, chopped 2 ounces soft cheese 1 ½ teaspoons gelatin, powdered 1 garlic clove, minced 1 teaspoon poblano pepper, deveined and minced Sea salt and pepper, to taste 3 tablespoons water 3 tablespoons mayonnaise 1/4 cup scallions, chopped

Directions Dissolve the gelatin in water for about 10 minutes. Warm the soft cheese over low heat heat; fold in the gelatin and whisk until it is well incorporated. Let it cool to room temperature. Add in the other ingredients and mix to combine. Spoon the mixture into ramekins and place in your refrigerator until set.

956.   Pecan Cream Pie

(Ready in about 30 minutes + chilling time | Servings 6) Per serving: 305 Calories; 30.6g Fat; 4.7g Carbs; 4.6g Protein; 0.5g Fiber

Ingredients

For the Crust:

3/4 cup almond meal 1/3 cup coconut flour 1/4 cup coconut oil 1/3 cup Swerve

For the Custard:

3 egg yolks 1/3 cup almond meal 1 ¼ cups whipping cream 1/3 cup Swerve 3/4 cup water 1/2 teaspoon ground cinnamon 1 teaspoon vanilla essence For the Topping: 1 cup whipping cream 2 tablespoons pecans, chopped

Directions Microwave the coconut oil; add in 1/3 cup of Swerve and whisk until it has dissolved completely. Stir in the almond meal and coconut flour and mix again. Press the crust mixture into the bottom of a parchment-lined baking pan. Place in your refrigerator to harden. Melt the whipping cream and egg yolks until everything is well incorporated. Whisk in the remaining ingredients for custard. Spread the custard mixture over the crust and place in your refrigerator for at least 1 hour. Beat 1 cup of whipping cream using an electric mixer until peaks are completely stiff. Top your pie with the cream and garnish with chopped pecans.Bon appétit!

957.   Decadent Omelet with Blueberries

(Ready in about 10 minutes | Servings 1) Per serving: 488 Calories; 42g Fat; 8g Carbs; 15.3g Protein; 0.3g Fiber

Ingredients

2 eggs, whisked 2 tablespoons double cream 1/2 teaspoon ground cardamom 1 tablespoon coconut oil 2 tablespoons soft cheese 6 fresh blueberries, sliced

Directions

Beat the eggs with the cream and cardamom until well combined. In a saucepan, melt the coconut oil over a medium-high flame. Now, cook the egg mixture for 3 to 4 minutes.Bon appétit!

958.   Pizza Dipping Sauce

(Ready in about 20 minutes | Servings 10) Per serving: 160 Calories; 12.7g Fat; 2.4g Carbs; 8.9g Protein; 0.8g Fiber

Ingredients

8 ounces pepperoni, chopped 1 cup marinara sauce 1 teaspoon dried basil Salt and black pepper, to taste 1/2 cup black olives, to garnish 1/2 teaspoon cayenne pepper 1/2 teaspoon dried oregano 8 ounces cream cheese, room

temperature 2 ounces Parmesan cheese, shredded

Directions

Begin by preheating your oven to 365 degrees F. Mix the cheese, marinara sauce, and spices in a bowl. Place the mixture in a lightly oiled baking dish. Top with the pepperoni and olives and bake for 15 to 18 minutes or until hot and bubbly on top.Enjoy!

959.   Cheese Chicken Tenders

(Ready in about 20 minutes | Servings 4) Per serving: 416 Calories; 26g Fat; 3.2g Carbs; 40.7g Protein; 0.3g Fiber

Ingredients

1 pound chicken tenders 1 tablespoon butter 1/3 cup chicken stock 2 tablespoon tomato paste 1 cup Cheddar cheese, shredded 1 teaspoon garlic, minced 1/2 cup double cheese

Directions

In a frying pan, melt the butter over a moderately-high flame; cook the chicken for 5 to 6 minutes until no longer pink. Add in the garlic and continue to sauté for 1 minuet or so; reserve. Cook the cream, stock, and tomato paste until it has reduced by half. Remove from the heat. Add in the reserved chicken and garlic; scatter the cheese over the top. Cover and let it sit for about 10 minutes.Bon appétit!

960.   Comte Cheese Custard with Chanterelles

(Ready in about 45 minutes | Servings 6) Per serving: 263 Calories; 22.4g Fat; 6.1g Carbs; 10g Protein; 0.2g Fiber

Ingredients

1 tablespoon ghee, room temperature 4 ounces Chanterelle mushrooms, chopped 1/2 teaspoon fresh garlic, minced 1 ½ cups double cream 4 ounces Comté cheese, crumbled 3 eggs, whisked Salt and pepper, to taste

Directions

Melt the cream and add in the cheese; stir until melted. Add in the whisked eggs, salt, and pepper; continue to stir for about 2 minutes or until well combined. Spoon the mixture into 6 ramekins; place the ramekins into a large pan with hot water (depth of about 1-inch). Bake in the preheated oven at 310 degrees F for about 35 minutes or until set. Sauté the mushrooms in hot ghee until they release liquid; add in the garlic and continue to sauté a minute more or until aromatic. Top each custard with sautéed chanterelles.Enjoy!

961. Classic Egg, Chèvre and Salami Breakfast

(Ready in about 5 minutes | Servings 3) Per serving: 303 Calories; 22.4g Fat; 3.6g Carbs; 21.6g Protein; 0.4g Fiber

Ingredients

3 teaspoons olive oil 3 slices salami, chopped Salt and pepper, to taste 1 teaspoon deli mustard 6 eggs 1/2 cup Chèvre cheese, shredded 1/2 cup soft cheese Salt and pepper, to taste

Directions

Brush three mason jars with olive oil. Crack two eggs into each jar. Add the other ingredients to your jars and cover them. Shake until everything is well combined. Uncover and microwave for 2 minutes on high.

962. Smoked Fish Pâté

(Ready in about 10 minutes + chilling time | Servings 12) Per serving: 64 Calories; 2.9g Fat; 1.3g Carbs; 7.9g Protein; 0.2g Fiber

Ingredients

3/4 cup soft cheese 2 ounces coriander, finely chopped Salt and pepper, to taste 1/2 teaspoon cayenne pepper 2 tablespoons butter 1/2 teaspoon deli mustard 12 ounces smoked salmon, skinned, deboned, and flaked

Directions

Pulse all of the above ingredients in your food processor and place in your refrigerator.

963. Fluffy Almond Bars

(Ready in about 20 minutes | Servings 4) Per serving: 278 Calories; 30.1g Fat; 2.2g Carbs; 2.2g Protein; 0.1g Fiber

Ingredients

1 cup whipped cream 2 tablespoons almond butter 1/2 cup almonds, chopped 1/4 teaspoon nutmeg 1/4 teaspoon cinnamon 2 tablespoons butter

Directions Beat the cream with nutmeg and cardamom, and spread the mixture on the bottom of a foil-lined baking pan. Then, mix the regular butter and almond butter. Spread this mixture over the creamed mixture. Scatter the chopped almonds over the top. Cut into bars.Enjoy!

964. Breakfast Nut Granola & Smoothie Bowl

Ready in about: 5 minutes | Serves: 4 Per serving: Kcal 361, Fat 31.2g, Net Carbs 2g, Protein 13g

Ingredients

6 cups Greek yogurt 4 tbsp almond butter A handful toasted walnuts 3 tbsp unsweetened cocoa powder 4 tsp swerve brown sugar 2 cups nut granola for topping

Directions

Combine the Greek yogurt, almond butter, walnuts, cocoa powder, and swerve brown sugar in a smoothie maker. Puree at high speed until smooth and well mixed. Share the smoothie into four breakfast bowls, top with a half cup of granola each one, and serve.

965.   Chocolate Protein Coconut Shake

Ready in about: 5 minutes | Serves: 4 Per serving: Kcal 265, Fat: 15.5g, Net Carbs: 4g, Protein: 12g

Ingredients

3 cups flax milk, chilled 3 tsp unsweetened cocoa powder 1 medium avocado, peeled, sliced 1 cup coconut milk, chilled 3 mint leaves + extra to garnish 3 tbsp erythritol 1 tbsp low carb protein powder Whipping cream for topping

Directions

Combine the flax milk, cocoa powder, avocado, coconut milk, 3 mint leaves, erythritol, and protein powder into the smoothie maker, and blend for 1 minute to smooth. Pour the drink into serving glasses, lightly add some whipping cream on top, and garnish with 1 or 2 mint leaves. Serve immediately.

966.   Chocolate Smoothie

Ready in about: 10 minutes | Serves: 2 Per serving: Kcal 335; Fat: 31.7g Net Carbs: 12.7g, Protein:

Ingredients

7g ½ cup pecans ¾ cup coconut milk ¼ cup water 4 oz watercress 1 tsp low carb protein powder 1 tbsp chia seeds 1 tbsp unsweetened cocoa powder 4 fresh dates, pitted

Directions

In a blender, add all ingredients and process until creamy and uniform. Chill and serve in glasses.

967.   Almond Waffles with Cinnamon Cream

Ready in about: 25 minutes | Serves: 6 Per serving: Kcal 307, Fat 24g, Net Carbs 8g, Protein 12g

Ingredients

Cinnamon cream 8 oz cream cheese, softened 1 tsp cinnamon powder 3 tbsp swerve brown sugar 2 tbsp cinnamon Waffles 5 tbsp butter, melted 1 ½ cups unsweetened almond milk 7 large eggs ¼ tsp liquid stevia ½ tsp baking powder 1 ½ cups almond flour

Directions

Combine cream cheese, cinnamon, and swerve with a mixer until smooth. Cover and chill until ready to use. To make the waffles, whisk the butter, milk, and eggs in a medium bowl. Add the stevia and baking powder and mix. Stir in the almond flour and combine until no lumps exist. Let the batter sit for 5 minutes to thicken. Spritz a waffle iron with a cooking spray. Ladle a ¼ cup of the batter into the waffle iron and cook according to the manufacturer's instructions until golden, about 10 minutes in total. Repeat with the remaining batter. Slice the waffles into quarters. Apply the cinnamon spread in between each of two waffles and snap. Serve.

968.   Avocado & Kale Eggs

Ready in about: 20 minutes | Serves: 4 Per serving: Kcal 274, Fat 23g, Net Carbs 4g, Protein 13g

Ingredients

2 tbsp ghee 1 red onion, sliced 4 oz chorizo, cut into thin rounds 1 cup kale, chopped 1 ripe avocado, peeled and chopped 4 eggs Preheat oven to 370°F.

Directions

Melt ghee in a cast iron pan over medium heat and sauté the onion for 2 minutes. Add the chorizo and cook for 2 minutes more, stirring occasionally. Introduce the kale with a splash of water, stir, and cook for 3 minutes until it is wilted. Mix in the avocado and turn the heat off. Create four holes in the mixture, crack the eggs into each hole, and slide the pan into the preheated oven. Bake for 6 minutes until the egg whites are set or firm and yolks still runny. Serve right away.

969.   Ricotta Cloud Pancakes with Whipped Cream

Ready in about: 20 minutes | Serves: 4 Per serving: Kcal 407, Fat 30.6g, Net Carbs 6.6g, Protein 11.5g

Ingredients

1 cup almond flour 1 tsp baking powder 2 ½ tbsp erythritol ⅓ tsp salt 1 ¼ cups ricotta cheese ⅓ cup coconut milk 2 large eggs 1 cup heavy whipping cream

Directions

In a bowl, whisk the almond flour, baking powder, erythritol, and salt. Crack the eggs into the blender and process for 30 seconds. Add the ricotta cheese, continue processing it, and gradually pour the coconut milk in while you keep on blending. In about 90 seconds, the mixture will be creamy and smooth. Pour it into the dry ingredients and whisk to combine. Set a skillet over medium heat and let it heat for a minute. Then, fetch a soup spoonful of mixture into the skillet and cook it for 1 minute. Flip the pancake and cook further for 1 minute. Remove onto a plate and repeat the cooking process until the batter is exhausted. Serve the pancakes with whipping cream.

970.   Giant Egg Quiche

Ready in about: 60 minutes | Serves: 6 Per serving: Kcal 485, Fat 39.7g, Net Carbs 6.3g, Protein 24.5g

Ingredients

12 eggs, beaten 1 ½ cups cheddar cheese, shredded 1 ½ cups almond milk ½ tsp dried thyme Salt to taste ¼ cup mushrooms, sliced ½ cup broccoli, chopped 1 clove garlic, minced Quiche crust ¾ cup almond flour A pinch of salt 2 oz cold butter ½ tsp baking powder 1 tbsp cold water 2 eggs Preheat oven to 370⁰F.

Directions

In a bowl, mix all the crust ingredients until dough is formed. Press it into a greased baking dish and bake for 20-25 minutes until lightly golden. Spread the cheddar cheese on the crust. Mix the eggs, almond milk, thyme, salt, mushrooms, broccoli, and garlic in a bowl. Pour the ingredients over the pie crust and bake in the oven for 35 minutes until the quiche is set. Remove and serve sliced.

971.   Cauliflower & Cheese Burgers

Ready in about: 35 minutes | Serves: 6 Per serving: Kcal 416; Fat: 33.8g, Net Carbs: 7.8g, Protein: 13g

Ingredients

3 tbsp olive oil 1 onion, chopped 1 garlic clove, minced 1 lb cauliflower, grated 6 tbsp coconut flour ½ cup gruyere cheese, shredded 1 cup Parmesan cheese, grated 2 eggs, beaten Sea salt and black pepper to taste

Directions

Warm the olive oil in a skillet over medium heat. Add in garlic and onion and cook until soft, about 3 minutes. Stir in cauliflower and cook for a minute. Allow cooling and set aside. Add in the rest of the ingredients. Form balls from the mixture, then press them to form burger patties. Preheat oven to 400⁰F. Bake the burgers for 20 minutes, flipping once until the top is golden brown. Serve warm.

972. Carrot Zucchini Bread

Ready in about: 70 minutes | Serves: 4 Per serving: Kcal 175, Fat 10.5g, Net Carbs 1.8g, Protein 11.6g

Ingredients

1 cup shredded carrots 1 cup shredded zucchini, squeezed ⅓ cup coconut flour 1 tsp vanilla extract 6 eggs 1 tbsp coconut oil ¾ tsp baking soda 1 tbsp cinnamon powder ½ tsp salt ½ cup Greek yogurt 1 tsp apple cider vinegar ½ tsp nutmeg powder Preheat the oven to 350°F.

Directions

Mix the carrots, zucchini, coconut flour, vanilla extract, eggs, coconut oil, baking soda, cinnamon, salt, Greek yogurt, vinegar, and nutmeg. Pour the batter into a greased loaf pan. Bake for 55 minutes. Remove the bread after and let cool for 5 minutes. Preserve the bread and use it for toasts, sandwiches, or served with soups and salads.

973. Cheesy Zucchini Balls with Bacon

Ready in about: 20 minutes + chilling time | Serves: 6 Per serving: Kcal 407; Fat: 26.8g, Net Carbs: 5.8g, Protein: 33.4g

Ingredients

2 lb zucchinis, chopped ½ lb bacon, chopped 6 oz cottage cheese, crumbled 6 oz cream cheese, softened 1 cup fontina cheese, grated ½ cup dill pickles, chopped 2 cloves garlic, crushed 1 cup Parmesan cheese, grated ½ tsp caraway seeds ¼ cup olive oil Salt and black pepper to taste 1 cup pork rinds, crushed

Directions

In a bowl, mix zucchini, cottage cheese, dill pickles, ½ cup of Parmesan cheese, garlic, cream cheese, bacon, and fontina cheese until well combined. Shape the mixture into balls. Refrigerate for 3 hours. In another bowl, mix the remaining Parmesan cheese, pork rinds, black pepper, caraway seeds, and salt. Remove the balls from the fridge and roll them in the Parmesan mixture. Warm the olive oil in a skillet over medium heat. Fry the balls until browned on all sides. Set on a paper towel to soak up any excess oil.

974. Mushroom & Cheese Lettuce Wraps

Ready in about: 20 minutes | Serves: 4 Per serving: Kcal 472; Fat: 44g, Net Carbs: 5.4g, Protein: 19.5g

Ingredients

Wraps 6 eggs 2 tbsp almond milk 1 tbsp olive oil Sea salt to taste Filling 2 tbsp olive oil 1 cup mushrooms, sliced ½ tsp cayenne pepper 8 fresh lettuce leaves 4 gruyere cheese slices 2 tomatoes, sliced

Directions

Mix all the ingredients for the wraps thoroughly. Set a frying pan over medium heat. Add in ¼ of the mixture and cook for 4 minutes on both sides. Do the same with the remaining mixture. Set aside. In the same pan, warm the remaining olive oil over medium heat. Cook the mushrooms for 5 minutes until they are browned and softened. Stir in cayenne pepper, black pepper, and salt. Set 2 lettuce leaves onto every egg wrap and top with the mushrooms. Arrange the tomato and cheese slices on top to serve.

975. Italian Sausage Stacks

Ready in about: 20 minutes | Serves: 6 Per serving: Kcal 378, Fat 23g, Net Carbs 5g, Protein 16g

Ingredients

6 Italian sausage patties 4 tbsp olive oil 2 ripe avocados, pitted Salt and black pepper to taste 6 fresh eggs Red pepper flakes to garnish

Directions In a skillet, warm the oil over medium heat and fry the sausage patties about 8 minutes until lightly browned and firm. Remove the patties to a plate. Spoon the avocado into a bowl and mash it with a fork. Season with salt and black pepper. Spread the mash on the sausages. Boil 3 cups of water in a wide pan over high heat and reduce to simmer (don't boil). Crack each egg into a small bowl and gently put the egg into the simmering water. Poach for 2-3 minutes. Use a perforated spoon to remove from the water on a paper towel to dry. Repeat with the other 5 eggs. Top each stack with a poached egg and sprinkle with chili flakes. Serve with turnip wedges.

976. Cheese & Aioli Eggs

Ready in about: 20 minutes | Serves: 4 Per serving: Kcal: 355; Fat 22.5g, Net Carbs 1.8g, Protein 29.5g

Ingredients 4 eggs, hard-boiled and chopped 14 oz tuna in brine, drained ¼ lettuce head, torn into pieces 2 green onions, finely chopped ½ cup feta cheese, crumbled ⅓ cup sour cream Aioli 1 cup mayonnaise 2 cloves garlic, minced 1 tbsp lemon juice Salt and black pepper to taste

Directions Set the eggs in a serving bowl. Place in tuna, onion, feta cheese, lettuce, and sour cream. In a bowl, mix the mayonnaise, lemon juice, and garlic. Season with salt and pepper. Pour the aioli into the serving bowl and stir to incorporate everything. Serve with pickles.

977. Baked Quail Eggs in Avocados

Ready in about: 15 minutes | Serves: 4 Per serving: Kcal 234, Fat 19.1g, Net Carbs 2.2g, Protein 8.2g

Ingredients

2 large avocados, halved and pitted 4 small eggs Salt and black pepper to taste Preheat oven to 400°F.

Directions Crack the quail eggs into the avocado halves and place them on a greased baking sheet. Bake the filled avocados in the oven for 8-10 minutes until eggs are cooked. Season and serve.

978. Mascarpone Snapped Amaretti Biscuits

Ready in about: 25 minutes | Serves: 6 Per serving: Kcal 165, Fat 13g, Net Carbs 3g, Protein 9g

Ingredients

egg whites 1 egg yolk, beaten 1 tsp vanilla bean paste 4 tbsp swerve sugar A pinch of salt ¼ cup ground fragrant almonds 1 lemon juice 7 tbsp sugar-free amaretto liquor ¼ cup mascarpone cheese ¼ cup butter, room temperature ¾ cup swerve confectioner's sugar Peheat oven to 300°F.

Directions Line a baking sheet with parchment paper. In a bowl, beat egg whites, salt, and vanilla paste with a hand mixer while you gradually spoon in the swerve sugar until stiff. Add in almonds and fold in the egg yolk, lemon juice, and amaretto liquor. Spoon mixture into a piping bag. Press out 50 mounds on the baking sheet. Bake the biscuits for 15 minutes until golden brown. Transfer to a wire rack to cool. Whisk the mascarpone cheese, butter, and swerve confectioner's sugar with the cleaned electric mixer. Spread a scoop of mascarpone cream onto the case of half of the biscuits and snap with the remaining biscuits. Dust with some swerve confectioner's sugar and serve.

979. Cheese Stuffed Avocados

Ready in about: 20 minutes | Serves: 4 Per serving: Kcal 342; Fat: 30.4g, Net Carbs: 7.5g, Protein: 11.1g

Ingredients

3 avocados, halved, pitted, skin on ½ cup feta cheese, crumbled ½ cup cheddar cheese, grated 2 eggs, beaten Salt and black pepper to taste 1 tbsp fresh basil, chopped Preheat oven to 360°F.

Directions

Lay avocado halves in a baking dish. In a bowl, mix both types of cheeses, pepper, eggs, and salt. Split the mixture into the avocado halves. Bake for 15 minutes. Top with basil and serve.

980. Cheese Ciabatta with Pepperoni

Ready in about: 30 minutes | Serves: 6 Per serving: Kcal 464, Fat: 33.6g, Net Carbs: 9.1g, Protein: 31.1g

Ingredients

10 oz cream cheese, melted 2 ½ cups mozzarella, shredded 4 large eggs, beaten 3 tbsp Romano cheese, grated ½ cup pork rinds, crushed 2 tsp baking powder ½ cup tomato puree 12 pepperoni slices

Directions

In a bowl, combine eggs, mozzarella cheese, cream cheese, baking powder, pork rinds, and Romano cheese. Form into 6 chiabatta shapes. Set a pan over medium heat. Cook each ciabatta for 2 minutes per side. Sprinkle tomato puree over each one and top with pepperoni slices to serve.

981. Breakfast Buttered Eggs

Ready in about: 15 minutes | Serves: 2 Per serving: Kcal 321, Fat: 21.5g, Net Carbs: 2.5g, Protein: 12.8g

Ingredients

1 tbsp coconut oil 1 tbsp butter 1 tsp fresh thyme, chopped 4 eggs 1 garlic clove, minced 1 tsp fresh parsley, chopped ¼ tsp cumin ¼ tsp cayenne pepper Salt and black pepper to taste

Directions

Put the coconut oil and butter in a skillet over medium heat. Add in the garlic and thyme and cook for 30 seconds. Sprinkle with parsley and cook for 2 minutes, until crisp. Carefully crack the eggs into the skillet. Lower the heat and cook for 4-6 minutes. Season with salt, black pepper, cumin, and cayenne pepper. When the eggs are just set, turn the heat off and serve.

982. Hashed Zucchini & Bacon Breakfast

Ready in about: 25 minutes | Serves: 2 Per serving: Kcal 340, Fat: 26.8g, Net Carbs: 6.6g, Protein: 17.4g

Ingredients

1 medium zucchini, diced 2 bacon slices 2 eggs 1 tbsp coconut oil ½ small onion, chopped 1 tbsp fresh parsley, chopped

Directions

Place the bacon in a skillet and cook for 5 minutes until crispy. Set aside. Warm the coconut oil and cook the onion until soft for about 3 minutes, stirring occasionally. Add in the zucchini and cook for 10 more minutes until zucchini is brown and tender, but not mushy. Transfer to a plate. Crack the eggs into the same skillet and fry over medium heat. Top the zucchini mixture with the bacon slices and fried eggs. Serve hot sprinkled with parsley.

983. Cheesy Sausage Quiche

Ready in about: 55 minutes | Serves: 6 Per serving: Kcal 340, Fat: 28g, Net Carbs: 3g, Protein: 17g

Ingredients

6 eggs 12 oz raw sausage roll 10 cherry tomatoes, halved 2 tbsp heavy cream 2 tbsp Parmesan cheese Salt and black pepper to taste 2 tbsp chopped parsley 5 eggplant slices Preheat oven to 370°F.

Directions

Press the sausage roll at the bottom of a greased pie dish. Arrange the eggplant slices over the sausage and nd top with cherry tomatoes. Whisk the eggs with heavy cream, salt, Parmesan cheese, and pepper. Spoon the mixture over the sausage. Bake for about 40 minutes until browned around the edges. Serve sprinkled with parsley.

984. Peanut Butter Fudge

(Ready in about 3 hours | Servings 8) Per serving: 180 Calories; 18.3g Fat; 4.5g Carbs; 1g Protein; 1.1g Fiber

Ingredients

3/4 cup peanut butter 1/4 cup Swerve 1/8 teaspoon salt 3 tablespoons coconut butter, melted 1 teaspoon vanilla 3 tablespoons cocoa powder, unsweetened 1/2 cup ghee 1/3 cup almond milk 1 tablespoon liquid Stevia

Directions

Melt the peanut butter and ghee in your microwave. Add in the almond milk, 1/4 cup Swerve, and salt; stir to combine well and scrape the base into a foil-lined baking pan. Refrigerate for about 3 hours or until set. Now, make the sauce by whisking the other ingredients until well combined. Spread the sauce over your fudge. Cut into squares.Enjoy!

985. Perfect Family Steak

(Ready in about 20 minutes + marinating time | Servings 6) Per serving: 350 Calories; 17.3g Fat; 2.1g Carbs; 42.7g Protein; 0.4g Fiber

Ingredients

1 ½ tablespoons canola oil 2 tablespoons coconut aminos 2 garlic cloves, minced 1/2 cup white onions, chopped 1 tablespoon white vinegar 1/4 cup dry red wine 2 pounds skirt steak 1/2 teaspoon ground bay leaf Salt and pepper, to taste

Directions

Combine the oil, coconut aminos, garlic, onions, vinegar, and red wine in a ceramic dish. Add in the steak, ground bay leaf, salt, and pepper. Let it marinate overnight. Sear the steak in a nonstick skillet over a moderately-high flame. Sear the steak for 8 to 11 minutes per side.Bon appétit!

986. Beef Salad Bowl

(Ready in about 15 minutes | Servings 4) Per serving: 404 Calories; 32.9g Fat; 8g Carbs; 12.8g Protein; 6g Fiber

Ingredients

1/2 pound flank steak, cut into strips 1 cucumber, sliced 1 celery, sliced 1 tablespoon fresh basil, snipped 1 poblano chili, minced Sea salt and ground black pepper, to taste 2 tablespoons olive oil 1 teaspoon coconut aminos 2 tablespoons lime juice, freshly squeezed 1 tablespoon fresh lime juice 1/4 cup sesame seeds, lightly toasted 1 shallot, peeled and sliced 1/2 teaspoon ginger-garlic paste 2 avocados, pitted, peeled and sliced

Directions

In a large frying pan, heat the oil over medium-low flame. Sauté the shallot until tender or about 3 minutes. Add in the steak and cook for 5 to 6 minutes per side. Season the steak with salt and pepper.Enjoy!

987. Thai-Style Sausage and Vegetable Bowl

(Ready in about 40 minutes | Servings 4) Per serving: 250 Calories; 17.5g Fat; 5.4g Carbs; 6.8g Protein; 2.1g Fiber

Ingredients

4 beef sausages, sliced 1 cup tomato Nam Prik, no sugar added 2 tablespoons sesame oil 1 medium onion, chopped 1 tablespoon lemongrass, sliced Salt and pepper, to taste 1 Bird's eye chili, deveined and chopped 1 parsnip, chopped 1 ½ cups chicken broth 1/4 cup Marsala wine 1 teaspoon fresh turmeric 2 rosemary sprigs 1 teaspoon garlic, minced 1 green bell pepper, deveined and chopped

Directions

Ina wok, heat the sesame oil over a moderately-high heat. Sear the sausage for about 3 minutes or until no longer pink. Add in the onion, garlic, peppers, parsnip, lemongrass, salt, and pepper. Cook an additional 6 to 7 minutes. Add in the remaining ingredients and bring it to a rapid boil. Reduce the heat to a simmer. Continue to simmer for 20 to 25 minutes.Bon appétit!

988. Coconut Ice Cream

(Ready in about 10 minutes + chilling time | Servings 4) Per serving: 260 Calories; 24.3g Fat; 6.5g Carbs; 2.5g Protein; 2.7g Fiber

Ingredients

1 ¼ cups coconut milk 17 drops liquid Monk fruit 1/2 cup coconut flakes 1/2 teaspoon xanthan gum 1/3 cup double cream

Directions

Thoroughly combine all ingredients, except for the xanthan gum, using your electric mixer. Add in the xanthan gum, mixing constantly, until the mixture has thickened. Prepare your ice cream in a machine following the manufacturer's instructions.Bon appétit!

989. Mustard Bacon Chips

(Ready in about 15 minutes | Servings 6) Per serving: 409 Calories; 31.6g Fat; 1.1g Carbs; 28g Protein; 0g Fiber

Ingredients

1 tablespoon deli mustard 1 pound bacon, cut into small squares 1 tablespoon cayenne pepper

Directions

Toss all ingredients in a rimmed baking pan. Bake in the preheated oven at 365 degrees F for about 15 minutes.Enjoy!

990. Flank Steak with Eggs

(Ready in about 30 minutes | Servings 6) Per serving: 429 Calories; 27.8g Fat; 3.2g Carbs; 39.1g Protein; 0.6g Fiber

Ingredients

2 tablespoons lard, melted 1 ½ pounds flank steak, cut into strips Salt and black pepper, to taste 1/2 teaspoon cayenne pepper 1/2 cup onions, finely chopped 2 garlic cloves, minced 2 Spanish peppers, chopped 6 eggs

Directions

In a nonstick skillet, melt the lard over a moderately-high heat. Sear the steak for 10 minutes, stirring frequently to ensure even cooking. Season with salt, black pepper, and cayenne pepper and set aside. In the same skillet, sauté the onion, garlic, and peppers for about 4 minutes or until they are tender and fragrant. Add the meat back to the skillet. Create six indentions in the sautéed mixture. Crack an egg into each indention. Cover and continue to cook for about 5 minutes or until the eggs are set.Enjoy!

991.   Blade Roast with Cheese

(Ready in about 8 hours | Servings 6) Per serving: 397 Calories; 31.4g Fat; 3.9g Carbs; 23.5g Protein; 0.5g Fiber

Ingredients

1 ½ pounds boneless blade roast 2 tablespoons olive oil 1/4 cup red wine 1 cup chicken stock 1 teaspoon garlic, minced 1 teaspoon coriander seeds 1/2 teaspoon mustard seeds 6 ounces goat cheese, crumbled 1 onion, chopped

Directions

In a frying pan, heat the oil over medium-high heat. Cook the onion until tender and translucent. Add in the garlic and continue to sauté for a further 30 seconds; transfer the sautéed mixture to your slow cooker. Sear the beef until golden-brown and transfer to the slow cooker. Add in the remaining ingredients, except for cheese. Cover and cook on Low heat setting for about 7 hours or until the meat has softened.Serve topped with goat cheese.

992.   Rum Spiked Chocolates

(Ready in about 25 minutes + chilling time | Servings 10) Per serving: 119 Calories; 11.7g Fat; 5.2g Carbs; 1.1g Protein; 4g Fiber

Ingredients

1 cup coconut flour 1/2 stick cold butter 1 ½ cups whipped cream 8 ounces chocolate chips, unsweetened 1/2 cup almond meal 1/4 teaspoon cinnamon 1 teaspoon pure vanilla extract 1 tablespoon rum A pinch of grated nutmeg 2 packets stevia

Directions

Begin by preheating your oven to 340 degrees F. Mix the coconut flour, almond meal, nutmeg, stevia, cinnamon, vanilla, and rum in your blender or food processor. Cut in the cold butter and mix again. Press the mixture into molds. Bake for about 10 minutes and place on a wire rack. Heat the double cream over medium-low flame; once it is warmed, fold in the chocolate and stir to combine well. Spread the filling over the base and place in your refrigerator.Bon appétit!

993.   Hot and Spicy Mexican Wings

(Ready in about 50 minutes | Servings 6) Per serving: 236 Calories; 13.5g Fat; 6g Carbs; 19.4g Protein; 1.7g Fiber

Ingredients

12 chicken wings Salt and red pepper, to taste For the Dip: 1 cup tomatillos, peeled 2 tablespoons lime juice, freshly squeezed 1 Habanero pepper, minced 2 tablespoons coriander, minced 4 ripe tomatoes 1 shallot, finely chopped

Directions

Toss the chicken wings with salt and red pepper; brush them with a nonstick spray. Bake in the preheated oven at 396 degrees F for 45 to 50 minutes or until they're crispy. In your blender, process the remaining ingredients to make the sauce.Enjoy!

994.   Coconut Cream Mocha Espresso

(Ready in about 10 minutes + chilling time | Servings 6) Per serving: 218 Calories; 24.7g Fat; 1.1g Carbs; 0.4g Protein; 0g Fiber

Ingredients

1 teaspoon instant espresso powder 1/2 teaspoon pure coconut extract 1/2 teaspoon pure vanilla extract 3 tablespoons erythritol A pinch of salt 4 ounces coconut oil 5 ounces coconut cream

Directions

Melt the coconut oil in a double boiler; add in the remaining ingredients. Remove from heat and stir to combine well. Pour into a silicone mold and place in your freezer.

995. Chicken Salad with Avocado

(Ready in about 20 minutes | Servings 4) Per serving: 408 Calories; 34.2g Fat; 4.8g Carbs; 22.7g Protein; 3.1g Fiber

Ingredients

2 chicken breasts Sea salt and red pepper, to taste 1/2 teaspoon deli mustard 1/3 cup extra-virgin olive oil 1 tablespoon soy sauce 1/2 teaspoon Italian seasoning mix 1 tablespoon lemon juice 1 avocado, pitted and sliced 2 egg yolks

Directions

Toss the chicken breasts with salt, red pepper and Italian seasoning mix. Cook the chicken on the preheated grill for 4 minutes per side. Cut the chicken into the strips.Dress your salad and serve!

996. Chicken with Mustard Sauce

(Ready in about 25 minutes | Servings 4) Per serving: 311 Calories; 16.9g Fat; 2.1g Carbs; 33.6g Protein; 0.9g Fiber

Ingredients

1 pound chicken breasts Salt and red pepper, to season 1 tablespoon olive oil 1/2 cup onions, chopped 2 garlic cloves, minced 1/2 cup low-sodium chicken broth 1/2 cup whipped cream 2 tablespoons deli mustard 1/2 cup fresh chives, chopped

Directions

Rub the chicken with salt and pepper. Heat the oil in a frying pan over a moderately-high heat. Sear the chicken for about 8 minutes and set aside. Then, sauté the onion and garlic for about 3 minutes until aromatic. Pour in the broth and cook until the liquid has reduced by half. Stir in the whipped cream and mustard. Add the sauce and chives to the reserved chicken.Bon appétit!

997. Turkey and Vegetable Kebabs

(Ready in about 30 minutes | Servings 6) Per serving: 293 Calories; 13.8g Fat; 5.7g Carbs; 34.5g Protein; 1g Fiber

Ingredients

1 cup red onion, cut into wedges 1 ½ cups grape tomatoes, sliced 1 tablespoon fresh cilantro, chopped 1 ½ pounds turkey breast, cubed 1 tablespoon Italian seasoning mix 1 cup bell peppers, sliced 1 cup zucchini, cut into thick slices 2 tablespoons olive oil

Directions

Toss the turkey breast with olive oil and Italian seasoning mix. Thread the turkey onto skewers, alternating them with the vegetables. Continue until all the ingredients are used up. Grill the kebabs for about 10 minutes, turning them occasionally to ensure even cooking. Toss the kebabs with the cilantro.Bon appétit!

998. Vegetable and Mushroom Medley

(Ready in about 30 minutes | Servings 4) Per serving: 133 Calories; 3.7g Fat; 6.7g Carbs; 14g Protein; 1g Fiber

Ingredients

1/2 pound button mushrooms, chopped 1 cup onion, chopped Salt and pepper, to taste 1/2 teaspoon ground allspice 1 teaspoon ground bay leaves 1/3 cup fresh parsley, chopped 1 teaspoon jalapeno pepper, finely minced 2 garlic cloves, minced 2 celery stalks, chopped 1 tablespoon lard, melted 3 cups vegetable broth 1 cup tomato puree

Directions

In a heavy-bottomed pot, melt the lard over medium-high heat. Cook the onion, jalapeno pepper, garlic, celery, and mushrooms for 7 to 8 minutes. Add in the vegetable broth, tomato puree, and spices, and bring to a boil. Turn the heat to a simmer; cover and let it cook for about 20 minutes. Bon appétit!

999.   Cheesy Meatloaf in a Mug

(Ready in about 10 minutes | Servings 2) Per serving: 327 Calories; 16.6g Fat; 5.8g Carbs; 40g Protein; 1.8g Fiber

Ingredients

1/2 pound ground pork 1/2 cup marinara sauce Salt and pepper, to season 2 garlic cloves, minced 1/2 cup Swiss cheese, shredded 1/2 teaspoon mustard powder 1/2 teaspoon red pepper flakes 1 teaspoon shallot powder

Directions

In a mixing bowl, combine all ingredients until everything is well combined. Spoon the mixture into two microwave-safe mugs. Microwave at 70 percent power for about 6 minutes until no longer pink in the center

1000.   Herring Salad Boats

(Ready in about 10 minutes | Servings 4) Per serving: 120 Calories; 5.4g Fat; 5.8g Carbs; 12.3g Protein; 1.4g Fiber

Ingredients

7 ounces canned herring, chopped Salt and black pepper, to taste 1 tablespoon fresh cilantro, chopped 4 red pickled peppers, slice into halves 1 teaspoon Dijon mustard 2 tablespoons lemon juice 1 celery, chopped 1/2 cup onions, chopped

Directions

Thoroughly combine the herring, Dijon mustard, celery, onions, lemon juice, salt, black pepper, and fresh cilantro. Mix until everything is well combined. Spoon the herring mixture into the pickle boats.

1001.   Hot and Spicy Egg Salad

(Ready in about 15 minutes | Servings 8) Per serving: 174 Calories; 13g Fat; 2.7g Carbs; 7.4g Protein; 0.6g Fiber

Ingredients

10 eggs 1 teaspoon lemon juice Salt and pepper, to season 1 head butterhead lettuce, torn into pieces 1 tablespoon Dijon mustard 1/2 cup onions 1/2 stalk of celery, minced 3/4 cup mayonnaise 1 teaspoon hot sauce

Directions

Place the eggs in a saucepan and cover them with water by 1 inch. Cover and bring the water to a boil over high heat. Boil for 6 to 7 minutes over medium-high heat. Peel the eggs and chop them coarsely. Add in the remaining ingredients and toss to combine well.Bon appétit!

CPSIA information can be obtained
at www.ICGtesting.com
Printed in the USA
LVHW100119100221
678894LV00019B/1193